Rheumatoid Arthritis: Clinical Updates on Diagnosis and Treatment

Rheumatoid Arthritis: Clinical Updates on Diagnosis and Treatment

Guest Editor

Shunsuke Mori

MDPI

Basel • Beijing • Wuhan • Barcelona • Belgrade • Novi Sad • Cluj • Manchester

Guest Editor
Shunsuke Mori
Department of Rheumatology
National Hospital
Organization Kumamoto
Saishun Medical Center
Kumamoto
Japan

Editorial Office
MDPI AG
Grosspeteranlage 5
4052 Basel, Switzerland

This is a reprint of the Special Issue, published open access by the journal *Journal of Clinical Medicine* (ISSN 2077-0383), freely accessible at: https://www.mdpi.com/journal/jcm/special_issues/1D32Y0W831.

For citation purposes, cite each article independently as indicated on the article page online and as indicated below:

Lastname, A.A.; Lastname, B.B. Article Title. *Journal Name* **Year**, *Volume Number*, Page Range.

ISBN 978-3-7258-7164-3 (Hbk)
ISBN 978-3-7258-7165-0 (PDF)
https://doi.org/10.3390/books978-3-7258-7165-0

Contents

About the Editor

Shunsuke Mori

Shunsuke Mori is a director of the Clinical Research Center for Rheumatic Diseases, National Hospital Kumamoto Saishun Medical Center in Kumamoto, Japan. He completed his MD and PhD at Kumamoto University Medical School and has previously worked at the UCLA School of Medicine (Los Angeles, CA, USA) and Kumamoto University Medical School. His research has focused on comprehending the pleiotropic effects of cytokine networks in chronic inflammation and antitumor immunity, and he has a particular interest in therapeutically targeting cytokine pathways in inflammatory and tumor cells. Currently, his research aim is to explore the optimal management of patients with rheumatoid arthritis (RA) who have significant complications, such as RA-associated lung diseases, chronic kidney disease, malignancy, and chronic infectious diseases. He is also exploring the optimal positioning of biological and nonbiological targeted disease-modifying antirheumatic drugs in the treatment algorithm for RA.

Preface

Rheumatoid arthritis (RA) is a chronic immune-mediated inflammatory disease characterized by persistent synovitis and progressive damage to multiple joints. Joint damage is related to physical function and health-related quality of life. In addition to joint damage, RA-associated systemic inflammation can cause medical problems in multiple tissues and organs. Over the past two decades, significant advances have been made in the management of RA. Early diagnosis, prompt initiation of pharmaceutical therapies, and application of a treat-to-target strategy with tight disease control have greatly improved long-term outcomes of patients with RA. A growing array of conventional, biological, and nonbiological targeted disease-modifying antirheumatic drugs (DMARDs) are currently available.

Despite this remarkable therapeutic revolution, we are confronted by many difficulties in our daily practice of managing patients with RA. Some patients remain unresponsive to current DMARD therapies or experience disease flares after achieving a state of remission or low disease activity. Additionally, the presence of persistent subclinical inflammation may induce progressive damage of joints, even after patients have achieved clinical remission. Currently, we lack reliable biomarkers by which to select optimal DMARD therapies and predict the patient response to individual treatments. RA-related extra-articular manifestations, such as respiratory, cardiovascular, and renal disease, osteoporosis, and malignancy, contribute greatly to the diminished quality of life and mortality of RA patients. Poor control of disease activity can increase the risk of death. Thus, we need to improve our overall approach to RA patients who are at increased risk of extra-articular manifestations.

The aim of this Special Issue is to highlight up-to-date information on concepts in RA pathogenesis and new advances in diagnostic and therapeutic strategies for RA, with a particular focus on the abovementioned unmet clinical needs in patients with RA. We hope that this collection will stimulate further investigation, facilitate multidiscipline collaboration, and inspire new perspectives in the study of RA.

Shunsuke Mori
Guest Editor

Journal of
Clinical Medicine

MDPI

Review

Unmet Needs and Current Challenges of Rheumatoid Arthritis: Difficult-to-Treat Rheumatoid Arthritis and Late-Onset Rheumatoid Arthritis

Satoshi Takanashi and Yuko Kaneko *

Division of Rheumatology, Department of Internal Medicine, Keio University School of Medicine, 35 Shinanomachi, Shinjuku-ku, Tokyo 160-8582, Japan
* Correspondence: ykaneko.z6@keio.jp; Tel.: +81-3-5363-3786; Fax: +81-3-5379-5037

Abstract: Despite remarkable advances in the management of RA, there are still unmet needs that rheumatologists need to address. In this review, we focused on difficult-to-treat RA (D2T RA) and late-onset RA (LORA), and summarized their characteristics and management. The prevalence of D2T RA is reported to be 6–28% and many factors have been identified as risk factors for D2T RA, including female sex, long disease duration, seropositivity for rheumatoid factor and anti-cyclic citrullinated peptide antibody and their high titer, baseline high disease activity, and comorbidities. D2T RA is broadly divided into inflammatory and non-inflammatory conditions, and clinical features differ according to background. A proportion of D2T RA can be managed with treatment modification, mainly with interleukin-6 receptor inhibitors or Janus kinase inhibitors, but some D2T RA patients have a poor prognosis; thus, the implementation of precision medicine by stratifying patients according to disease status is needed. In the aging society, the epidemiology of RA is changing and the prevalence of LORA is increasing worldwide. LORA has distinct clinical features compared with young-onset RA, such as acute onset, low seropositivity, and high inflammation. The pathogenesis of LORA remains to be elucidated, but proinflammatory cytokines, including interleukin-6, have been reported to be significantly elevated. LORA has several management concerns other than RA itself, such as geriatric syndrome and multimorbidity. The treat-to-target strategy is effective for LORA, but the evidence is still lacking; thus, it is important to accumulate clinical and related basic data to establish the optimal treatment strategy for LORA.

Keywords: rheumatoid arthritis; difficult-to-treat rheumatoid arthritis (D2T RA); JAK inhibitors; late-onset rheumatoid arthritis; elderly; aging

1. Introduction

The landscape of rheumatoid arthritis (RA) has changed dramatically in recent decades. The development of the 2010 American College of Rheumatology (ACR)/European Alliance of Associations for Rheumatology (EULAR) classification criteria [1], which allows for the early diagnosis of RA; the treat-to-target (T2T) strategy [2]; novel treatments, such as biologic disease-modifying anti-rheumatic drugs (bDMARDs) and Janus kinase inhibitors (JAKis) (Table 1) [3,4]; and the widespread use of evidence-based EULAR recommendations for RA [5] have contributed to a paradigm shift in the management of RA. As a result, the achievement rate of the treatment goal has improved remarkably [6], and the life expectancy of patients with RA is increasing [7]. Furthermore, research is underway to establish disease prevention and chronicity techniques in preclinical RA [8,9]. Despite the remarkable progress in the management of RA, there are several unmet needs that rheumatologists need to address in the future, such as difficult-to-treat RA (D2T RA), in which treatment goals are not achieved for multifactorial reasons [10,11], as well as late-onset RA (LORA) in the super-aging society [12,13].

In this review, we focus on these unresolved issues in the field of RA and discuss how they can be addressed in the future.

Table 1. Molecular targeted therapy for rheumatoid arthritis.

TNF inhibitors	Infliximab
	Etanercept
	Adalimumab
	Golimumab
	Certolizumab pegol
	Ozoralizumab
T cell co-stimulation modulator	Abatacept
IL-6 receptor inhibitors	Tocilizumab
	Sarilumab
B cell depletion	Rituximab
JAK inhibitors	Tofacitinib
	Baricitinib
	Peficitinib
	Upadacitinib
	Filgotinib

IL-6: interleukin-6; JAK: Janus kinase; TNF: tumor necrosis factor.

2. Difficult-to-Treat Rheumatoid Arthritis (D2T RA)

2.1. Concept and Definition of Difficult-to-Treat RA (D2T RA)

There is a proportion of patients who remain symptomatic after several cycles of treatment based on EULAR recommendation and who fail to achieve the treatment goal; this population has been recognized as a significant clinical problem [10]. They have been described as refractory, treatment-resistant, severe, complex, or difficult-to-treat, but there has been a lack of consistent terminology to define this population. To address the great unmet need, the EULAR Task Force conducted an international survey among rheumatologists to provide terminology and a definition of D2T RA as an essential first step. This international survey on the disease characteristics of D2T RA was conducted among 410 rheumatologists in 2018. In the survey, 50% of them answered 'disease activity score assessing 28 joints using erythrocyte sedimentation rate (DAS28-ESR) >3.2 or presence of signs suggestive of active inflammatory disease activity with a DAS28-ESR $\leq$ 3.2' as being characteristics of D2T RA [11]. Also, 62% answered '$\geq$1 or 2 conventional synthetic (cs) DMARDs and $\geq$2 b DMARDs or targeted synthetic (ts) DMARDs with different modes of action' as being the minimum number of inadequately effective DMARDs that should have been applied. Based on the results, EULAR proposed a definition of D2T RA in 2021 [14] (Table 2). Briefly, all three criteria need to be present in D2T RA, as follows: first, a treatment failure of 2 $\geq$ bDMARDs with a different mechanism of action after failing csDMARDs treatment; second, signs suggestive of active or progressive disease, such as moderate or high disease activity according to the validated composite measures, inability to taper glucocorticoid treatment, rapid radiographic progression, and symptoms that are causing a reduction in quality of life; third, the perception of the rheumatologist and/or patients that the management of RA is problematic.

Table 2. EULAR definition of difficult-to-treat rheumatoid arthritis (D2T RA).

1	Treatment according to European League Against Rheumatism recommendation and failure of ≥2 b/tsDMARDs (with different mechanisms of action) * after failing csDMARD therapy (unless contraindicated).†
2	Signs suggestive of active/progressive disease, defined as ≥1 of: a. At least moderate disease activity (according to validated composite measures including joint counts; for example, DAS28-ESR > 3.2 or CDAI > 10). b. Signs (including acute phase reactants and imaging) and/or symptoms suggestive of active disease (joint related or other). c. Inability to taper glucocorticoid treatment (below 7.5 mg/day prednisone or equivalent). d. Rapid radiographic progression (with or without signs of active disease). ‡ e. Well-controlled disease according to above standards, but still having RA symptoms that are causing a reduction in quality of life.
3	The management of signs and/or symptoms is perceived as problematic by the rheumatologist and/or the patient.

All three criteria need to be present in D2T RA. * Unless restricted by access to treatment due to socioeconomic factors. † If csDMARD treatment is contraindicated, a failure of ≥2 b/tsDMARDs with different mechanisms of action is sufficient. ‡ Rapid radiographic progression: change in van der Heijde-modified Sharp score ≥5 points at 1 year. Abbreviations—b: biological; CDAI: clinical disease activity index; cs: conventional synthetic; DAS28-ESR: disease activity score assessing 28 joints using erythrocyte sedimentation rate; DMARD: disease-modifying antirheumatic drug; mg: milligram; RA: rheumatoid arthritis; ts: targeted synthetic.

2.2. Prevalence of Difficult-to-Treat RA

At the time the concept of D2T RA was developed, its prevalence was estimated to be around 3–10% of all RA patients [10]. Since the EULAR definition of D2T RA has been proposed, several real-world studies of D2T RA have been published and the actual prevalence of D2T RA ranges from 5.9 to 27.5% in clinical practice (Table 3) [15–31]. The reasons for the variation in the prevalence of D2T RA may be due to differences in the patient populations included (proportion of early RA, established RA), healthcare systems, type of institute (academic hospital, general hospital, clinic), and access to drugs.

Table 3. Prevalence and clinical characteristics of D2T RA.

Reference	Prevalence % (n)	Relevant Factors
Roodenrijs NMT [15]	N/A	Low socioeconomic status Young onset Multiple comorbidities Fibromyalgia Depression/anxiety Non-adherence Alcohol use Limited drug option
Takanashi S [16]	10.1 (173/1709)	Female Long disease duration Delayed bDMARDs/JAKis initiation Low body weight RF positivity Anti-CCP positivity Contraindication or intolerance to MTX Admission history of infection Multiple comorbidities Chronic kidney disease Lung disease
Watanabe R [17]	7.9 (53/672)	High RF titer (≥156.4 IU/mL) High baseline disease activity Lung disease
Messelink MA [18]	6.6 (123/1873)	N/A
Ochi S [19]	16.6 (353/2128)	N/A

Table 3. *Cont.*

Reference	Prevalence % (n)	Relevant Factors
Yoshii I [20]	21.5 (71/330)	Young onset Long disease duration High RF titer High anti-CCP titer High RDCI High baseline disease activity Worse QOL score Worse radiological progression
Giollo A [21]	24.9 (48/193)	Delayed MTX treatment Long-term glucocorticoid use
Novella-Navarro M [22]	13.7 (122/893)	Young onset
Leon L [23]	5.9 (35/631)	Young onset RF positivity High baseline DAS28 High baseline HAQ Dyslipidemia Liver disease DMARD monotherapy
Hecquet S [24]	23.8 (76/320)	Low socioeconomic status Long disease duration RF positivity Diabetes mellitus Interstitial lung disease Non-MTX use
Garcia-Salinas R [25]	27.5 (76/276)	High RF titer Anti-CCP positivity/ high titer Bad baseline HAQ Presence of erosion
Jung JY [26]	11.7 (271/2321)	Young age Long disease duration Low RF Non-csDMARDs use Rheumatoid nodule Cardiovascular disease Worse RAPID3
David P [27]	16.8 (247/1469)	N/A
Michitsuji T [28]	14.0 (43/307)	N/A
Bertsias A [29]	19.9 (251/12664)	Female Young age at bDMARDs/JAKis initiation RF negativity Shorter disease duration Osteoarthritis DAS28 at bDMARDs/JAKis initiation
Alp G [30]	8.9 (27/302)	Young onset Long disease duration Sjögren syndrome Extra-articular manifestation Comorbidity Fibromyalgia High RF

Table 3. *Cont.*

Reference	Prevalence % (n)	Relevant Factors
Watanabe R [31]	12.4 (450/3623)	Young onset High RF Comorbidity High disease activity Diabetes mellitus

Anti-CCP: ant-cyclic citrullinated peptide antibody; bDMARDs: biological disease-modifying anti-rheumatic drugs; csDMARDs: conventional synthetic disease-modifying anti-rheumatic drugs; DAS: disease activity score; D2T RA: difficult-to-treat rheumatoid arthritis; HAQ: health assessment questionnaire; JAKi: Janus kinase inhibitor; MTX: methotrexate; N/A; not available; RAPID3: Routine Assessment of Patient Index Data 3; QOL: quality of life; RDCI: rheumatic disease comorbidity index; RF: rheumatoid factor.

The accumulation of evidence has revealed several concerns about the definition of D2T RA. Firstly, how to deal with older patients with comorbidities. We verified the definition in our institution, where approximately 60% of 1700 patients were treated with b/tsDMARDs, resulting in approximately 85% achieving target (60% in remission and 25% in low disease activity), and revealed that 10% are classified as D2T RA [16]. In the process of this research, we also identified 77 patients (5%) who were non-D2T RA despite being in moderate or high disease activity due to the non-fulfillment of the criterion of the failure of two b/tsDMARDs with different mechanisms of action [32]. This population was older at diagnosis and last visit (62.3 and 77.5 years, respectively), and had more comorbidities, including lung and kidney disease (41.6 and 50.6%, respectively), which made them or their attending physicians reluctant to intensify or change the treatment. These data suggested that we should pay more attention to patients with RA who do not meet the current criteria because of safety concerns.

Secondly, how to deal with the patients who have limited access to bDMARDs or JAKi due to the socioeconomic reasons [16]. Because of the high cost of the drugs, some patients with an inadequate response to methotrexate (MTX) are unable to try bDMARDs or JAKi. In the definition of D2T RA, the following is described in the footnote: "failure of $\geq$2 b/tsDMARDs unless restricted by access to treatment due to socioeconomic factors"; therefore, these patients are also included as having D2T RA. The definition of D2T RA is a broad concept that includes social factors, so it is necessary to recognize that D2T RA is a heterogeneous condition.

These real-world data highlight the performance and concerns of the EULAR definition in clinical practice.

2.3. Clinical Characteristics and Risk Factors for D2T RA

In general, many factors may be complicatedly associated with the condition of D2T RA, such as immunologic mechanism, pharmacogenetics, smoking, immunogenicity of bDMARDs, adverse drug reactions, medication non-adherence, and inappropriate medication use [10]. In addition, factors surrounding the patients such as comorbidities, obesity, and joint damage may affect the signs and symptoms of RA. We have summarized the factors contributing to D2T RA from the real-world data in Table 3 [15–31]. There are many factors including female sex; young onset; long disease duration; treatment delay; seropositivity for rheumatoid factor (RF) and anti-cyclic citrullinated peptide antibody (anti-CCP); multiple comorbidities, especially lung disease, chronic kidney disease, and fibromyalgia; and baseline high disease activity. These data suggested that D2T RA is a highly heterogeneous and multifactorial condition. Interestingly, these factors have been shown to work synergistically to increase the risk of D2T RA. In one study, RF titer, baseline DAS28, and co-existing pulmonary disease were extracted as risk factors of D2T RA, and the combinational score of the three factors was positively correlated with the futuristic development of D2T RA [17]. Another study showed that treatment delay, female gender, and higher disease activity were independent predictors of refractory disease course and that a matrix risk model using these factors efficiently predicts patients' progression to D2T RA [33].

2.4. Subgroup of D2T RA

As D2T RA is a heterogeneous condition, it is important to stratify patients appropriately for optimal treatment (Table 4). At first, patients are usually divided into two groups according to the presence or absence of inflammation [34]. Inflammatory D2T RA is characterized by a lack of response to multiple DMARDs and persistent signs of inflammation. On the other hand, non-inflammatory D2T RA has also been exposed to multiple DMARDs and remains symptomatic, but there is little objective inflammation. In this condition, the effects of accumulated damage and/or secondary osteoarthritis, functional decline, chronic pain syndrome and/or fibromyalgia, as well as central sensitization, also modify the symptoms of RA. In a cross-sectional study comparing the clinical features of inflammatory and non-inflammatory D2T RA based on ultrasound findings, 57% of patients with D2T RA had residual synovitis in one or more joints, while the remaining 40% had no detectable inflammation. These two groups were clinically distinct—the inflammatory group had an increased swollen joint count (5.0), high CRP levels (1.0 mg/dL), and high DAS28-CRP (5.3), while the non-inflammatory group had a higher proportion of obesity (55%) and fibromyalgia (15%) [27]. A previous study suggested that such residual pain in non-inflammatory D2T RA is attributable to persistent central sensitization and the development of maladaptive pain processing [35]. Another study reported that synovial fibroblast lining cells may be involved in dorsal root ganglion axonal growth and cause low inflammatory intractable pain [36]. Further detailed elucidation of the mechanism is required for appropriate treatment.

Table 4. Subgroup of D2T RA.

Reference	Subgroup and Characteristics
Roodenrijs NMT [15]	Non-adherence and dissatisfaction - Treatment non-adherence - Depression Pain syndrome and obesity - Smoking - Obesity - Fibromyalgia - Anxiety - High tender joint count True refractory RA - Erosion - Rheumatologist's with to intensify treatment (where no further treatment options exist)
Takanashi S [16]	Multidrug resistance - Failure to 3 ≥ bDMARDs/JAKis - High tender joint count - High physician global assessment Comorbidity - Older age - History of admission due to infection - High RDCI - Long disease duration - Small physique Socioeconomic - Difficulty in initiation of bDMARDs/JAKi due to economic reason

Table 4. *Cont.*

Reference	Subgroup and Characteristics
David P [27]	Persistent inflammatory refractory RA (PIRRA) - High swollen joint count - High CRP - Worse DAS28-CRP Non-inflammatory refractory RA (NIRRA) - High BMI and more obese people - High fibromyalgia prevalence

BMI: body mass index; bDMARDs: biologic disease-modifying anti-rheumatic drugs; CRP: C-reactive protein; DAS: disease activity score; JAKi: Janus kinase inhibitor; RA: rheumatoid arthritis; RDCI: rheumatic disease comorbidity index.

There are several reports on subgroups of D2T RA from real-world cohort studies. In our study, we divided into three groups based on medical record information and the opinion of attending rheumatologists—the multidrug resistance group, the comorbidity group, and the socioeconomic group [16]. We found that the clinical characteristics differed between the groups. The multidrug resistance group had the highest tender joint count (3.4 joints) and evaluator global assessment score (21.9 mm) of the three groups, despite having tried an average of 3.9 different bDMARDs/JAKis. The patients in the comorbidity group showed the highest rate of admission due to infection (64.7%), the highest score of rheumatic disease comorbidity index (1.9), and the most frequent comorbidities of lung involvement (52.9%). They were also significantly older (75.3 years), had the longest disease duration (18.4 years), and showed the smallest physique.

The other study that conduced cluster analysis using the clinical characteristics of D2T RA showed that there are three subgroups—non-adherence and dissatisfaction group, pain syndromes and obesity group, and true refractory RA [15]. This study showed that co-existing factors not directly related to the pathology of RA, such as obesity, anxiety, depression, fibromyalgia, and treatment non-adherence, were also important in stratifying D2T RA.

Therefore, D2T RA can be stratified according to its clinical features, reflecting the heterogeneity of this state, and a personalized approach will be needed to resolve the D2T RA.

2.5. Management and Treatment Strategy of Difficult-to-Treat RA

EULAR has proposed points to consider and an algorithm for the management of D2T RA [37]. This algorithm proposes a multifaceted approach, including not only pharmacological but also non-pharmacological intervention, because the reasons for the difficulties in the management are different for each individual. First, this proposal emphasizes the need to reassess the diagnosis of RA from other diseases. If a patient is suspected of having D2T RA, the possibility of misdiagnosis and/or the presence of a co-existing mimicking disease should be considered. Once the diagnosis of RA has been re-confirmed, a treat-to-target strategy should be implemented in accordance with the EULAR recommendation and also the residual inflammation should be assessed using ultrasound. Regarding the choice of treatment among bDMARDs and JAKis, it is recommended to switch to the other mode of action, and there are also some real-life data to support this strategy [16,38]. Additionally, it was mentioned that the maximum dose acceptable from a safety point of view should be used. In addition to pharmacological treatment, we should focus on non-pharmacological management, including education, exercise, and self-management, to optimize the management of functional disability, pain, and fatigue.

We have reported the long-term follow-up data of patients with D2T RA [39]. Our data showed that patients who resolved D2T RA more frequently underwent treatment changes, suggesting that further treatment modification was important for the management of D2T RA. In this study, 80% of patients who resolved D2T RA were treated with IL-6i or JAKis, and logistic analysis showed that the use of IL-6i was a relevant factor for the resolution of

D2T RA. Another study demonstrated that JAKi treatment had the highest CDAI remission rate in patients with D2T RA compared to TNFi, IL-6i, and CTLA4-Ig [18]. A further study revealed that JAKi and RTX showed the highest DAS28-ESR remission rate in patients with D2T RA [24]. A recent study involving 450 patients with D2T RA revealed that IL-6i and JAKi were associated with fewer discontinuations due to ineffectiveness compared to TNFi [31]. These data suggest that IL-6i and JAKi may be the preferred choice for the management of D2T RA. Recently, the overexpression of the type 1 interferon signature has been suggested as one of the key cytokines involved in D2T RA [40,41]. Several data have suggested that JAKis, which can suppress the interferon pathway, and IL-6is show the preferred treatment response in patients with type 1 interferon overexpression [19,42]. However, as the pathophysiology of RA is heterogeneous and the optimal treatment target may differ among individuals, it is necessary to establish an appropriate method to stratify patients with D2T RA based on their immune status using transcriptome, gene expression, cytokines, or clinical data, which can lead to precise treatment to overcome D2T RA.

Evidence for non-pharmacological interventions in D2T RA is limited. It would be difficult to accumulate and assess the data on non-pharmacological interventions in retrospective studies; therefore, prospective non-pharmacological interventional programs should be conducted that could help to optimize the management of D2T RA in terms of pain, fatigue, and functional disability.

2.6. Outcome of D2T RA

There are few reports on the outcome of D2T RA. We identified 173 patients with D2T RA [16], followed them for 5 years, and investigated their outcome [39]. During the 5-year follow-up, 23 patients were lost to follow-up. Of the 150 patients with D2T RA, 45% resolved D2T RA, 50% had persistent D2T RA, and 5% deceased. Patients who resolved D2T RA significantly changed their treatment during the five years, and the use of IL-6 receptor inhibitors was associated with preferable outcomes. On the other hand, the relevant factors for poor prognosis in D2T RA were multiple comorbidities and glucocorticoid dose escalation. Multimorbidity was known to be a strong predictor of a poor outcome of RA from the cluster analysis based on the number of comorbidities [43]. Indeed, Watanabe et al. also demonstrated that the use of oral glucocorticoids is associated with a risk of toxic side effects in patients with D2T RA [31]. Glucocorticoid use is known to be associated with numerous side effects, including infection, cardiovascular disease, and osteoporosis [44,45]. These results suggested that a portion of patients with D2T RA can be managed by further treatment modification and that a treatment strategy without glucocorticoids is important to overcome D2T RA.

Another study investigated the long-term functional trend in D2T RA [29]. Trajectory analysis revealed four distinct functional HAQ trends. About 20% of D2T RA patients had a more favorable function, with mHAQ scores of 0.41 that remained stable during follow-up. Approximately 40% of the D2T RA patients showed a gradual improvement (mHAQ from 1.21 to 0.87). On the contrary, two groups with unfavorable functional status were identified, of which about 30% had a gradual worsening of functional status (mHAQ from 0.68 to 1.10) and 10% had stable and significant functional limitations throughout follow-up, with mHAQ scores > 1.5. The presence of mental health- and pain-related conditions or metabolic diseases had a significant contribution to the worsening of the mHAQ, suggesting that a special focus on comorbidities, together with better control of the inflammatory burden, could improve the outcome of patients with D2T RA.

Inadequate disease control of RA is strongly associated with all-cause mortality, cardiovascular disease, cancer, and respiratory disease [46]. Co-existing comorbidities also have a strong impact on the prognosis of D2T RA; it is necessary to manage and try to escape D2T RA by adapting the appropriate treatment and thorough management of comorbidities to improve their outcome.

We summarize the clinical characteristics and management of D2T RA in Figure 1.

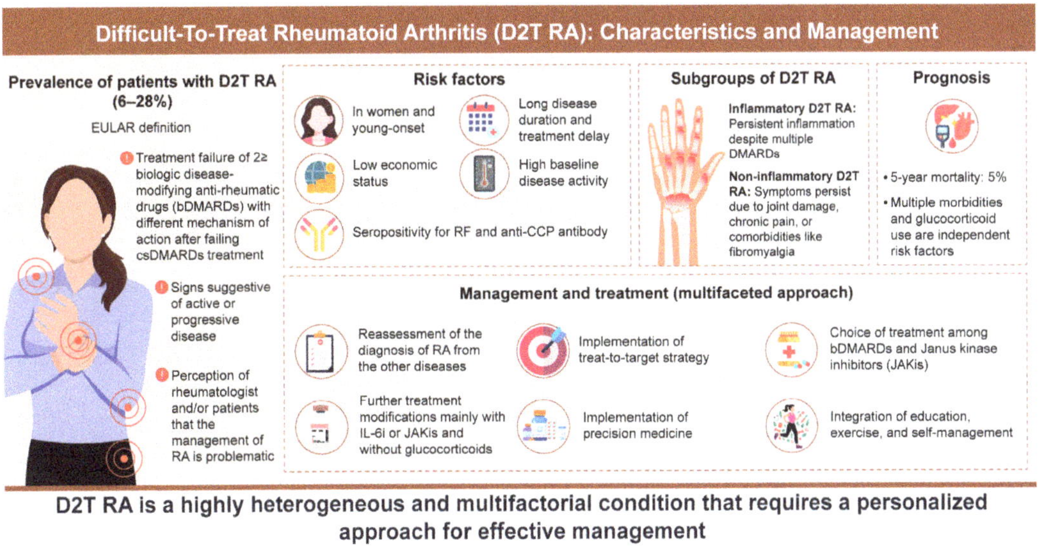

Figure 1. Clinical characteristics and management of difficult-to-treat rheumatoid arthritis (D2T RA). The prevalence of D2T RA is 6–28% in the real-world, and female, young onset, long disease duration, treatment delay, high disease activity, low economic status, and seropositivity are risk factors. D2T RA can be divided into two groups with or without residual inflammation. The 5-year mortality is 5%, and comorbidity and glucocorticoid use are risk factors. D2T RA is a highly heterogeneous and multifactorial condition that requires a personalized approach for effective management.

2.7. Future Prospectives for Preventing D2T RA

There have been no clinical trials in D2T RA to date and this should be considered in the future. However, ideally, preventive strategies should be implemented to avoid increasing levels of D2T RA in the future. It is crucial to identify the optimal therapeutic target molecule at an early stage of RA. Currently, it is difficult to predict an individual's response to targeted therapy, so treatment guidelines are based on a trial-and-error approach, in which a molecular targeted treatment is given and if it does not work, the therapeutic target is changed. However, repeated treatment failures are known to lead to the development of D2T RA, so the implementation of precision medicine by stratifying patients according to disease status and using state-of-the-art methods such as identifying the molecular biology of RA; machine learning will improve treatment response rates. In particular, basic research on synovial fibroblasts and dendritic cell precursors should be targeted to address this condition [36,47].

3. Late-Onset Rheumatoid Arthritis (LORA)

3.1. Epidemiology and Clinical Characteristics of LORA

The epidemiology of RA is changing and its prevalence has increased in recent decades [48]. In particular, autoantibody-negative, so-called 'seronegative', RA is increasing, and the majority of this population suffers from late-onset rheumatoid arthritis (LORA) [49]. In line with this trend, the age at onset of RA has been increasing worldwide, and the onset age in the histogram demonstrated a major peak around the ages of 60 to 70 [50,51]. Given the aging society worldwide, the number of LORA patients is expected to increase in the future [49]. However, there is no consensus on the definition of LORA, with many using 60 or 65 years as a common cut-off [13].

LORA has been reported to differ from young-onset RA (YORA), which is generally defined as an age of onset of RA of less than 60 or 65 years and does not include juvenile idiopathic arthritis, not only in age of onset but also in several clinical features [51–56]. Specifically, patients with LORA are known to be typically negative for autoantibodies including anti-CCP and RF, and have a more acute onset, proximal joint involvement, and higher inflammatory markers, making it sometimes difficult to distinguish from polymyalgia rheumatica (Table 5). Multivariate analysis showed that cases with three factors extracted as independently associated with LORA—anti-CCP antibody negativity, acute onset, and high erythrocyte sedimentation rate—were considered typical of LORA, with the number of relevant cases gradually increasing from 65 years of age. When LORA was defined as a patient fulfilling all three factors, a cut-off age of 68–73 years was found using receiver operating curve analysis [51].

Table 5. Clinical characteristics of late-onset rheumatoid arthritis.

	Young-Onset RA	Late-Onset RA
Sex (female), (%)	70–85	50–80
Acute onset, (%)	5–10	20–65
Proximal joint involvement, (%)	35–50	50–80
Positivity for anti-CCP, (%)	60–85	40–70
Positivity for RF, (%)	70–85	45–75
TJC	2–6	5–6
SJC	2–4	4–8
PGA, mm	35–50	35–65
EGA, mm	30–60	30–60
ESR, mm/h	20–35	40–60
CRP, mg/dL	0.5–1.5	0.8–4.5
CDAI	10–17	15–20
DAS28-ESR	4–5.5	5–6
HAQ-DI	0.4–0.7	0.7–1.5

Anti-CCP: anti-cyclic citrullinated peptide; CDAI: clinical disease activity index; CRP: C-reactive protein; DAS: disease activity score; EGA: evaluator global assessment; ESR: erythrocyte sedimentation rate; HAQ: health assessment questionnaire—disability index; RF: rheumatoid factor; SJC: swollen joint count; TJC: tender joint count; PGA: patient global assessment.

LORA has also been reported to be more prone to progressive bone destruction [53,54]. One study reported that the improvement in DAS28-ESR at 12 months was as good in LORA as in YORA, but residual synovial thickening and power Doppler signals assessed using ultrasounds and radiographic progression were significantly worse in LORA [53]. Similarly, in a study comparing the proportion of radiological progression in LORA and YORA that was free of bone erosions at the time of RA diagnosis and achieved remission after a further 1–2 years, bone erosions were significantly more common in LORA [54]. In addition, patients with bone erosions had a significantly higher disease activity at diagnosis. These results suggest that LORA differs from YORA not only in the age of onset but also in the clinical features of RA itself, and that even if disease activity can be controlled, there is a high risk of radiological progression; therefore, early diagnosis and treatment is needed.

3.2. Pathogenesis of Late-Onset Rheumatoid Arthritis

Although the clinical features of LORA are distinct from those of YORA, the underlying immune status remains unclear. A study using synovial biopsy revealed that the baseline synovial pathotype, including lympho-myeloid, diffuse-myeloid, and pauci-immune-fibroid, did not differ between LORA and YORA [53]. After 6 months of treatment, there was a trend towards a higher frequency of the pauci-immune-fibroid pathotype in YORA, coupled with a reduction in the frequency of the lympho-myeloid pathotype. In addition to the synovial pathotype, the overall synovitis inflammatory score and macrophage (lining/sublining), T cell, B cell, and plasma cell infiltration did not differ between the two groups at baseline and 6 months. However, YORA patients demonstrated a significant decrease in all synovial inflammatory parameters, whereas LORA presented only mild, albeit significant, decreases in synovitis, sublining macrophage, and T cell scores, with no significant changes in lining macrophages, B cells, and plasma cells. To summarize, although no obvious difference between LORA and YORA was detected via the immunostaining of bulk synovial tissue at baseline, differences in synovial tissue changes after treatment were observed, with a reduced inflammatory cell infiltration in YORA, suggesting that more high-resolution strategies, such as single-cell analysis, may help to elucidate and understand the differences in the pathogenesis of LORA and YORA.

With regard to serum cytokines, significantly higher levels of IL-6 were found in patients with LORA, especially in those with polymyalgia rheumatica-like symptoms, compared to those with YORA [57]. On the other hand, levels of serum tumor necrosis factor-α were significantly lower in patients with LORA than in those with YORA. Studies using synovial fluid have also reported significantly higher levels of IL-6 in LORA compared to YORA. It is known that there is a chronic inflammatory state called 'inflammageing', which is associated with increased IL-6 in older people [58]. In addition, cellular stress responses with the release of IL-6 increase with age, contributing to the persistent inflammation seen in older people [59,60]. As the fundamental differences between late-onset and young-onset RA are poorly understood, a multifaceted analysis combining immunophenotyping and cytokine analysis using synovial tissue and peripheral blood with clinical features and treatment response data would contribute to a detailed understanding of the pathogenesis and to the establishment of optimal treatment strategies for LORA.

3.3. *Management of Late-Onset Rheumatoid Arthritis*

In the management of LORA, there are many issues other than RA itself, including geriatric syndromes such as frailty, dementia, physical function, and organ dysfunction, as well as comorbidity, which are complex and intertwined with each other, making it a very difficult condition to address, which has been referred to as the 'spaghetti model' [61]. To manage the complex 'spaghetti model', the 5Ms approach—Mind, Mobility, Medication, Multicomplexity, and Matters Most—is proposed, which focuses on geriatric care and can help to develop a management plan tailored to the needs of older people.

Regarding the treatment of RA, a consensus statement on LORA has now been published [62], recommending methotrexate as primary treatment, with consideration of molecular-targeted agents if treatment goals cannot be achieved. Achieving a treat-to-target strategy has been shown to be associated with high remission rates without increasing the rate of adverse events in patients with LORA [63]. In this study, the presence of lung lesions and malignancy were independent risk factors for adverse events, while age, methotrexate use, and bDMARDs use were not extracted as relevant factors; therefore, a treatment strategy similar to YORA is desirable, with due consideration for safety. The Glucocorticoid Low-dose in Rheumatoid Arthritis (GLORIA) trial, a recent pragmatic randomized trial, investigated the efficacy and safety of add-on low-dose prednisolone (5 mg/day) in patients aged 65 years with established RA [64]. Add-on low-dose prednisolone therapy shows beneficial long-term effects in older patients with RA, with a trade-off of a 24% increase in adverse events, which mainly consisted of infection. However, this study did not focus on newly onset LORA, and long-term glucocorticoid use (>2 years) is associated with cardiovascular diseases [44], osteoporosis [45], severe infectious adverse events [65], and sarcopenia [66]; thus, we need to be careful about glucocorticoid use, and it is mentioned that the glucocorticoid dose should be kept at a minimum and should be discontinued within 6 months whenever possible in the consensus statement [63].

With regard to geriatric syndromes, the progression of frailty is a strong predictor for subsequent hospitalization and mortality in patients with LORA, and once it has progressed, frailty is difficult to reverse even after an improvement in the disease activity of RA [67]. Comprehensive strategies such as diet, exercise, and vaccination to prevent frailty are considered as important as RA management [68].

Multimorbidity is also an important aspect in the management of LORA; for instance, chronic kidney disease and lung disease may limit the use of methotrexate. An observational study has shown that a group of patients with the highest number of complications had a higher mortality rate when categorized by the number of comorbidities [43]. In addition, a higher number of complications leads to a higher number of drugs administered, and polypharmacy, especially the administration of more than 10 drugs, is associated with difficulties in controlling disease activity in RA and a higher incidence of adverse events [69]. Uncontrolled RA activity is also known to lead to complications such as infection, respiratory disease, and renal dysfunction [46,70,71]; thus, the appropriate control of RA disease activity is also linked to the prevention and management of complications. Therefore, LORA requires a more multifaceted approach than YORA.

We summarize the clinical characteristics and management of LORA in Figure 2.

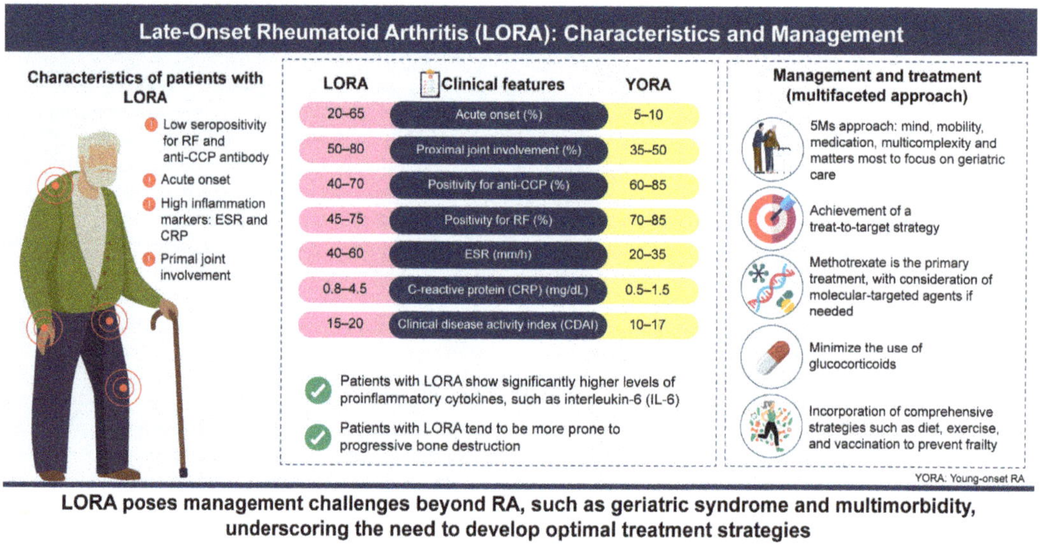

Figure 2. Clinical characteristics and management of late-onset rheumatoid arthritis (LORA). LORA tends to have low seropositivity, acute onset, high inflammation makers, and proximal joint involvement. LORA poses management challenges beyond RA, such as geriatric syndrome and multimorbidity, underscoring the need to develop optimal treatment strategies.

3.4. Future Prospectives for LORA

Although the number of patients with LORA is increasing rapidly with the aging society and is expected to increase further in the future, there are many unresolved issues relating to LORA. Remarkable advances have been made in the treatment of RA, but the evidence is mainly based on studies focused on patients with YORA and there is an urgent need to establish evidence for LORA. In the future, randomized controlled studies focusing on newly onset LORA and the accumulation of real-world data on LORA are needed to determine the optimal strategy. We have already initiated a registry study of LORA [72], which will provide information on the actual treatment situation and problems in LORA. In addition to clinical data, accompanying basic research, such as single-cell analysis using synovial specimens or focusing on immunosenescence in patients with RA, will help determine optimal treatment strategies by elucidating the pathological differences between LORA and YORA.

Funding: This work was supported by JSPS KAKENHI; grant number JP 22K16350 for S.T.

Conflicts of Interest: S.T. has received speaking fees from Asahi-Kasei, Astellas, Bristol-Myers Squibb, Eisai, Eli Lilly, Janssen, Mitsubishi-Tanabe, Pfizer, Taisho, and UCB. Y.K. has received research grants from AbbVie, Eisai, Sanofi, Chugai, Mitsubishi-Tanabe, and Taisho, and has received scholarship grants from Asahi-Kasei, Eisai, Boehringer Ingelheim, and Taisho, as we as receiving speaking fees from AbbVie, Asahi-Kasei, Astellas, Ayumi Pharmaceutical Corporation, Boehringer Ingelheim, Bristol-Myers Squibb, Chugai, Eisai, Eli Lilly, Glaxo Smith Kline, Novartis, Pfizer, Janssen, UCB, and Gilead Sciences.

References

1. Aletaha, D.; Neogi, T.; Silman, A.J.; Funovits, J.; Felson, D.T.; Bingham, C.O., III; Birnbaum, N.S.; Burmester, G.R.; Bykerk, V.P.; Cohen, M.D.; et al. 2010 rheumatoid arthritis classification criteria: An American College of Rheumatology/European League Against Rheumatism collaborative initiative. *Ann. Rheum. Dis.* **2010**, *69*, 1580–1588. [CrossRef] [PubMed]
2. Smolen, J.S.; Aletaha, D.; Bijlsma, J.W.J.; Breedveld, F.C.; Boumpas, D.; Burmester, G.; Combe, B.; Cutolo, M.; de Wit, M.; Dougados, M.; et al. Treating rheumatoid arthritis to target: Recommendations of an international task force. *Ann. Rheum. Dis.* **2010**, *69*, 631–637. [CrossRef] [PubMed]
3. Burmester, G.R.; Bijlsma, J.W.J.; Cutolo, M.; McInnes, I.B. Managing rheumatic and musculoskeletal diseases—Past, present and future. *Nat. Rev. Rheumatol.* **2017**, *13*, 443–448. [CrossRef] [PubMed]
4. Virtanen, A.; Spinelli, F.R.; Telliez, J.B.; O'Shea, J.J.; Silvennoinen, O.; Gadina, M. JAK inhibitor selectivity: New opportunities, better drugs? *Nat. Rev. Rheumatol.* **2024**, *20*, 649–665. [CrossRef]
5. Smolen, J.S.; Landewé, R.B.M.; Bergstra, S.A.; Kerschbaumer, A.; Sepriano, A.; Aletaha, D.; Caporali, R.; Edwards, C.J.; Hyrich, K.L.; Pope, J.E.; et al. EULAR recommendations for the management of rheumatoid arthritis with synthetic and biological disease-modifying antirheumatic drugs: 2022 update. *Ann. Rheum. Dis.* **2023**, *82*, 3–18. [CrossRef]
6. Takanashi, S.; Kaneko, Y.; Takeuchi, T. CDAI and DAS28 in the management of rheumatoid arthritis in clinical practice. *Ann. Rheum. Dis.* **2020**, *79*, 671–674. [CrossRef] [PubMed]
7. Chiu, Y.M.; Lu, Y.P.; Lan, J.L.; Chen, D.Y.; Wang, J.D. Lifetime Risks, Life Expectancy, and Health Care Expenditures for Rheumatoid Arthritis: A Nationwide Cohort Followed Up From 2003 to 2016. *Arthritis Rheumatol.* **2021**, *73*, 750–758. [CrossRef] [PubMed]
8. Krijbolder, D.I.; Verstappen, M.; van Dijk, B.T.; Dakkak, Y.J.; Burgers, L.E.; Boer, A.C.; Park, Y.J.; de Witt-Luth, M.E.; Visser, K.; Kok, M.R.; et al. Intervention with methotrexate in patients with arthralgia at risk of rheumatoid arthritis to reduce the development of persistent arthritis and its disease burden (TREAT EARLIER): A randomised, double-blind, placebo-controlled, proof-of-concept trial. *Lancet* **2022**, *400*, 283–294. [CrossRef]
9. Rech, J.; Tascilar, K.; Hagen, M.; Kleyer, A.; Manger, B.; Schoenau, V.; Hueber, A.J.; Kleinert, S.; Baraliakos, X.; Braun, J.; et al. Abatacept inhibits inflammation and onset of rheumatoid arthritis in individuals at high risk (ARIAA): A randomised, international, multicentre, double-blind, placebo-controlled trial. *Lancet* **2024**, *403*, 850–859. [CrossRef] [PubMed]
10. de Hair, M.J.H.; Jacobs, J.W.G.; Schoneveld, J.L.M.; van Laar, J.M. Difficult-to-treat rheumatoid arthritis: An area of unmet clinical need. *Rheumatology* **2018**, *57*, 1135–1144. [PubMed]
11. Roodenrijs, N.M.T.; de Hair, M.J.H.; van der Goes, M.C.; Jacobs, J.W.G.; Welsing, P.M.J.; van der Heijde, D.; Aletaha, D.; Dougados, M.; Hyrich, K.L.; McInnes, I.B.; et al. Characteristics of difficult-to-treat rheumatoid arthritis: Results of an international survey. *Ann. Rheum. Dis.* **2018**, *77*, 1705–1709. [CrossRef] [PubMed]
12. Nawrot, J.; Boonen, A.; Peeters, R.; Starmans, M.; van Onna, M. Rheumatologists' Views and Experiences in Managing Rheumatoid Arthritis in Elderly Patients: A Qualitative Study. *J. Rheumatol.* **2018**, *45*, 590–594. [CrossRef]
13. Takanashi, S.; Kaneko, Y.; Kawahito, Y.; Kida, T.; Sugihara, T.; Kojima, T.; Harada, R.; Ishitoku, M.; Hirata, S.; Hashimoto, M.; et al. A preliminary survey of rheumatologists on the management of late-onset rheumatoid arthritis in Japan. *Intern. Med.* **2024**. *ahead of print*. [CrossRef] [PubMed]
14. Nagy, G.; Roodenrijs, N.M.T.; Welsing, P.M.; Kedves, M.; Hamar, A.; van der Goes, M.C.; Kent, A.; Bakkers, M.; Blaas, E.; Senolt, L.; et al. EULAR definition of difficult-to-treat rheumatoid arthritis. *Ann. Rheum. Dis.* **2021**, *80*, 31–35. [CrossRef]
15. Roodenrijs, N.M.T.; van der Goes, M.C.; Welsing, P.M.J.; Tekstra, J.; Lafeber, F.P.J.G.; Jacobs, J.W.G.; van Laar, J.M. Difficult-to-treat rheumatoid arthritis: Contributing factors and burden of disease. *Rheumatology* **2021**, *60*, 3778–3788. [CrossRef]
16. Takanashi, S.; Kaneko, Y.; Takeuchi, T. Characteristics of patients with difficult-to-treat rheumatoid arthritis in clinical practice. *Rheumatology* **2021**, *60*, 5247–5256. [CrossRef] [PubMed]
17. Watanabe, R.; Hashimoto, M.; Murata, K.; Murakami, K.; Tanaka, M.; Ohmura, K.; Ito, H.; Matsuda, S. Prevalence and predictive factors of difficult-to-treat rheumatoid arthritis: The KURAMA cohort. *Immunol. Med.* **2022**, *45*, 35–44. [CrossRef] [PubMed]
18. Messelink, M.A.; Roodenrijs, N.M.T.; van Es, B.; Hulsbergen-Veelken, C.A.R.; Jong, S.; Overmars, L.M.; Reteig, L.C.; Tan, S.C.; Tauber, T.; van Laar, J.M.; et al. Identification and prediction of difficult-to-treat rheumatoid arthritis patients in structured and unstructured routine care data: Results from a hackathon. *Arthritis Res. Ther.* **2021**, *23*, 184. [CrossRef] [PubMed]
19. Ochi, S.; Sonomoto, K.; Nakayamada, S.; Tanaka, Y. Preferable outcome of Janus kinase inhibitors for a group of difficult-to-treat rheumatoid arthritis patients: From the FIRST Registry. *Arthritis Res. Ther.* **2022**, *24*, 61. [CrossRef]
20. Yoshii, I.; Sawada, N.; Chijiwa, T. Clinical characteristics and variants that predict prognosis of difficult-to-treat rheumatoid arthritis. *Rheumatol. Int.* **2022**, *42*, 1947–1954. [CrossRef]
21. Giollo, A.; Zen, M.; Larosa, M.; Astorri, D.; Salvato, M.; Calligaro, A.; Botsios, K.; Bernardi, C.; Bianchi, G.; Doria, A. Early characterization of difficult-to-treat rheumatoid arthritis by suboptimal initial management: A multicentre cohort study. *Rheumatology* **2023**, *62*, 2083–2089. [CrossRef]

22. Novella-Navarro, M.; Ruiz-Esquide, V.; Torres-Ortiz, G.; Chacur, C.A.; Tornero, C.; Fernández-Fernández, E.; Monjo, I.; Sanmartí, R.; Plasencia-Rodríguez, C.; Balsa, A. A paradigm of difficult-to-treat rheumatoid arthritis: Subtypes and early identification. *Clin. Exp. Rheumatol.* **2023**, *41*, 1114–1119.
23. Leon, L.; Madrid-Garcia, A.; Lopez-Viejo, P.; González-Álvaro, I.; Novella-Navarro, M.; Freites Nuñez, D.; Rosales, Z.; Fernandez-Gutierrez, B.; Abasolo, L. Difficult-to-treat rheumatoid arthritis (D2T RA): Clinical issues at early stages of disease. *RMD Open* **2023**, *9*, e002842. [CrossRef]
24. Hecquet, S.; Combier, A.; Steelandt, A.; Pons, M.; Wendling, D.; Molto, A.; Miceli-Richard, C.; Allanore, Y.; Avouac, J. Characteristics of patients with difficult-to-treat rheumatoid arthritis in a French single-centre hospital. *Rheumatology* **2023**, *62*, 3866–3874. [CrossRef] [PubMed]
25. Garcia-Salinas, R.; Sanchez-Prado, E.; Mareco, J.; Ronald, P.; Ruta, S.; Gomez, R.; Magri, S. Difficult to treat rheumatoid arthritis in a comprehensive evaluation program: Frequency according to different objective evaluations. *Rheumatol. Int.* **2023**, *43*, 1821–1828. [CrossRef] [PubMed]
26. Jung, J.Y.; Lee, E.; Kim, J.W.; Suh, C.H.; Shin, K.; Kim, J.; Kim, H.A. Unveiling difficult-to-treat rheumatoid arthritis: Long-term impact of biologic or targeted synthetic DMARDs from the KOBIO registry. *Arthritis Res. Ther.* **2023**, *25*, 174. [CrossRef]
27. David, P.; Di Matteo, A.; Hen, O.; Dass, S.; Marzo-Ortega, H.; Wakefield, R.J.; Bissell, L.A.; Nam, J.; Mankia, K.; Emery, P.; et al. Poly-Refractory Rheumatoid Arthritis: An Uncommon Subset of Difficult to Treat Disease With Distinct Inflammatory and Noninflammatory Phenotypes. *Arthritis Rheumatol.* **2024**, *76*, 510–521. [CrossRef]
28. Michitsuji, T.; Fukui, S.; Morimoto, S.; Endo, Y.; Nishino, A.; Nishihata, S.; Tsuji, Y.; Shimizu, T.; Umeda, M.; Sumiyoshi, R.; et al. Clinical and ultrasound features of difficult-to-treat rheumatoid arthritis: A multicenter RA ultrasound cohort study. *Scand. J. Rheumatol.* **2024**, *53*, 123–129. [CrossRef] [PubMed]
29. Bertsias, A.; Flouri, I.D.; Repa, A.; Avgoustidis, N.; Kalogiannaki, E.; Pitsigavdaki, S.; Bertsias, G.; Sidiropoulos, P. Patterns of comorbidities differentially affect long-term functional evolution and disease activity in patients with 'difficult to treat' rheumatoid arthritis. *RMD Open* **2024**, *10*, e003808. [CrossRef]
30. Alp, G.; Cinakli, H.; Kurut Aysin, İ.; Solmaz, D.; Akar, S. Challenges and insights in managing difficult-to-treat rheumatoid arthritis: Real-world clinical perspectives. *Clin. Exp. Rheumatol.* **2024**, *42*, 1398–1406. [CrossRef]
31. Watanabe, R.; Ebina, K.; Gon, T.; Okano, T.; Murata, K.; Murakami, K.; Maeda, Y.; Jinno, S.; Shirasugi, I.; Son, Y.; et al. Predictive factors and treatment outcomes associated with difficult-to-treat rheumatoid arthritis conditions: The ANSWER cohort study. *Rheumatology* **2024**, *9*, 2418–2426. [CrossRef] [PubMed]
32. Takanashi, S.; Kaneko, Y.; Takeuchi, T. Elderly patients with comorbidities in the definition of difficult-to-treat rheumatoid arthritis. *Ann. Rheum. Dis.* **2021**, *80*, 1491–1493. [CrossRef] [PubMed]
33. Bécède, M.; Alasti, F.; Gessl, I.; Haupt, L.; Kerschbaumer, A.; Landesmann, U.; Loiskandl, M.; Supp, G.M.; Smolen, J.S.; Aletaha, D. Risk profiling for a refractory course of rheumatoid arthritis. *Semin. Arthritis Rheum.* **2019**, *49*, 211–217. [CrossRef] [PubMed]
34. Buch, M.H.; Eyre, S.; McGonagle, D. Persistent inflammatory and non-inflammatory mechanisms in refractory rheumatoid arthritis. *Nat. Rev. Rheumatol.* **2021**, *17*, 17–33. [CrossRef]
35. Sluka, K.A.; Clauw, D.J. Neurobiology of fibromyalgia and chronic widespread pain. *Neuroscience* **2016**, *338*, 114–129. [CrossRef] [PubMed] [PubMed Central]
36. Bai, Z.; Bartelo, N.; Aslam, M.; Murphy, E.A.; Hale, C.R.; Blachere, N.E.; Parveen, S.; Spolaore, E.; DiCarlo, E.; Gravallese, E.M.; et al. Synovial fibroblast gene expression is associated with sensory nerve growth and pain in rheumatoid arthritis. *Sci. Transl. Med.* **2024**, *16*, eadk3506. [CrossRef] [PubMed]
37. Nagy, G.; Roodenrijs, N.M.T.; Welsing, P.M.J.; Kedves, M.; Hamar, A.; van der Goes, M.C.; Kent, A.; Bakkers, M.; Pchelnikova, P.; Blaas, E.; et al. EULAR points to consider for the management of difficult-to-treat rheumatoid arthritis. *Ann. Rheum. Dis.* **2022**, *81*, 20–33. [CrossRef] [PubMed]
38. Takanashi, S.; Kondo, Y.; Saito, S.; Kikuchi, J.; Hanaoka, H.; Takeuchi, T.; Kaneko, Y. Effectiveness and safety of rituximab in special types of rheumatoid arthritis. *Int. J. Rheum. Dis.* **2023**, *26*, 2240–2247. [CrossRef] [PubMed]
39. Takanashi, S.; Takeuchi, T.; Kaneko, Y. Five-year follow-up of patients with difficult-to-treat rheumatoid arthritis. *Rheumatology* **2024**. *ahead of print*. [CrossRef]
40. Duquesne, J.; Bouget, V.; Cournède, P.H.; Fautrel, B.; Guillemin, F.; de Jong, P.H.P.; Heutz, J.W.; Verstappen, M.; van der Helm-van Mil, A.H.M.; Mariette, X.; et al. Machine learning identifies a profile of inadequate responder to methotrexate in rheumatoid arthritis. *Rheumatology* **2023**, *62*, 2402–2409. [CrossRef]
41. Cooles, F.A.H.; Tarn, J.; Lendrem, D.W.; Naamane, N.; Lin, C.M.; Millar, B.; Maney, N.J.; E Anderson, A.; Thalayasingam, N.; Diboll, J.; et al. Interferon-α-mediated therapeutic resistance in early rheumatoid arthritis implicates epigenetic reprogramming. *Ann. Rheum. Dis.* **2022**, *81*, 1214–1223. [CrossRef] [PubMed]
42. Sanayama, Y.; Ikeda, K.; Saito, Y.; Kagami, S.; Yamagata, M.; Furuta, S.; Kashiwakuma, D.; Iwamoto, I.; Umibe, T.; Nawata, Y.; et al. Prediction of therapeutic responses to tocilizumab in patients with rheumatoid arthritis: Biomarkers identified by analysis of gene expression in peripheral blood mononuclear cells using genome-wide DNA microarray. *Arthritis Rheumatol.* **2014**, *66*, 1421–1431. [CrossRef]
43. Crowson, C.S.; Atkinson, E.J.; Kronzer, V.L.; Kimbrough, B.A.; Arment, C.A.; Peterson, L.S.; Wright, K.; Mason, T.G., II; Bekele, D.I.; Davis, J.M., III; et al. Comorbidity clusters in patients with rheumatoid arthritis identify a patient phenotype with a favourable prognosis. *Ann. Rheum. Dis.* **2024**, *83*, 556–563. [CrossRef] [PubMed] [PubMed Central]

44. Ocon, A.J.; Reed, G.; Pappas, D.A.; Curtis, J.R.; Kremer, J.M. Short-term dose and duration-dependent glucocorticoid risk for cardiovascular events in glucocorticoid-naive patients with rheumatoid arthritis. *Ann. Rheum. Dis.* **2021**, *80*, 1522–1529. [CrossRef] [PubMed]
45. Wiebe, E.; Huscher, D.; Schaumburg, D.; Palmowski, A.; Hermann, S.; Buttgereit, T.; Biesen, R.; Burmester, G.R.; Palmowski, Y.; Boers, M.; et al. Optimising both disease control and glucocorticoid dosing is essential for bone protection in patients with rheumatic disease. *Ann. Rheum. Dis.* **2022**, *81*, 1313–1322. [CrossRef]
46. England, B.R.; Sayles, H.; Michaud, K.; Caplan, L.; Davis, L.A.; Cannon, G.W.; Sauer, B.C.; Solow, E.B.; Reimold, A.M.; Kerr, G.S.; et al. Cause-Specific Mortality in Male US Veterans with Rheumatoid Arthritis. *Arthritis Care Res.* **2016**, *68*, 36–45. [CrossRef] [PubMed]
47. Yamada, S.; Nagafuchi, Y.; Wang, M.; Ota, M.; Hatano, H.; Takeshima, Y.; Okubo, M.; Kobayashi, S.; Sugimori, Y.; Masahiro, N.; et al. Immunomics analysis of rheumatoid arthritis identified precursor dendritic cells as a key cell subset of treatment resistance. *Ann. Rheum. Dis.* **2023**, *82*, 809–819. [CrossRef]
48. Conrad, N.; Misra, S.; Verbakel, J.Y.; Verbeke, G.; Molenberghs, G.; Taylor, P.N.; Mason, J.; Sattar, N.; McMurray, J.J.V.; McInnes, I.B.; et al. Incidence, prevalence, and co-occurrence of autoimmune disorders over time and by age, sex, and socioeconomic status: A population-based cohort study of 22 million individuals in the UK. *Lancet* **2023**, *401*, 1878–1890. [CrossRef] [PubMed]
49. Matthijssen, X.M.E.; Huizinga, T.W.J.; van der Helm-van Mil, A.H.M. Increasing incidence of autoantibody-negative RA is replicated and is partly explained by an aging population. *Ann. Rheum. Dis.* **2022**, *81*, e69. [CrossRef] [PubMed]
50. Kato, E.; Sawada, T.; Tahara, K.; Hayashi, H.; Tago, M.; Mori, H.; Nishino, J.; Matsui, T.; Tohma, S. The age at onset of rheumatoid arthritis is increasing in Japan: A nationwide database study. *Int. J. Rheum. Dis.* **2017**, *20*, 839–845. [CrossRef] [PubMed]
51. Uchiyama, S.; Takanashi, S.; Takeno, M.; Gono, T.; Kaneko, Y.; Takeuchi, T.; Kuwana, M. Should we reconsider the definition of elderly-onset rheumatoid arthritis in an ageing society? *Mod. Rheumatol.* **2022**, *32*, 323–329. [CrossRef] [PubMed]
52. Takanashi, S.; Takeuchi, T.; Kaneko, Y. Effects of Aging on Rheumatoid Factor and Anticyclic Citrullinated Peptide Antibody Positivity in Patients with Rheumatoid Arthritis. *J. Rheumatol.* **2023**, *50*, 330–334. [CrossRef]
53. Romão, V.C.; Humby, F.; Kelly, S.; Di Cicco, M.; Mahto, A.; Lazarou, I.; Hands, R.; Rocher-Ros, V.; van der Heijde, D.; Fonseca, J.E.; et al. Treatment-resistant synovitis and radiographic progression are increased in elderly-onset rheumatoid arthritis patients: Findings from a prospective observational longitudinal early arthritis cohort study. *Semin. Arthritis Rheum.* **2020**, *50*, 735–743. [CrossRef]
54. Murata, K.; Ito, H.; Hashimoto, M.; Nishitani, K.; Murakami, K.; Tanaka, M.; Yamamoto, W.; Mimori, T.; Matsuda, S. Elderly onset of early rheumatoid arthritis is a risk factor for bone erosions, refractory to treatment: KURAMA cohort. *Int. J. Rheum. Dis.* **2019**, *22*, 1084–1093. [CrossRef]
55. Hao, N.; Ishikawa, H.; Abe, A.; Sudo, M.; Takamura, S.; Otani, H.; Ito, S.; Nakazono, K.; Murasawa, A. Unveiling the arthritis divide: Exploring treatment response and impact in late-onset vs. young-onset rheumatoid arthritis. *Mod. Rheumatol.* **2024**. *ahead of print*. [CrossRef] [PubMed]
56. Asai, S.; Suzuki, M.; Hara, R.; Hirano, Y.; Nagamine, S.; Kaneko, T.; Suto, T.; Okano, T.; Yoshioka, Y.; Hirao, M.; et al. Comparison of effectiveness of methotrexate in patients with late-onset versus younger-onset rheumatoid arthritis: Real-world data from an inception cohort in Japan (NICER-J). *Mod. Rheumatol.* **2024**, *34*, 892–899. [CrossRef] [PubMed]
57. Chen, D.Y.; Hsieh, T.Y.; Chen, Y.M.; Hsieh, C.W.; Lan, J.L.; Lin, F.J. Proinflammatory cytokine profiles of patients with elderly-onset rheumatoid arthritis: A comparison with younger-onset disease. *Gerontology* **2009**, *55*, 250–258. [CrossRef]
58. Boren, E.; Gershwin, M.E. Inflamm-aging: Autoimmunity, and the immune-risk phenotype. *Autoimmun. Rev.* **2004**, *3*, 401–406. [CrossRef] [PubMed]
59. Franceschi, C.; Bonafè, M.; Valensin, S.; Olivieri, F.; De Luca, M.; Ottaviani, E.; De Benedictis, G. Inflamm-aging: An evolutionary perspective on immunosenescence. *Ann. N. Y. Acad. Sci.* **2000**, *908*, 244–254. [CrossRef] [PubMed]
60. Kirkland, J.L. The biology of senescence: Potential for prevention of disease. *Clin. Geriatr. Med.* **2002**, *18*, 383–405. [CrossRef]
61. van Onna, M.; Boonen, A. Challenges in the management of older patients with inflammatory rheumatic diseases. *Nat. Rev. Rheumatol.* **2022**, *18*, 326–334. [CrossRef] [PubMed]
62. Kojima, M.; Sugihara, T.; Kawahito, Y.; Kojima, T.; Kaneko, Y.; Ishikawa, H.; Abe, A.; Matsui, K.; Hirata, S.; Kishimoto, M.; et al. Consensus statement on the management of late-onset rheumatoid arthritis. *Mod. Rheumatol.* **2024**, *34*, 1095–1102. [CrossRef]
63. Sugihara, T.; Ishizaki, T.; Onoguchi, W.; Baba, H.; Matsumoto, T.; Iga, S.; Kubo, K.; Kamiya, M.; Hirano, F.; Hosoya, T.; et al. Effectiveness and safety of treat-to-target strategy in elderly-onset rheumatoid arthritis: A 3-year prospective observational study. *Rheumatology* **2021**, *60*, 4252–4261. [CrossRef]
64. Boers, M.; Hartman, L.; Opris-Belinski, D.; Bos, R.; Kok, M.R.; Da Silva, J.A.; Griep, E.N.; Klaasen, R.; Allaart, C.F.; Baudoin, P.; et al. Low dose, add-on prednisolone in patients with rheumatoid arthritis aged 65+: The pragmatic randomised, double-blind placebo-controlled GLORIA trial. *Ann. Rheum. Dis.* **2022**, *81*, 925–936. [CrossRef]
65. Barbulescu, A.; Sjölander, A.; Delcoigne, B.; Askling, J.; Frisell, T. Glucocorticoid exposure and the risk of serious infections in rheumatoid arthritis: A marginal structural model application. *Rheumatology* **2023**, *62*, 3391–3399. [CrossRef] [PubMed]
66. Yamada, Y.; Tada, M.; Mandai, K.; Hidaka, N.; Inui, K.; Nakamura, H. Glucocorticoid use is an independent risk factor for developing sarcopenia in patients with rheumatoid arthritis: From the CHIKARA study. *Clin. Rheumatol.* **2020**, *39*, 1757–1764. [CrossRef] [PubMed]

67. Hanlon, P.; Morton, F.; Siebert, S.; Jani, B.D.; Nicholl, B.I.; Lewsey, J.; McAllister, D.; Mair, F.S. Frailty in rheumatoid arthritis and its relationship with disease activity, hospitalisation and mortality: A longitudinal analysis of the Scottish Early Rheumatoid Arthritis cohort and UK Biobank. *RMD Open* **2022**, *8*, e002111. [CrossRef]
68. Kim, D.H.; Rockwood, K. Frailty in Older Adults. *N. Engl. J. Med.* **2024**, *391*, 538–548. [CrossRef] [PubMed]
69. Bechman, K.; Clarke, B.D.; Rutherford, A.I.; Yates, M.; Nikiphorou, E.; Molokhia, M.; Norton, S.; Cope, A.P.; Hyrich, K.L.; Galloway, J.B. Polypharmacy is associated with treatment response and serious adverse events: Results from the British Society for Rheumatology Biologics Register for Rheumatoid Arthritis. *Rheumatology* **2019**, *58*, 1767–1776. [CrossRef] [PubMed]
70. Hanaoka, H.; Kikuchi, J.; Hiramoto, K.; Saito, S.; Kondo, Y.; Kaneko, Y. Decreased chronic kidney disease in rheumatoid arthritis in the era of biologic disease-modifying anti-rheumatic drugs. *Clin. Kidney J.* **2022**, *15*, 1373–1378. [CrossRef] [PubMed]
71. Fukui, S.; Winkelmayer, W.C.; Tedeschi, S.K.; Marrugo, J.; Guan, H.; Harrold, L.; Litman, H.J.; Shinozaki, T.; Solomon, D.H. Disease activity of rheumatoid arthritis and kidney function decline: A large prospective registry study. *Ann. Rheum. Dis.* **2024**. *ahead of print*. [CrossRef] [PubMed]
72. Kojima, M.; Kawahito, Y.; Sugihara, T.; Kojima, T.; Harada, R.; Hirata, S.; Hashimoto, M.; Hidaka, T.; Ishikawa, H.; Ito, H.; et al. Late-onset rheumatoid arthritis registry study, LORIS study: Study protocol and design. *BMC Rheumatol.* **2022**, *6*, 90. [CrossRef] [PubMed]

Journal of
Clinical Medicine

MDPI

Review

Osteoporosis and Rheumatoid Arthritis: Mechanisms Underlying Osteoclast Differentiation and Activation or Factors Associated with Hip Fractures

Takeshi Miyamoto

Department of Orthopedic Surgery, Faculty of Life Sciences, Kumamoto University, 1-1-1 Honjo, Chuo-ku, Kumamoto 860-8556, Japan; miyamoto.takeshi@kuh.kumamoto-u.ac.jp; Tel.: +81-96-373-5226

Abstract: Osteoporosis is defined as a condition of increased risk of fracture due to decreased bone strength. In developed countries, the number of patients with osteoporosis and fragility fractures has been increasing in recent years due to the growing elderly population, posing a social challenge not only to fracture patients and their families but also to the social healthcare economy. Osteoporosis can be divided into two categories: primary osteoporosis caused by aging or menopause and secondary osteoporosis caused by metabolic or inflammatory diseases or drugs such as glucocorticoids. The majority of patients have primary osteoporosis, and the pathogenesis of postmenopausal osteoporosis and factors associated with fragility fractures in the elderly have been elucidated. On the other hand, rheumatoid arthritis (RA) is one of the causes of secondary osteoporosis. RA is a chronic inflammatory disease characterized by joint swelling and destruction. Most often, treatment focuses on suppressing these symptoms. However, physicians should be aware of the risk of osteoporosis in RA patients, because (1) RA is a chronic inflammatory disease, which itself can be a risk factor for osteoporosis; (2) glucocorticoids, which are sometimes administered to treat RA, can be a risk factor for osteoporosis; and (3) patients with RA are becoming older, and aging is an osteoporosis risk factor. A comprehensive understanding of the pathogenesis of osteoporosis and its fragility fractures requires elucidating the mechanisms underlying osteoclast activation, which drives their development. Furthermore, identifying the factors associated with fragility fractures is essential. This review summarizes the pathogenesis of osteoporosis, the factors associated with fragility fractures, and the associations between RA and osteoporosis development.

Keywords: rheumatoid arthritis (RA); osteoporosis; chronic inflammation; glucocorticoid; aging

1. Introduction

Osteoporosis is defined as a condition of increased risk of fracture due to decreased bone strength. Bone mineral density is responsible for about 70% of bone strength and structural and material bone quality for the remaining 30%. Bone mineral density (BMD) can be quantitatively measured by dual energy X-Ray absorptiometry (DXA), and diagnostic reference values have been established. On the other hand, the remaining 30% is defined by structural bone quality, such as bone microstructure, and material quality, such as the extracellular matrix protein composition. Structural bone quality is measured by micro-CT, high-resolution peripheral quantitative CT (HR-pQCT), or trabecular bone score (TBS), while material quality is measured by urinary pentosidine, but no diagnostic criteria to start drug treatment have been established. Osteoporosis can be classified as either primary osteoporosis, which is caused by aging or menopause, or secondary osteoporosis, which is caused by factors such as metabolic disease, inflammatory diseases such as rheumatoid arthritis (RA), and some medications. Osteoporosis is one of the typical age-related diseases whose prevalence increases with aging. In a survey conducted from 2015–2016, the number of patients with osteoporosis diagnosed by decreased bone mineral density over 40 years of age was estimated to be 15.9 million in Japan (4.1 million men and 11.8 million women), and the prevalence of osteoporosis in different age groups shows a clear increase with increasing age [1]. In addition, the 15.9 million patients with osteoporosis from 2015–2016 is a significant increase from the 12.8 million (3.0 million men and 9.6 million women) from 2005–2007 [2]. The increase in the number of osteoporosis patients is thought to be due to the increase in the geriatric population [1].

RA has complications [3], among them, osteoporosis, which should not be overlooked as it is directly related to bone fractures and to the resulting decreases in activity level of daily living (ADL) and quality of life (QOL). Additionally, there are various risks associated with osteoporosis, including RA [4]. RA patients can develop various risks of developing osteoporosis, including elevated levels of inflammatory cytokines in the blood or joints, glucocorticoid use, and aging. Bone alterations in patients with rheumatoid arthritis (RA) are basically assessed by bone mineral density loss, existing fragility fractures, and the Fracture Risk Assessment tool (FRAX) developed by the WHO for patients with primary osteoporosis [5], but in RA patients, joint erosion and/or destruction/deformation are also critical indicators for the local activation of osteoclasts.

RA patients have been shown to have a higher risk of fragility fractures than non-RA patients. A cohort study showed that the incidence rate (IR) per 1000 person years (PY) with 95% confidence intervals (CI) for the first fracture in RA patients was 18.3 (15.7–21.2) and the incidence rate ratio (IRR) was 1.32 (1.10–1.60) [6]. In addition, RA is listed as a risk for osteoporosis in FRAX [5], and many reports indicate that RA is a risk for osteoporosis [7,8]. However, despite the fact that RA patients are at high risk of fractures, osteoporosis is currently not adequately treated [8]. Physicians should always be aware that RA carries the risk of osteoporosis and fragility fractures.

To understand the pathogenesis of the disease, it is first necessary to understand how physiological bone metabolism is regulated. These mechanisms and pathways are essential for the regulation of bone homeostasis, and their disruptions can lead directly to changes in bone mass. Understanding the regulatory mechanisms of bone homeostasis has led to the discoveries of the receptor activator of the nuclear factor kappa B ligand (RANKL) as a therapeutic target for osteoporosis and bone erosion, Sclerostin as a target for osteogenesis-promoting drugs, and the mechanism underlying postmenopausal osteoporosis development [9–11]. Furthermore, the elucidation of the mechanism by which inflammatory cytokines cause bone erosion suggests the need to regulate inflammatory cytokines and related cellular activities in order to suppress bone erosion. Knowing the mechanisms underlying the osteoclast activation that causes osteoporosis development and fragility fractures and the factors associated with hip fractures in patients who actually developed hip fractures are mandatory for developing a way to prevent their developments. In the development of fragility fractures such as hip fracture, various factors play a role in the loss of bone mineral density and bone strength, including osteoclast activation. However, there are few reviews that introduce physiological osteoclast differentiation as well as osteoclast differentiation and activation under inflammatory conditions such as RA in a unified manner. In addition, there are no reviews that include factors that are characteristic of patients who actually developed hip fractures. This review aims to discuss the various factors and mechanisms involved in osteoclast activation, which causes bone loss and joint erosion, and the factors associated with fractures in patients with fragility fractures.

This manuscript mainly overviews and focuses on the literature related to the pathogenesis of osteoporosis and the mechanisms underlying the development of osteoporosis and joint erosion in RA. To highlight the importance of understanding the pathogenesis of osteoporosis and joint erosion, clinical articles showing the clinical aspects of RA, osteoporosis, and fragility fracture patients or cohort studies, together with the molecular mechanisms underlying these clinical outcomes, are alternately discussed.

2. Regulation of Bone Homeostasis

Bone homeostasis is mainly regulated by two cell types: osteoclasts, which are responsible for bone resorption, and osteoblasts, which are responsible for bone formation. Bone is not a static tissue with no metabolism, but bone homeostasis is continuously and dynamically regulated by bone resorption by osteoclasts and bone formation by osteoblasts. When the activities of osteoclasts and osteoblasts are balanced, bone is in a state of dynamic equilibrium and bone mass is maintained at a constant level. However, with menopause and aging, osteoclast activity relatively exceeds osteoblast activity, resulting in bone loss and osteoporosis.

Osteoclasts are terminally differentiated cells of the monocyte–macrophage lineage derived from hematopoietic stem cells and are the unique cells in the body responsible for bone resorption. The discovery of the receptor activator of the nuclear factor kappa B ligand the (RANKL)-RANK system has rapidly advanced our understanding of the mechanisms underlying osteoclast differentiation [12–15]. RANKL is a member of the tumor necrosis factor alpha (TNFα) superfamily of cytokines [16], and the osteoprotegerin (OPG)/osteoclastogenesis inhibitory factor (OCIF), a decoy receptor for RANKL, masks RANKL under normal conditions and prevents osteoclast differentiation [17,18]. Denosumab, a RANKL-neutralizing antibody, is used as a therapeutic agent for osteoporosis [9], a giant cell tumor of bone; metastatic bone tumors; and other diseases in which osteoclast activity is increased, resulting in decreased bone density and bone destruction. In Japan, denosumab is also used to inhibit joint erosion in RA [19].

After binding to its receptor RANK, RANKL activates various signals in osteoclast progenitor cells to promote osteoclast differentiation. The transcription factor c-Fos is essential for osteoclast differentiation [20]. c-Fos-deficient mice completely lacked osteoclasts, and the mice developed osteopetrosis [20]. Downstream from c-Fos, a transcription factor identified as essential for osteoclast differentiation is a nuclear factor of the activated T cells 1 (NFATc1) [21]. NFATc1 binds to the transcriptional regulatory regions of various osteoclast-specific molecules such as Cathepsin K and directly regulates their expressions [21]. NFATc1 also drives osteoclast differentiation positively by upregulating NFATc1 expression through auto-amplification, which induces NFATc1's own expression [22]. RANKL stimulation activates calcium signaling through spleen tyrosine kinase (Syk) and Phospholipase gamma (PLCγ) from the immunoreceptor's tyrosine-based activation-motif (ITAM) signal FcRγ and the DNAX activation protein of 12 kDa (DAP12), resulting in the expression and activation of NFATc1 [23]. Administration of FK506, an inhibitor of calcineurin also used as a treatment for RA, has been shown to suppress osteoclast differentiation by the suppression of NFATc1 but also suppresses osteoblast activity, resulting in decreased bone density [24].

3. Multinucleation of Osteoclasts by a Cell–Cell Fusion

It has long been known that osteoclasts become multinucleated by the cell–cell fusion of mononuclear osteoclasts. It was formerly believed that the multinucleation of osteoclasts requires cells to increase in size by fusion in order to form structures such as ruffled boarders and sealing zones, which are considered essential for osteoclasts to exhibit bone resorption capacity. Although various molecules have been reported to be involved in the cell–cell fusion of osteoclasts, an analysis of dendritic cell-specific transmembrane protein (DC-STAMP)-deficient mice showed that DC-STAMP is essential for the multinucleation of osteoclasts by cell–cell fusion of mononuclear osteoclasts [25]. Although osteoclasts from DC-STAMP-deficient mice were mononuclear, the expression of differentiation markers was similar to that of multinuclear osteoclasts from wild-type mice, indicating that DC-STAMP functions specifically for cell–cell fusion rather than differentiation [25]. Subsequently, the cell–cell fusion of osteoclasts was also demonstrated to be strongly inhibited in mice lacking v-ATPase V0 subunit d2 (Atp6v0d2), one of the subunits of the proton pump, and CD200-deficient mice [26,27]. Furthermore, the cell–cell fusion of osteoclasts was demonstrated to be completely inhibited in osteoclast stimulatory transmembrane protein (OC-STAMP)-deficient mice without affecting osteoclast differentiation [28]. An analysis of mice in which the cell–cell fusion of osteoclasts was inhibited has shown that although the cell–cell fusion of osteoclasts is not essential for resorption, it does increase its efficiency [25,28]. DC-STAMP and OC-STAMP were also shown to be essential for the cell–cell fusion of foreign-body giant cells (FBGCs), which are differentiated from the progenitor cells common to osteoclasts and become multinucleated by the cell–cell fusion of mononuclear FBGCs [25,28]. FBGCs are formed in artificial joints and other medical devices that are placed in the body. Both DC-STAMP and OC-STAMP have also been shown to be transcriptional targets of NFATc1 in osteoclasts [28,29].

4. Regulation of Osteoclast Differentiation by Transcriptional Repressors

As described above, osteoclast differentiation is positively regulated downstream of RANKL by the transcription factor c-Fos-NFATc1 axis [20,21]. MAF bZIP transcription factor B (MafB), interferon regulatory factor 8 (Irf8), and B cell lymphoma 6 (Bcl6), all of which are transcriptional repressors, have also been identified as negative regulators of osteoclast differentiation [30–32]. As negative regulators of osteoclast differentiation, they play an inhibitory role in NFATc1, the accelerator of osteoclast differentiation. Mice deficient in either Irf8 or Bcl6 have been shown to exhibit a constant increase in osteoclast differentiation and activation, which in turn exhibits a decrease in bone mineral density [30,32]. The RANKL-RANK axis induces the expression and activation of NFATc1, a master transcription factor for osteoclast differentiation, via calcium signaling (Figure 1). However, NFATc1 expression and activation alone are not sufficient to promote osteoclast differentiation. Bcl6 is a transcriptional repressor that negatively regulates osteoclast differentiation (Figure 1). Indeed, the overexpression of Bcl6 inhibits osteoclast differentiation [32]. Meanwhile, B lymphocyte-induced maturation protein-1 (Blimp1) (also called PR domain containing 1, Prdm1), a transcriptional repressor downstream of RANKL, directly suppresses Bcl6 expression, resulting in inducing osteoclast differentiation (Figure 1) [32]. Blimp1 global knockout mice are embryonic lethal, but in conditional knockout mice lacking osteoclast-specific Blimp1, increased bone mass was observed due to inhibition of osteoclastogenesis [32,33]. Furthermore, Blimp1 conditional knockout mice, which are systemically deficient in Blimp1 after adulthood, also show an increase in bone mass due to the inhibition of osteoclastogenesis [34]. This suggests that Blimp1 may be a potential therapeutic target for increasing bone mass by inhibiting osteoclastogenesis [34].

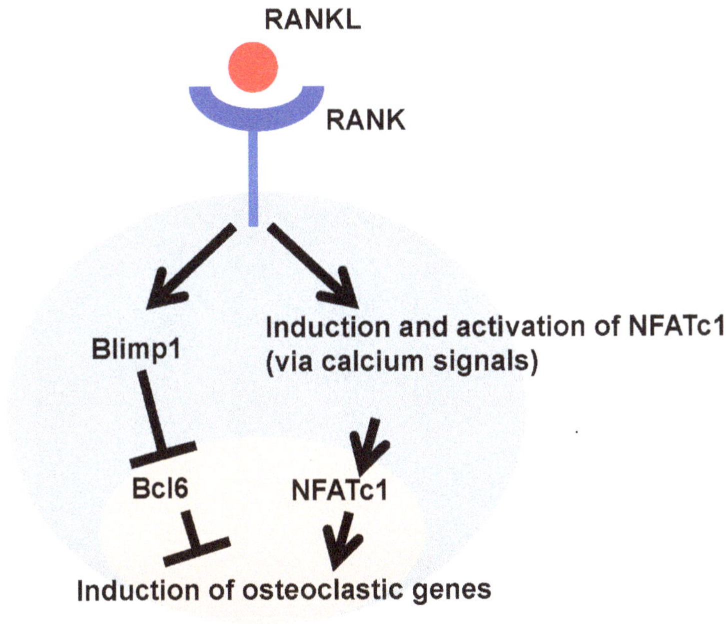

Figure 1. Regulation of osteoclastogenesis: NFATc1 and Blimp1-Bcl6 axis.

5. Mechanisms Underlying Postmenopausal Osteoporosis

In postmenopausal individuals, estrogen deficiency increases the activity of osteoclasts, which are responsible for bone resorption, leading to osteoporosis that is attributable to decreased bone mass. Moreover, menopause-related decreases in blood estrogen levels are known to increase levels of bone resorption markers in blood. Osteoclasts are found only on the bone's surface in hypoxic regions marked by an extremely low oxygen concentration [35]. We have shown that osteoclasts express hypoxia inducible factor 1 alpha (HIF1α), a transcription factor that regulates responses to hypoxia, and that in the premenopausal estrogen-sufficiency state, HIF1α expression by osteoclasts is suppressed by estrogen in those hypoxic regions (Figure 2) [11]. The osteoclastic bone resorptive activity required for physiological bone remodeling is independent of HIF1α (Figure 2). However, in estrogen-deficient conditions following menopause onset, HIF1α expression and activity increases, promoting osteoclastic bone resorption and leading to osteoporosis development (Figure 2) [11]. In mice genetically engineered to lack HIF1α in osteoclasts, no bone loss occurs in a postmenopausal osteoporosis model (ovariectomy, OVX) in which both ovaries are removed [11]. Furthermore, after a screen for HIF1α-inhibiting agents, we identified a small molecule that efficiently inhibits HIF1α expression in osteoclasts [30]. When we administered it to OVX mice, bone loss caused by estrogen deficiency was completely inhibited [11]. We also found that testosterone inhibits HIF1α expression in osteoclasts [36]. We then found that, in a male osteoporosis model in which bilateral testes were removed (orchiectomy, ORX), the administration of our HIF1α inhibitor completely blocked bone loss in ORX mice as well [36]. We also demonstrated that the treatment of mice with either selective estrogen-receptor modulators (SERMs), such as raloxifene, bazedoxifene, or tamoxifen, or the activated vitamin D3 analogue eldecalcitol, inhibited HIF1α expression in osteoclasts [37–39].

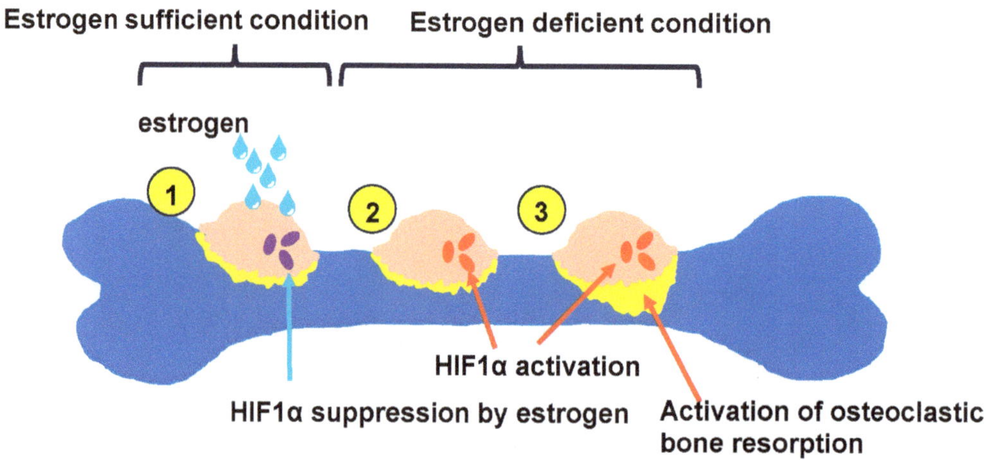

Figure 2. A mechanism underlying osteoclast activation in an estrogen-deficient condition. During the premenopausal estrogen sufficiency state, HIF1α, a transcriptional factor in osteoclasts, is continuously suppressed by estrogen (1). When estrogen deficiency occurs due to menopause, estrogen no longer suppresses HIF1α, and HIF1α is activated (2), which in turn the activation of osteoclasts leading to the development of osteoporosis (3).

6. Bone Remodeling

Bone metabolism can be divided into two major types: bone remodeling, in which bone formation is activated after resorption, and bone modeling, in which bone is formed without resorption. Remodeling is seen in areas where osteoclasts are present, such as trabecular bone, while modeling is seen mainly in membranous ossification. Classically, the growth factors such as transforming growth factor beta 1 (TGFβ) and insulin-like growth factor 1 (IGF1), which accumulate in the bone matrix, are released and activated by osteoclast bone resorption, and in turn, stimulate bone remodeling by activating osteoblasts to stimulate bone formation (refs. [40,41], Figure 3). TGFβ is stored in the bone extracellular matrix protein in an inactive latent form (ref. [40], Figure 3), and latent-TGFβ is known to be converted to the active form by acid. During bone resorption, this acid is secreted by osteoclasts, and the active form of TGFβ acts as a remodeling factor that activates osteoblasts following bone resorption (ref. [40], Figure 3). However, some factors have been reported to act on the osteoblast side via factors expressed by differentiated osteoclasts (Figure 3) rather than on bone resorption (Figure 3). The concept of bone remodeling has diversified, as ephrin B2 expressed on osteoclasts stimulates Eph B4 expressed on osteoblasts to promote bone formation [42], semaphorin 4D (Sema4D) expressed on osteoclasts conversely inhibits bone formation [43], and PDGF BB expressed on osteoclasts promotes bone formation through angiogenesis [44]. The concept of bone remodeling has diversified (Figure 3).

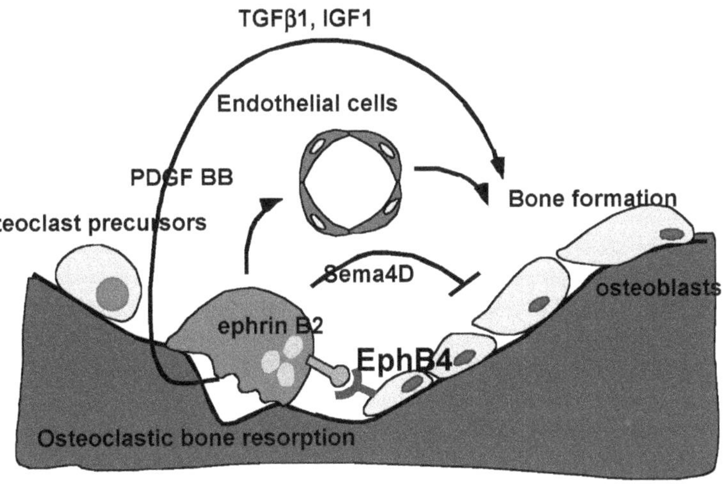

Figure 3. Regulation of bone remodeling. Bone remodeling is thought to be regulated by the activation of mesenchymal stem cells and osteoblasts by growth factors such as TGFβ1 and IGF1 released from the bone matrix by osteoclastic bone resorption. It has also been reported that ephrin B2, a membrane-bound ligand expressed by osteoclasts, stimulates Eph B4, a receptor expressed on osteoblasts. Semaphorin 4D (Sema 4D) secreted by osteoclasts inhibits bone formation, and PDGF BB secreted by osteoclasts promotes bone formation via angiogenesis.

7. Coupling and Uncoupling of Bone Metabolisms

In primary osteoporosis, a typical bone disease, both osteoclast and osteoblast activities are elevated, and when osteoclasts are suppressed with bisphosphonates or other bone resorption inhibitors, bone formation is also suppressed. Bone resorption inhibitors are currently the most commonly used drugs in the treatment of osteoporosis, as they suppress bone formation but increase bone mass by inhibiting excessive osteoclast activity. On the other hand, it has been suggested that the long-term administration of potent bone resorption inhibitors leads to the suppression of bone turnover, called severely suppressed bone turnover (SSBT), which may cause osteonecrosis of the jaw and atypical femur fractures [45–48]. Semaphorin 3a expressed by osteoblasts suppresses osteoclasts while activating osteoblasts, and it has been shown that both osteoclasts and osteoblasts can contribute to increased bone mass by creating an uncoupling state where the activities of the two cells are not synchronized [49]. Cathepsin K, a proteolytic enzyme that is activated under acidic conditions characteristic of osteoclasts and is used as a marker of osteoclast differentiation, has been reported to exhibit an uncoupling phenotype in an autosomal recessive genetic disease called pycnodysostosis and in gene-deficient mice, in which osteoclast activity increases rather than decreases [50,51]. A Cathepsin K inhibitor was previously developed as a therapeutic agent for increasing bone mass, although it was not launched due to an adverse effect. It has also been reported that the signal transducer and activator of transcription 1 (Stat1) acts to inhibit differentiation in both osteoclasts and osteoblasts, and although both cells are activated by Stat1 loss, osteoblast activation is relatively more dominant than osteoclast activation, resulting in increased bone mass [52, 53]. Mutations in the SOST gene encoding the Sclerostin protein result in a disease that causes increased bone mass [54,55]. Similarly, mice lacking the SOST gene have an increased bone mass phenotype with elevated bone formation [56]. Treatment with Romosozumab, a neutralizing antibody against Sclerostin, increases bone mass by uncoupling the transient activation of osteoblasts with the sustained inhibition of osteoclast activity in osteoporosis patients [10]. Romosozumab treatment has been shown to significantly prevent fragility fractures as a treatment for osteoporosis [57].

8. Treatment Strategy for Osteoporosis

Osteoporosis drugs increase bone mineral density (BMD) and reduce fragility fractures by intervening in bone metabolism. In women aged 55–81 years, alendronate, which is a bisphosphonate, significantly reduced the incidence of clinical vertebral fractures (hazard reduction 55%, $p < 0.001$) compared with a placebo for 3 years of treatment, and also significantly reduced hip fractures, which are difficult to prevent (relative hazard 0.49, $p = 0.047$). [58]. Denosumab, a neutralizing antibody against RANKL, significantly reduced the risk of new vertebral fracture (hazard ratio, 0.32; $p < 0.001$) and hip fracture (hazard ratio, 0.60; $p = 0.04$) in osteoporotic women aged 60 to 90 years after 3 years of treatment with denosumab versus placebo (hazard ratio, 0.60; $p = 0.04$). [9]. Teriparatide (PTH 1–34) has been shown to significantly reduce the risk of vertebral fracture versus placebo in postmenopausal osteoporotic patients treated for an average of 21 months (relative risk 0.35: $p < 0.001$). [59].

A potential limitation of osteoporosis drugs is that some have a limited duration of administration and others do not, making it difficult to compare long-term outcomes for differences in efficacy between these drugs. In postmenopausal women with low bone mineral density, romosozumab was superior to alendronate, a bisphosphonate, and teriparatide, an osteogenic agent, at 6 and 12 months after treatment, and BMD has been shown to increase significantly in the lumbar spine, proximal femur, and femoral neck at 6 and 12 months after treatment with romosozumab. [10]. Abaloparatide and teriparatide, both of which are bone-forming agents, also significantly reduced the incidences of new morphometric vertebral fractures in postmenopausal women with osteoporosis in both groups, as compared to the placebo (Abaloparatide group: relative risk, 0.14 [95% CI, 0.05 to 0.39]; $p < 0.001$, teriparatide group: relative risk, 0.20 [95% CI, 0.08 to 0.47]; $p < 0.001$), but there was no significant difference between the two groups [60].

On the other hand, the fact that the majority of hip fracture patients were not receiving treatment for osteoporosis at the time of fracture [61] makes it more important to ensure that drugs reach patients who need treatment than to develop drugs with high efficacy.

9. Joint Erosion and Osteoclasts in RA

In RA, in addition to the chronic inflammation of the joints, the activation of osteoclasts has been known to occur locally in the joints. In addition, when the types of T cell subsets were still poorly known, arthritis was thought to be caused by the activity of TH1 cells, which induce inflammation. However, because TH1 cells produce interferon gamma (IFNγ), a strong osteoclast suppressor, the activation of osteoclasts in a TH1-activated environment is inconsistent. TH17 cells, which produced IL-17 but not IFNγ, have been identified, and IL-17-deficient mice have been shown to exhibit improved pathogenesis of arthritis [62,63]. The TH17 cell is now considered to be an essential component in the pathogenesis of arthritis. Nowadays, single RNA sequencing or genome-wide studies using RA patient samples are being used to further elucidate the pathogenesis of the disease [64,65].

Osteoclasts play a major role in joint erosion and destruction in RA patients. This evidence has been shown in several osteoclast-deficient mouse models of arthritis. It has been reported that joint destruction in the human TNFα transgenic (hTNF Tg) was reportedly abolished by crossing it with c-Fos-deficient mice, in which osteoclasts were completely absent [66]. However, joint inflammation in the hTNF Tg/c-Fos-deficient mice was also observed in hTNF Tg mice, suggesting a distinction between arthritis and joint destruction [66]. In addition, an adjuvant-induced arthritis model in rats has shown that osteoprotegerin (OPG) administration can inhibit bone and cartilage destruction but not arthritis [67]. These findings indicate that joint destruction is caused by osteoclasts and that joint destruction can be prevented if osteoclasts can be suppressed even if inflammation remains severe. In RA patients, the administration of denosumab, a RANKL-neutralizing antibody, has been shown to significantly inhibit joint erosion by inhibiting osteoclast activity but not the joint-space narrowing caused by arthritis.

10. Chronic Inflammation in Rheumatoid Arthritis and Osteoporosis

In patients with RA, blood or local concentrations of inflammatory cytokines such as TNFα, IL-1, and IL-6 are generally elevated, particularly in older patients, causing joint swelling and destruction [68] via osteoclast activation. These factors are expressed by synovial fibroblasts and inflammatory cells infiltrating the joint synovium at the site of inflammation, and their concentration increases at the joint site, increasing osteoclast activity at that site and promoting pannus formation, joint destruction, and joint deformation (Figure 4) [69]. Together or alone, TNFα, IL-1 or IL-6 stimulate the expression of inflammatory cytokines, such as other IL-6 family proteins in synovial fibroblasts, thus promoting inflammatory cytokine expression in a positive feedback manner (Figures 4-1 and 5) [69]. This activity further promotes the expression of RANKL, which is essential for osteoclast differentiation, induction, and activation, to induce osteoclastogenesis (Figures 4-1 and 5) [69]. TNFα reportedly induces osteoclast activity directly (Figure 4-2) [70]. RANKL is a member of the TNFα superfamily, and some evidence suggests that intracellular signaling via RANKL or TNFα is similar. The TNF receptor-associated factor 6 (TRAF6) was demonstrated to be required for RANKL-induced osteoclastogenesis [71,72]. On the other hand, RANKL is required for osteoclast differentiation, while TNFα reportedly promotes the activation of osteoclast progenitor cells [73]. IL-1 is known to act directly on osteoclasts or osteoclast progenitors (Figure 4-2) [74], causing osteoclast activation and the prolonged survival of osteoclasts. Furthermore, TNFα, IL-1, and IL-6 induce RANKL expression by acting on osteoblasts (Figure 4) [69], thereby contributing to osteoclast induction. IL-6 also reportedly contributes to RANKL expression in T cells and osteoclast induction in synovial cells in joints (Figure 4-3) [75]. It is also possible that inflammatory cytokines expressed in joint tissues may increase IL-6 levels in the blood, resulting in a systemic increase in osteoclast activity. TNFα, IL-1, and IL-6 also activate signal transducer and activator of transcription factor 3 (STAT3), either directly (via IL-6) or indirectly (via TNFα and IL-1), and activated STAT3 promotes the expression of the IL-6 family cytokines and RANKL in fibroblasts (Figure 5) [69]. IL-6 family cytokines induced by activated STAT3 are known to enhance the expression of IL-6 family cytokines and RANKL, furthering inflammation and joint destruction (Figure 5) [69]. The induced IL-6 family cytokines further activate STAT3 to continuously induce IL-6 family cytokines and RANKL (Figure 5). We found that positive feedback loops of proinflammatory cytokines are not triggered by proinflammatory cytokines in Stat3-deficient cells, indicating that Stat3 induces the triggering of positive feedback loops of proinflammatory cytokines [69]. In Stat3-deficient cells, the induction of RANKL expression by inflammatory cytokines was also inhibited [69]. Furthermore, the conditional deletion of Stat3 at an adult stage was demonstrated to significantly inhibit arthritis development in RA mouse models [76]. RA susceptibility is also a risk factor for osteoporosis and fragility fractures, as RA is listed as a risk for osteoporosis in the Fracture Risk Assessment tool (FRAX) used to assess the risk of fragility fractures due to osteoporosis.

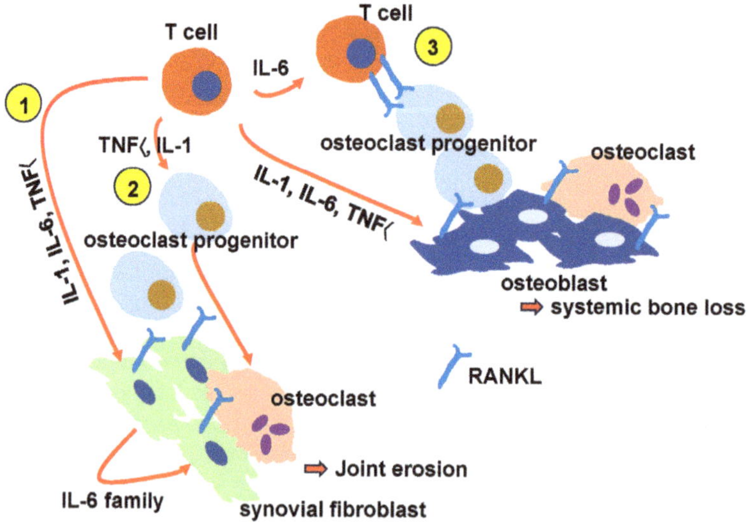

Figure 4. Inflammatory cytokine network for joint erosion and systemic bone loss in RA. T cells activated by antigen presentation, such as citrullinated proteins, secrete inflammatory cytokines such as TNFα, IL-6, and IL-1 (1). All of these inflammatory cytokines act on synovial fibroblasts to activate the expression of inflammatory cytokines such as the IL-6 family. These inflammatory cytokines also induce osteoclast differentiation by inducing RANKL expression in synovial fibroblasts (1). TNFα directly activates osteoclast differentiation, while IL-1 prolongs osteoclast survival (2). IL-6 also activates T cells and induces osteoclast differentiation by inducing RANKL expression (3).

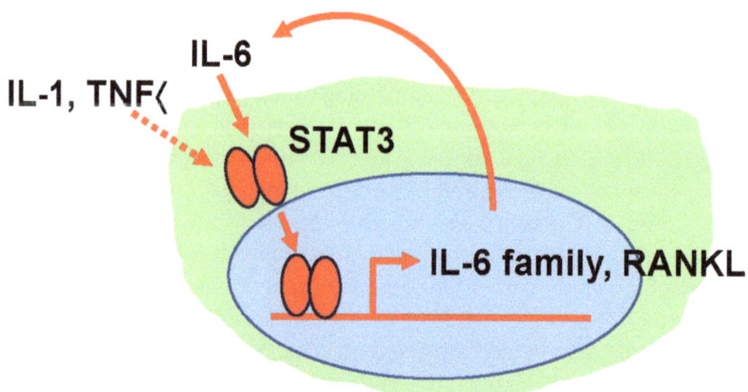

Figure 5. A positive feedback loop of inflammatory cytokine and RANKL expression. IL-6 directly activates and TNFα and IL-1 indirectly activate the transcription factor STAT3. The activated STAT3 induces the expression of inflammatory cytokines such as the IL-6 family, forming a positive feedback loop in which inflammatory cytokines are induced by inflammatory cytokines. The IL-6 family induced by the STAT3 activation further activates STAT3, thereby continuing this loop. The activated STAT3 also induces RANKL expression and activates osteoclast differentiation. This RANKL expression is also continued in a positive feedback loop by inflammatory cytokines.

By contrast, elevated levels of inflammatory cytokines contribute to bone loss not only by activating osteoclasts but by suppressing bone formation by inhibiting osteoblast activity [77]. Some reports state that in RA patients, joint erosion can be rescued by blocking inflammation with biologics [78]. In RA patients, the induction of factors that suppress the

Wnt-β catenin signaling that promotes bone formation is also thought to contribute to bone loss [79,80].

11. Either Methotrexate (MTX) or CTLA4-Ig Directly Inhibit Osteoclast Differentiation

Methotrexate (MTX) is the anchor drug for RA therapy and is the first-line agent for patients with RA who are eligible for MTX. MTX was originally developed as an anticancer drug and was probably first administered to RA patients to suppress proliferating synovial cells. In fact, however, it has been shown to cause marked improvement of joint swelling and joint tenderness in RA patients [81]. We found that MTX significantly inhibited osteoclast differentiation in osteoclast cultures in vitro, and that MTX significantly inhibited calcium signaling and NFATC1 expression in the osteoclast progenitor cells induced by RANKL [82]. NFAT is also essential for T cell activation, and stimulation from the T cell receptor (TCR) activates NFAT. MTX is considered to exert its osteoclast-differentiation inhibitory and immunosuppressive effects by suppressing NFAT in osteoclasts and T cells, respectively.

Similarly, we demonstrated that CTLA4-Ig, which suppresses co-stimulatory signaling, also significantly inhibited osteoclast differentiation in vitro [83]. We showed that CTLA4-Ig significantly inhibited calcium signaling and NFATC1 expression in osteoclast progenitor cells induced by RANKL via FcRγ, an ITAM signaling molecule [83]. Thus, CTLA4-Ig also directly inhibits both osteoclasts and T cells, and it may exert joint-erosion inhibitory and immunosuppressive activity.

12. Glucocorticoid-Induced Osteoporosis

Although glucocorticoid treatment has long been essential in treating RA, particularly in patients who cannot tolerate MTX [84], it also could induce secondary osteoporosis [85]. Glucocorticoid administration induces bone loss by transiently activating osteoclasts early in the course of treatment, which thereby inhibits bone formation in mid- to long-term treatment stages. Glucocorticoid administration also reportedly increases the risk of fractures at various sites throughout the body [86,87], an effect more pronounced in women than in men [86]. Patients with RA who are treated with glucocorticoids reportedly have a higher risk of fracture than those not treated with glucocorticoids [88]. On the other hand, fracture risk gradually decreases when glucocorticoid administration is discontinued, often disappearing about a year later [86]. Fracture risk with glucocorticoid administration is also dose-dependent, with prednisolone doses equivalent to 7.5 mg/day or higher greatly increasing fracture risk [86]. Increased age and the presence of preexisting fractures also increase fracture risk with glucocorticoid administration [88]. On the other hand, high lumbar bone density and treatment with bisphosphonates can reduce fracture risk [85]. In various countries, approaches have been proposed to assess risk based on age, bone density, existing fractures, and glucocorticoid dosage and to recommend medication for fracture prevention.

13. Aging of RA Patients and Risk of Osteoporosis

Interestingly, the age of RA onset has increased in recent years, although the causes are not well understood [89]. Potentially relevant to this observation is the fact that RA treatment advances have improved the prognosis of RA patients. Although not limited to RA patients, it is well known that aging is a risk factor for osteoporosis in general, and its prevalence increases with age [2]. Osteoporosis is a risk for fragility fractures; therefore, the occurrence of fragility fractures should be noted in RA patients. Osteoporosis is also associated with sarcopenia [90–92]; thus, one should be aware of events such as falls that are related to the development of fragility fractures.

Among fragility fractures caused by osteoporosis, hip fractures are the most serious. According to a survey of conducted by Kumamoto University Hospital, the average age of hip fracture patients is approximately 85 years [61]. In addition, most of the patients enrolled in the hip fracture study had hip fractures due to falls. In our study, decreased grip strength, a diagnostic criterion for sarcopenia, was also identified as a factor significantly associated with hip fracture (Tables 1 and 2) [61]. Thus, in the condition known as rheumatoid sarcopenia [93], attention should be paid to the occurrence of fragility fractures such as hip fractures due to falls.

Table 1. Scores for the categories of each risk factor including items that need to be measured in the hospital.

Features	Features Importance	Score [a]
Serum 25OHD (ng/mL)		
10≥		0
10<	0.659	7
Femoral neck T-score		
≥−3.0		0
<−3.0	0.459	5
Total Barthel index score		
100		0
<100	0.349	3
Maximal handgrip strength (kg)		
18≥		0
18<	0.334	3
Locomotive syndrome		
<24		0
≥24	0.218	2
History of falls within 1 year		
<2		0
≥3	0.209	2
sIGF-1		
≥50		0
<50	0.189	2
Tea (cups/day)		
≤4		0
=5	−0.189	−2 [b]
Osteoporosis drugs		
No		0
Yes	−0.179	−1 [b]
Body mass index		
≥18.5		0
<18.5	0.070	1

[a] Calculated 10 times for each parameter estimate and decimals rounded off. [b] The scores of the protective factors (tea and osteoporosis drug) were expressed by negative numbers.

Table 2. Scores for the categories of each risk factor not including items that need to be measured in the hospital.

Features	Features Importance	Score [a]
Total Barthel index score		
100		0
<100	0.505	5
Locomotive syndrome		
<24		0
≥24	0.433	4
History of falls within 1 year		
<2		0
≥3	0.243	2
Tea (cups/day)		
≤4		0
=5	−0.231	−2 [b]
Cognitive impairment		
None		0
Yes	0.161	2
Osteoporosis drugs		
No		0
Yes	−0.133	−1 [b]
Use of walking aid		
Yes		0
No	0.094	1
Walking habit		
No		0
Yes	0.053	1

[a] Calculated 8 times for each parameter estimate and decimals rounded off. [b] The scores of protective factors (tea and osteoporosis drug) were expressed by negative numbers.

14. Conclusive Remarks

The main focus of the present article is to introduce the mechanisms of osteoporosis development and bone erosion rather than to offer a systematic review or statement. Therefore, rather than presenting an introduction to the literature with an aligned methodology and population, as in a systematic review, the papers were selected to highlight why an understanding of the mechanism is necessary. Thus, there is the possibility of concerns about the limitations of this manuscript, including the potential risk of bias in the included studies, gaps in the evidence base due to the lack of condition-based selection from an extensive article search, and differences in methodology and population among the cited papers. In any case, this paper provides a comprehensive overview of the pathogenesis and regulation of osteoporosis, fragility fractures, and bone erosion in rheumatoid arthritis from various perspectives. RA and osteoporosis are closely related, and RA treatment requires constant vigilance to monitor patients for the development of osteoporosis. While both patients and physicians are very aware of joint pain, erosion, destruction, and deformity, they tend to be less aware of osteoporosis, which has fewer symptoms. In this article, we have introduced three key osteoporosis risk factors in the context of RA: inflammatory disease, glucocorticoid administration, and advanced age. In particular, elderly patients with RA often experience all three factors and require special attention. In any case, bone mineral density examination, checking for preexisting fractures, or utilizing FRAX are actionable strategies for assessing osteoporosis development in RA patients and should be performed as part of routine care. Basic science is an extremely useful tool for elucidating the molecular mechanisms underlying the regulation of bone homeostasis and the pathogenesis of bone erosion in RA patients, allowing us to do things that cannot be performed in patients, such as creating knockout mice that target specific molecules and then extrapolating the results to a clinical setting. In fact, basic science, including understanding molecular mechanisms, has led to the development of therapeutic agents such as denosumab. In RA and in osteoporosis, sarcopenia is of particular importance, and patients with RA who develop osteoporosis should be treated to prevent fall fractures due to rheumatoid sarcopenia. If patients are scheduled to receive oral glucocorticoid treatment for at least 3 months, they could be prescribed anti-osteoporosis drugs prophylactically if they will receive at least 7.5 mg/day of prednisolone, have an existing fracture, or are 65 or older. Overall, in this era, awareness of RA is required to protect patients from bone fractures.

15. Future Direction of Osteoporosis and Bone Erosion Management

The number of patients with osteoporosis is expected to continue to increase with the growth of the elderly population, and the number of patients with fragility fractures such as hip fractures is also expected to increase. More detailed bone evaluation may be possible currently or in the near future. HR-pQCT is useful in the evaluation of bone microstructure and is able to show in detail the differences in bone responses to different osteoporosis drugs in postmenopausal osteoporosis patients [94]. In RA patients, HR-pQCT can be a useful tool in the evaluation of bone erosion because it can target the small joints and metacarpals of the fingers [95,96]. However, there is currently a limit to the size of bone that can be analyzed with HR-pQCT, and the femur and lumbar spine cannot be analyzed. Evaluation of regional volumetric BMD and biomechanical parameters using the Quantitative Computed Tomography (QCT)-based Finite Element Method (FEM) has also been proposed [97]. In addition, although ultrasonography has been thought to be unsuitable for bone mass assessment, BMD assessment of the lumbar spine and femur using ultrasonography has been proposed, and consistency with BMD measured by DXA has been demonstrated [98]. In the future, it is expected to be a modality without X-Ray exposure, such as DXA, HR-pQCT, and QCT-based FEM. Neither modality is yet at a stage where it can be used for a large number of patients in terms of widespread use.

With the widespread use of detailed bone erosion assessment like HR-pQCT, it may become clinically feasible to quantify the volume of bone erosion and its changes during the treatment. The incorporation of AI methods such as machine learning may make it possible to automate the assessment of Sharp scores and joint space narrowing and their changes in a timely manner and reduce the time required for these measurements in the future. Accumulation of data from longitudinal studies and the long-term follow-up of changes in joint statuses in RA patients would also be useful in future studies to evaluate in detail the effect of drugs in preventing joint destruction. In addition, basic science is still considered necessary. If the etiology rather than the pathogenesis of RA is clarified, the subgrouping of RA patients and more fundamental treatment may become possible in the future.

Because osteoporosis is associated with sarcopenia and fragility fractures [90,92], it is necessary to provide total care for these conditions in the elderly. A total of 93% of hip fracture patients were not receiving treatment for osteoporosis at the time of fracture [61]. If individuals have RA or other diseases that cause osteoporosis, they should receive examination and treatment for osteoporosis in conjunction with treatment for the particular diseases. In addition, the average age of hip fracture patients is approximately 85 years old [61], and thus, it is necessary to anticipate and prevent future osteoporosis and fragility fractures earlier rather than taking action at age 85. Toward this end, it will be necessary to improve the accuracy of prediction tools for future osteoporosis and fragility fractures [91]. A longitudinal study will recommend whether intervening before fracture can prevent fracture by identifying older adults who are at high risk.

Funding: This research received no external funding.

Conflicts of Interest: The author declares no conflicts of interest.

References

1. Yoshimura, N.; Iidaka, T.; Horii, C.; Muraki, S.; Oka, H.; Kawaguchi, H.; Nakamura, K.; Akune, T.; Tanaka, S. Trends in osteoporosis prevalence over a 10-year period in Japan: The ROAD study 2005–2015. *J. Bone Miner. Metab.* **2022**, *40*, 829–838. [CrossRef] [PubMed]
2. Yoshimura, N.; Muraki, S.; Oka, H.; Mabuchi, A.; En-Yo, Y.; Yoshida, M.; Saika, A.; Yoshida, H.; Suzuki, T.; Yamamoto, S.; et al. Prevalence of knee osteoarthritis, lumbar spondylosis, and osteoporosis in Japanese men and women: The research on osteoarthritis/osteoporosis against disability study. *J. Bone Miner. Metab.* **2009**, *27*, 620–628. [CrossRef]
3. Gravallese, E.M.; Firestein, G.S. Rheumatoid Arthritis—Common Origins, Divergent Mechanisms. *N. Engl. J. Med.* **2023**, *388*, 529–542. [CrossRef] [PubMed]
4. Buttgereit, F.; Palmowski, A.; Bond, M.; Adami, G.; Dejaco, C. Osteoporosis and fracture risk are multifactorial in patients with inflammatory rheumatic diseases. *Nat. Rev. Rheumatol.* **2024**, *20*, 417–431. [CrossRef]
5. World Health Organization. WHO scientific group on the assessment of osteoporosis at primary health care level. In *Summary Meeting Report;* World Health Organization: Brussels, Belgium, 2004.
6. Taylor-Williams, O.; Keen, H.; Preen, D.B.; Nossent, J.; Inderjeeth, C.A. First fracture in rheumatoid arthritis: Analysis by fracture site, gender, age, and comorbidities. *Osteoporos. Int.* **2025**, *36*, 113–121. [CrossRef] [PubMed]
7. Wu, D.; Luo, Y.; Li, T.; Zhao, X.; Lv, T.; Fang, G.; Ou, P.; Li, H.; Luo, X.; Huang, A.; et al. Systemic complications of rheumatoid arthritis: Focus on pathogenesis and treatment. *Front. Immunol.* **2022**, *13*, 1051082. [CrossRef]
8. Furuya, T. Clinical observations of osteoporosis in Japanese patients with rheumatoid arthritis. *Mod. Rheumatol.* **2022**, *32*, 839–845. [CrossRef] [PubMed]
9. Cummings, S.R.; Martin, J.S.; McClung, M.R.; Siris, E.S.; Eastell, R.; Reid, I.R.; Delmas, P.; Zoog, H.B.; Austin, M.; Wang, A.; et al. Denosumab for prevention of fractures in postmenopausal women with osteoporosis. *N. Engl. J. Med.* **2009**, *361*, 756–765. [CrossRef] [PubMed]
10. McClung, M.R.; Grauer, A.; Boonen, S.; Bolognese, M.A.; Brown, J.P.; Diez-Perez, A.; Langdahl, B.L.; Reginster, J.Y.; Zanchetta, J.R.; Wasserman, S.M.; et al. Romosozumab in postmenopausal women with low bone mineral density. *N. Engl. J. Med.* **2014**, *370*, 412–420. [CrossRef] [PubMed]
11. Miyauchi, Y.; Sato, Y.; Kobayashi, T.; Yoshida, S.; Mori, T.; Kanagawa, H.; Katsuyama, E.; Fujie, A.; Hao, W.; Miyamoto, K.; et al. HIF1α is required for osteoclast activation by estrogen deficiency in postmenopausal osteoporosis. *Proc. Natl. Acad. Sci. USA* **2013**, *110*, 16568–16573. [CrossRef]
12. Yasuda, H.; Shima, N.; Nakagawa, N.; Yamaguchi, K.; Kinosaki, M.; Mochizuki, S.; Tomoyasu, A.; Yano, K.; Goto, M.; Murakami, A.; et al. Osteoclast differentiation factor is a ligand for osteoprotegerin/osteoclastogenesis-inhibitory factor and is identical to TRANCE/RANKL. *Proc. Natl. Acad. Sci. USA* **1998**, *95*, 3597–3602. [CrossRef]
13. Lacey, D.L.; Timms, E.; Tan, H.L.; Kelley, M.J.; Dunstan, C.R.; Burgess, T.; Elliott, R.; Colombero, A.; Elliott, G.; Scully, S.; et al. Osteoprotegerin ligand is a cytokine that regulates osteoclast differentiation and activation. *Cell* **1998**, *93*, 165–176. [CrossRef] [PubMed]
14. Kong, Y.Y.; Yoshida, H.; Sarosi, I.; Tan, H.L.; Timms, E.; Capparelli, C.; Morony, S.; Oliveira-dos-Santos, A.J.; Van, G.; Itie, A.; et al. OPGL is a key regulator of osteoclastogenesis, lymphocyte development and lymph-node organogenesis. *Nature* **1999**, *397*, 315–323. [CrossRef]
15. Dougall, W.C.; Glaccum, M.; Charrier, K.; Rohrbach, K.; Brasel, K.; De Smedt, T.; Daro, E.; Smith, J.; Tometsko, M.E.; Maliszewski, C.R.; et al. RANK is essential for osteoclast and lymph node development. *Genes Dev.* **1999**, *13*, 2412–2424. [CrossRef]
16. Anderson, D.M.; Maraskovsky, E.; Billingsley, W.L.; Dougall, W.C.; Tometsko, M.E.; Roux, E.R.; Teepe, M.C.; DuBose, R.F.; Cosman, D.; Galibert, L. A homologue of the TNF receptor and its ligand enhance T-cell growth and dendritic-cell function. *Nature* **1997**, *390*, 175–179. [CrossRef]

17. Tsuda, E.; Goto, M.; Mochizuki, S.; Yano, K.; Kobayashi, F.; Morinaga, T.; Higashio, K. Isolation of a novel cytokine from human fibroblasts that specifically inhibits osteoclastogenesis. *Biochem. Biophys. Res. Commun.* **1997**, *234*, 137–142. [CrossRef] [PubMed]
18. Simonet, W.S.; Lacey, D.L.; Dunstan, C.R.; Kelley, M.; Chang, M.S.; Lüthy, R.; Nguyen, H.Q.; Wooden, S.; Bennett, L.; Boone, T.; et al. Osteoprotegerin: A novel secreted protein involved in the regulation of bone density. *Cell* **1997**, *89*, 309–319. [CrossRef] [PubMed]
19. Takeuchi, T.; Tanaka, Y.; Soen, S.; Yamanaka, H.; Yoneda, T.; Tanaka, S.; Nitta, T.; Okubo, N.; Genant, H.K.; van der Heijde, D. Effects of the anti-RANKL antibody denosumab on joint structural damage in patients with rheumatoid arthritis treated with conventional synthetic disease-modifying antirheumatic drugs (DESIRABLE study): A randomised, double-blind, placebo-controlled phase 3 trial. *Ann. Rheum. Dis.* **2019**, *78*, 899–907.
20. Grigoriadis, A.E.; Wang, Z.Q.; Cecchini, M.G.; Hofstetter, W.; Felix, R.; Fleisch, H.A.; Wagner, E.F. c-Fos: A key regulator of osteoclast-macrophage lineage determination and bone remodeling. *Science* **1994**, *266*, 443–448. [CrossRef] [PubMed]
21. Takayanagi, H.; Kim, S.; Koga, T.; Nishina, H.; Isshiki, M.; Yoshida, H.; Saiura, A.; Isobe, M.; Yokochi, T.; Inoue, J. Induction and activation of the transcription factor NFATc1 (NFAT2) integrate RANKL signaling in terminal differentiation of osteoclasts. *Dev. Cell* **2002**, *3*, 889–901. [CrossRef] [PubMed]
22. Asagiri, M.; Sato, K.; Usami, T.; Ochi, S.; Nishina, H.; Yoshida, H.; Morita, I.; Wagner, E.F.; Mak, T.W.; Serfling, E.; et al. Autoamplification of NFATc1 expression determines its essential role in bone homeostasis. *J. Exp. Med.* **2005**, *202*, 1261–1269. [CrossRef] [PubMed]
23. Koga, T.; Inui, M.; Inoue, K.; Kim, S.; Suematsu, A.; Kobayashi, E.; Iwata, T.; Ohnishi, H.; Matozaki, T.; Kodama, T.; et al. Costimulatory signals mediated by the ITAM motif cooperate with RANKL for bone homeostasis. *Nature* **2004**, *428*, 758–763. [CrossRef] [PubMed]
24. Koga, T.; Matsui, Y.; Asagiri, M.; Kodama, T.; de Crombrugghe, B.; Nakashima, K.; Takayanagi, H. NFAT and Osterix cooperatively regulate bone formation. *Nat. Med.* **2005**, *11*, 880–885. [CrossRef] [PubMed]
25. Yagi, M.; Miyamoto, T.; Sawatani, Y.; Iwamoto, K.; Hosogane, N.; Fujita, N.; Morita, K.; Ninomiya, K.; Suzuki, T.; Miyamoto, K.; et al. DC-STAMP is essential for cell-cell fusion in osteoclasts and foreign body giant cells. *J. Exp. Med.* **2005**, *202*, 345–351. [CrossRef]
26. Lee, S.H.; Rho, J.; Jeong, D.; Sul, J.Y.; Kim, T.; Kim, N.; Kang, J.S.; Miyamoto, T.; Suda, T.; Lee, S.K.; et al. v-ATPase V0 subunit d2-deficient mice exhibit impaired osteoclast fusion and increased bone formation. *Nat. Med.* **2006**, *12*, 1403–1409. [CrossRef]
27. Cui, W.; Cuartas, E.; Ke, J.; Zhang, Q.; Einarsson, H.B.; Sedgwick, J.D.; Li, J.; Vignery, A. CD200 and its receptor, CD200R, modulate bone mass via the differentiation of osteoclasts. *Proc. Natl. Acad. Sci. USA* **2007**, *104*, 14436–14441. [CrossRef] [PubMed]
28. Miyamoto, H.; Suzuki, T.; Miyauchi, Y.; Iwasaki, R.; Kobayashi, T.; Sato, Y.; Miyamoto, K.; Hoshi, H.; Hashimoto, K.; Yoshida, S.; et al. Osteoclast stimulatory transmembrane protein and dendritic cell–specific transmembrane protein cooperatively modulate cell–cell fusion to form osteoclasts and foreign body giant cells. *J. Bone Miner. Res.* **2012**, *27*, 1289–1297. [CrossRef]
29. Yagi, M.; Ninomiya, K.; Fujita, N.; Suzuki, T.; Iwasaki, R.; Morita, K.; Hosogane, N.; Matsuo, K.; Toyama, Y.; Suda, T.; et al. Induction of DC-STAMP by alternative activation and downstream signaling mechanisms. *J. Bone Miner. Res.* **2007**, *22*, 992–1001. [CrossRef]
30. Zhao, B.; Takami, M.; Yamada, A.; Wang, X.; Koga, T.; Hu, X.; Tamura, T.; Ozato, K.; Choi, Y.; Ivashkiv, L.B.; et al. Interferon regulatory factor-8 regulates bone metabolism by suppressing osteoclastogenesis. *Nat. Med.* **2009**, *15*, 1066–1071. [CrossRef] [PubMed]
31. Kim, K.; Kim, J.H.; Lee, J.; Jin, H.M.; Kook, H.; Kim, K.K.; Lee, S.Y.; Kim, N. MafB negatively regulates RANKL-mediated osteoclast differentiation. *Blood* **2007**, *109*, 3253–3259. [CrossRef]
32. Miyauchi, Y.; Ninomiya, K.; Miyamoto, H.; Sakamoto, A.; Iwasaki, R.; Hoshi, H.; Miyamoto, K.; Hao, W.; Yoshida, S.; Morioka, H.; et al. The Blimp1-Bcl6 axis is critical to regulate osteoclast differentiation and bone homeostasis. *J. Exp. Med.* **2010**, *207*, 751–762. [CrossRef] [PubMed]
33. Nishikawa, K.; Nakashima, T.; Hayashi, M.; Fukunaga, T.; Kato, S.; Kodama, T.; Takahashi, S.; Calame, K.; Takayanagi, H. Blimp1-mediated repression of negative regulators is required for osteoclast differentiation. *Proc. Natl. Acad. Sci. USA* **2010**, *107*, 3117–3122. [CrossRef] [PubMed]
34. Miyauchi, Y.; Miyamoto, H.; Yoshida, S.; Mori, T.; Kanagawa, H.; Katsuyama, E.; Fujie, A.; Hao, W.; Hoshi, H.; Miyamoto, K.; et al. Conditional inactivation of Blimp1 in adult mice promotes increased bone mass. *J. Biol. Chem.* **2012**, *287*, 28508–28517. [CrossRef]
35. Guitart, A.V.; Hammoud, M.; Sbarba, P.D.; Ivanovic, Z.; Praloran, V. Slow-cycling/quiescence balance of hematopoietic stem cells is related to physiological gradient of oxygen. *Exp. Hematol.* **2010**, *38*, 847–851. [CrossRef] [PubMed]
36. Tando, T.; Sato, Y.; Miyamoto, K.; Morita, M.; Kobayashi, T.; Funayama, A.; Kanaji, A.; Hao, W.; Watanabe, R.; Oike, T.; et al. Hif1α is required for osteoclast activation and bone loss in male osteoporosis. *Biochem. Biophys. Res. Commun.* **2016**, *470*, 391–396. [CrossRef] [PubMed]

37. Sato, Y.; Miyauchi, Y.; Yoshida, S.; Morita, M.; Kobayashi, T.; Kanagawa, H.; Katsuyama, E.; Fujie, A.; Hao, W.; Tando, T.; et al. The Vitamin D Analogue ED71 but Not 1,25(OH)2D3 Targets HIF1α Protein in Osteoclasts. *PLoS ONE* **2014**, *9*, e111845. [CrossRef]
38. Morita, M.; Sato, Y.; Iwasaki, R.; Kobayashi, T.; Watanabe, R.; Oike, T.; Miyamoto, K.; Toyama, Y.; Matsumoto, M.; Nakamura, M.; et al. Selective Estrogen Receptor Modulators Suppress Hif1α Protein Accumulation in Mouse Osteoclasts. *PLoS ONE* **2016**, *11*, e0165922. [CrossRef]
39. Sato, Y.; Tando, T.; Morita, M.; Miyamoto, K.; Kobayashi, T.; Watanabe, R.; Oike, T.; Matsumoto, M.; Nakamura, M.; Miyamoto, T. Selective estrogen receptor modulators and the vitamin D analogue eldecalcitol block bone loss in male osteoporosis. *Biochem. Biophys. Res. Commun.* **2017**, *482*, 1430–1436. [CrossRef] [PubMed]
40. Tang, Y.; Wu, X.; Lei, W.; Pang, L.; Wan, C.; Shi, Z.; Zhao, L.; Nagy, T.R.; Peng, X.; Hu, J.; et al. TGF-beta1-induced migration of bone mesenchymal stem cells couples bone resorption with formation. *Nat. Med.* **2009**, *15*, 757–765. [CrossRef]
41. Xian, L.; Wu, X.; Pang, L.; Lou, M.; Rosen, C.J.; Qiu, T.; Crane, J.; Frassica, F.; Zhang, L.; Rodriguez, J.P.; et al. Matrix IGF-1 maintains bone mass by activation of mTOR in mesenchymal stem cells. *Nat. Med.* **2012**, *18*, 1095–1101. [CrossRef]
42. Zhao, C.; Irie, N.; Takada, Y.; Shimoda, K.; Miyamoto, T.; Nishiwaki, T.; Suda, T.; Matsuo, K. Bidirectional ephrinB2-EphB4 signaling controls bone homeostasis. *Cell Metab.* **2006**, *4*, 111–121. [CrossRef] [PubMed]
43. Negishi-Koga, T.; Shinohara, M.; Komatsu, N.; Bito, H.; Kodama, T.; Friedel, R.H.; Takayanagi, H. Suppression of bone formation by osteoclastic expression of semaphorin 4D. *Nat. Med.* **2011**, *17*, 1473–1480. [CrossRef]
44. Xie, H.; Cui, Z.; Wang, L.; Xia, Z.; Hu, Y.; Xian, L.; Li, C.; Xie, L.; Crane, J.; Wan, M.; et al. PDGF-BB secreted by preosteoclasts induces angiogenesis during coupling with osteogenesis. *Nat. Med.* **2014**, *20*, 1270–1278. [CrossRef] [PubMed]
45. Whyte, M.P.; McAlister, W.H.; Novack, D.V.; Clements, K.L.; Schoenecker, P.L.; Wenkert, D. Bisphosphonate-induced osteopetrosis: Novel bone modeling defects, metaphyseal osteopenia, and osteosclerosis fractures after drug exposure ceases. *J. Bone Miner. Res.* **2008**, *23*, 1698–1707. [CrossRef] [PubMed]
46. Edwards, B.J.; Bunta, A.D.; Lane, J.; Odvina, C.; Rao, D.S.; Raisch, D.W.; McKoy, J.M.; Omar, I.; Belknap, S.M.; Garg, V.; et al. Bisphosphonates and nonhealing femoral fractures: Analysis of the FDA Adverse Event Reporting System (FAERS) and international safety efforts: A systematic review from the Research on Adverse Drug Events And Reports (RADAR) project. *J. Bone Jt. Surg. Am.* **2013**, *95*, 297–307. [CrossRef] [PubMed]
47. Gedmintas, L.; Solomon, D.H.; Kim, S.C. Bisphosphonates and risk of subtrochanteric, femoral shaft, and atypical femur fracture: A systematic review and meta-analysis. *J. Bone Miner. Res.* **2013**, *28*, 1729–1737. [CrossRef]
48. Visekruna, M.; Wilson, D.; McKiernan, F.E. Severely suppressed bone turnover and atypical skeletal fragility. *J. Clin. Endocrinol. Metab.* **2008**, *93*, 2948–2952. [CrossRef] [PubMed]
49. Hayashi, M.; Nakashima, T.; Taniguchi, M.; Kodama, T.; Kumanogoh, A.; Takayanagi, H. Osteoprotection by semaphorin 3A. *Nature* **2012**, *485*, 69–74. [CrossRef]
50. Gelb, B.D.; Shi, G.P.; Chapman, H.A.; Desnick, R.J. Pycnodysostosis, a lysosomal disease caused by cathepsin K deficiency. *Science* **1996**, *273*, 1236–1238. [CrossRef] [PubMed]
51. Saftig, P.; Hunziker, E.; Wehmeyer, O.; Jones, S.; Boyde, A.; Rommerskirch, W.; Moritz, J.D.; Schu, P.; von Figura, K. Impaired osteoclastic bone resorption leads to osteopetrosis in cathepsin-K-deficient mice. *Proc. Natl. Acad. Sci. USA* **1998**, *95*, 13453–13458. [CrossRef]
52. Kim, S.; Koga, T.; Isobe, M.; Kern, B.E.; Yokochi, T.; Chin, Y.E.; Karsenty, G.; Taniguchi, T.; Takayanagi, H. Stat1 functions as a cytoplasmic attenuator of Runx2 in the transcriptional program of osteoblast differentiation. *Genes Dev.* **2003**, *17*, 1979–1991. [CrossRef]
53. Fujie, A.; Funayama, A.; Miyauchi, Y.; Sato, Y.; Kobayashi, T.; Kanagawa, H.; Katsuyama, E.; Hao, W.; Tando, T.; Watanabe, R.; et al. Bcl6 promotes osteoblastogenesis through Stat1 inhibition. *Biochem. Biophys. Res. Commun.* **2015**, *457*, 451–456. [CrossRef] [PubMed]
54. Brunkow, M.E.; Gardner, J.C.; Van Ness, J.; Paeper, B.W.; Kovacevich, B.R.; Proll, S.; Skonier, J.E.; Zhao, L.; Sabo, P.J.; Fu, Y.; et al. Bone dysplasia sclerosteosis results from loss of the SOST gene product, a novel cystine knot-containing protein. *Am. J. Hum. Genet.* **2001**, *68*, 577–589. [CrossRef] [PubMed]
55. Balemans, W.; Patel, N.; Ebeling, M.; Van Hul, E.; Wuyts, W.; Lacza, C.; Dioszegi, M.; Dikkers, F.G.; Hildering, P.; Willems, P.J.; et al. Identification of a 52 kb deletion downstream of the SOST gene in patients with van Buchem disease. *J. Med. Genet.* **2002**, *39*, 91–97. [CrossRef] [PubMed]
56. Ryan, Z.C.; Ketha, H.; McNulty, M.S.; McGee-Lawrence, M.; Craig, T.A.; Grande, J.P.; Westendorf, J.J.; Singh, R.J.; Kumar, R. Sclerostin alters serum vitamin D metabolite and fibroblast growth factor 23 concentrations and the urinary excretion of calcium. *Proc. Natl. Acad. Sci. USA* **2013**, *110*, 6199–6204. [CrossRef] [PubMed]
57. Geusens, P.; Oates, M.; Miyauchi, A.; Adachi, J.D.; Lazaretti-Castro, M.; Ebeling, P.R.; Perez Niño, C.A.; Milmont, C.E.; Grauer, A.; Libanati, C. The Effect of 1 Year of Romosozumab on the Incidence of Clinical Vertebral Fractures in Postmenopausal Women with Osteoporosis: Results From the FRAME Study. *JBMR Plus* **2019**, *3*, e10211. [CrossRef] [PubMed]

58. Black, D.M.; Cummings, S.R.; Karpf, D.B.; Cauley, J.A.; Thompson, D.E.; Nevitt, M.C.; Bauer, D.C.; Genant, H.K.; Haskell, W.L.; Marcus, R.; et al. Randomised trial of effect of alendronate on risk of fracture in women with existing vertebral fractures. Fracture Intervention Trial Research Group. *Lancet* **1996**, *348*, 1535–1541. [CrossRef] [PubMed]
59. Neer, R.M.; Arnaud, C.D.; Zanchetta, J.R.; Prince, R.; Gaich, G.A.; Reginster, J.Y.; Hodsman, A.B.; Eriksen, E.F.; Ish-Shalom, S.; Genant, H.K.; et al. Effect of parathyroid hormone (1-34) on fractures and bone mineral density in postmenopausal women with osteoporosis. *N. Engl. J. Med.* **2001**, *344*, 1434–1441. [CrossRef]
60. Miller, P.D.; Hattersley, G.; Riis, B.J.; Williams, G.C.; Lau, E.; Russo, L.A.; Alexandersen, P.; Zerbini, C.A.; Hu, M.Y.; Harris, A.G.; et al. ACTIVE Study Investigators. Effect of Abaloparatide vs Placebo on New Vertebral Fractures in Postmenopausal Women With Osteoporosis: A Randomized Clinical Trial. *JAMA* **2016**, *316*, 722–733. [CrossRef] [PubMed]
61. Uragami, M.; Matsushita, K.; Shibata, Y.; Takata, S.; Karasugi, T.; Sueyoshi, T.; Masuda, T.; Nakamura, T.; Tokunaga, T.; Hisanaga, S.; et al. A machine learning-based scoring system and ten factors associated with hip fracture occurrence in the elderly. *Bone* **2023**, *176*, 116865. [CrossRef] [PubMed]
62. Nakae, S.; Saijo, S.; Horai, R.; Sudo, K.; Mori, S.; Iwakura, Y. IL-17 production from activated T cells is required for the spontaneous development of destructive arthritis in mice deficient in IL-1 receptor antagonist. *Proc. Natl. Acad. Sci. USA* **2003**, *100*, 5986–5990. [CrossRef]
63. Nakae, S.; Nambu, A.; Sudo, K.; Iwakura, Y. Suppression of immune induction of collagen-induced arthritis in IL-17-deficient mice. *J. Immunol.* **2003**, *171*, 6173–6177. [CrossRef]
64. Nakajima, S.; Tsuchiya, H.; Ota, M.; Ogawa, M.; Yamada, S.; Yoshida, R.; Maeda, J.; Shirai, H.; Kasai, T.; Hirose, J.; et al. Synovial Tissue Heterogeneity in Japanese Patients With Rheumatoid Arthritis Elucidated Using a Cell-Type Deconvolution Approach. *Arthritis Rheumatol.* **2023**, *75*, 2130–2136. [CrossRef]
65. Ishigaki, K.; Sakaue, S.; Terao, C.; Luo, Y.; Sonehara, K.; Yamaguchi, K.; Amariuta, T.; Too, C.L.; Laufer, V.A.; Scott, I.C.; et al. Multi-ancestry genome-wide association analyses identify novel genetic mechanisms in rheumatoid arthritis. *Nat. Genet.* **2022**, *54*, 1640–1651. [CrossRef]
66. Redlich, K.; Hayer, S.; Ricci, R.; David, J.P.; Tohidast-Akrad, M.; Kollias, G.; Steiner, G.; Smolen, J.S.; Wagner, E.F.; Schett, G. Osteoclasts are essential for TNF-alpha-mediated joint destruction. *J. Clin. Investig.* **2002**, *110*, 1419–1427. [CrossRef] [PubMed]
67. Kong, Y.Y.; Feige, U.; Sarosi, I.; Bolon, B.; Tafuri, A.; Morony, S.; Capparelli, C.; Li, J.; Elliott, R.; McCabe, S.; et al. Activated T cells regulate bone loss and joint destruction in adjuvant arthritis through osteoprotegerin ligand. *Nature* **1999**, *402*, 304–309. [CrossRef]
68. Cutolo, M.; Montecucco, C.M.; Cavagna, L.; Caporali, R.; Capellino, S.; Montagna, P.; Fazzuoli, L.; Villaggio, B.; Seriolo, B.; Sulli, A. Serum cytokines and steroidal hormones in polymyalgia rheumatica and elderly-onset rheumatoid arthritis. *Ann. Rheum. Dis.* **2006**, *65*, 1438–1443. [CrossRef]
69. Mori, T.; Miyamoto, T.; Yoshida, H.; Asakawa, M.; Kawasumi, M.; Kobayashi, T.; Morioka, H.; Chiba, K.; Toyama, Y.; Yoshimura, A. IL-1β and TNFα-initiated IL-6-STAT3 pathway is critical in mediating inflammatory cytokines and RANKL expression in inflammatory arthritis. *Int. Immunol.* **2011**, *23*, 701–712. [CrossRef] [PubMed]
70. Kobayashi, K.; Takahashi, N.; Jimi, E.; Udagawa, N.; Takami, M.; Kotake, S.; Nakagawa, N.; Kinosaki, M.; Yamaguchi, K.; Shima, N.; et al. Tumor necrosis factor alpha stimulates osteoclast differentiation by a mechanism independent of the ODF/RANKL-RANK interaction. *J. Exp. Med.* **2000**, *191*, 275–286. [CrossRef] [PubMed]
71. Naito, A.; Azuma, S.; Tanaka, S.; Miyazaki, T.; Takaki, S.; Takatsu, K.; Nakao, K.; Nakamura, K.; Katsuki, M.; Yamamoto, T.; et al. Severe osteopetrosis, defective interleukin-1 signalling and lymph node organogenesis in TRAF6-deficient mice. *Genes Cells* **1999**, *4*, 353–362. [CrossRef]
72. Oya, A.; Katsuyama, E.; Morita, M.; Sato, Y.; Kobayashi, T.; Miyamoto, K.; Nishiwaki, T.; Funayama, A.; Fujita, Y.; Kobayashi, T.; et al. Tumor necrosis factor receptor-associated factor 6 is required to inhibit foreign body giant cell formation and activate osteoclasts under inflammatory and infectious conditions. *J. Bone Miner. Metab.* **2018**, *36*, 679–690. [CrossRef] [PubMed]
73. Hasegawa, T.; Kikuta, J.; Sudo, T.; Matsuura, Y.; Matsui, T.; Simmons, S.; Ebina, K.; Hirao, M.; Okuzaki, D.; Yoshida, Y.; et al. Identification of a novel arthritis-associated osteoclast precursor macrophage regulated by FoxM1. *Nat. Immunol.* **2019**, *20*, 1631–1643. [CrossRef]
74. Katsuyama, E.; Miyamoto, H.; Kobayashi, T.; Sato, Y.; Hao, W.; Kanagawa, H.; Fujie, A.; Tando, T.; Watanabe, R.; Morita, M.; et al. Interleukin-1 receptor-associated kinase-4 (IRAK4) promotes inflammatory osteolysis by activating osteoclasts and inhibiting formation of foreign body giant cells. *J. Biol. Chem.* **2015**, *290*, 716–726. [CrossRef]
75. Komatsu, N.; Okamoto, K.; Sawa, S.; Nakashima, T.; Oh-hora, M.; Kodama, T.; Tanaka, S.; Bluestone, J.A.; Takayanagi, H. Pathogenic conversion of Foxp3+ T cells into TH17 cells in autoimmune arthritis. *Nat. Med.* **2014**, *20*, 62–68. [CrossRef]
76. Oike, T.; Sato, Y.; Kobayashi, T.; Miyamoto, K.; Nakamura, S.; Kaneko, Y.; Kobayashi, S.; Harato, K.; Saya, H.; Matsumoto, M.; et al. Stat3 as a potential therapeutic target for rheumatoid arthritis. *Sci. Rep.* **2017**, *7*, 10965. [CrossRef] [PubMed]

77. Messina, O.D.; Vidal, M.; Adami, G.; Vidal, L.F.; Clark, P.; Torres, J.A.M.; Lems, W.; Zerbini, C.; Arguissain, C.; Reginster, J.Y.; et al. Chronic arthritides and bone structure: Focus on rheumatoid arthritis-an update. *Aging Clin. Exp. Res.* **2023**, *35*, 1405–1416. [CrossRef]
78. Finzel, S.; Kraus, S.; Figueiredo, C.P.; Regensburger, A.; Kocijan, R.; Rech, J.; Schett, G. Comparison of the effects of tocilizumab monotherapy and adalimumab in combination with methotrexate on bone erosion repair in rheumatoid arthritis. *Ann. Rheum. Dis.* **2019**, *78*, 1186–1191. [CrossRef] [PubMed]
79. Diarra, D.; Stolina, M.; Polzer, K.; Zwerina, J.; Ominsky, M.S.; Dwyer, D.; Korb, A.; Smolen, J.; Hoffmann, M.; Scheinecker, C.; et al. Dickkopf-1 is a master regulator of joint remodeling. *Nat. Med.* **2007**, *13*, 156–163. [CrossRef]
80. Walsh, N.C.; Reinwald, S.; Manning, C.A.; Condon, K.W.; Iwata, K.; Burr, D.B.; Gravallese, E.M. Osteoblast function is compromised at sites of focal bone erosion in inflammatory arthritis. *J. Bone Miner. Res.* **2009**, *24*, 1572–1585. [CrossRef]
81. Weinblatt, M.E.; Coblyn, J.S.; Fox, D.A.; Fraser, P.A.; Holdsworth, D.E.; Glass, D.N.; Trentham, D.E. Efficacy of low-dose methotrexate in rheumatoid arthritis. *N. Engl. J. Med.* **1985**, *312*, 818–822. [CrossRef] [PubMed]
82. Kanagawa, H.; Masuyama, R.; Morita, M.; Sato, Y.; Niki, Y.; Kobayashi, T.; Katsuyama, E.; Fujie, A.; Hao, W.; Tando, T.; et al. Methotrexate inhibits osteoclastogenesis by decreasing RANKL-induced calcium influx into osteoclast progenitors. *J. Bone Miner. Metab.* **2016**, *34*, 526–531. [CrossRef]
83. Okada, H.; Kajiya, H.; Omata, Y.; Matsumoto, T.; Sato, Y.; Kobayashi, T.; Nakamura, S.; Kaneko, Y.; Nakamura, S.; Koyama, T.; et al. CTLA4-Ig directly inhibits osteoclastogenesis by interfering with intracellular calcium oscillations in bone marrow macrophages. *J. Bone Miner. Res.* **2019**, *34*, 1744–1752. [CrossRef] [PubMed]
84. Smolen, J.S.; Landewé, R.B.M.; Bergstra, S.A.; Kerschbaumer, A.; Sepriano, A.; Aletaha, D.; Caporali, R.; Edwards, C.J.; Hyrich, K.L.; Pope, J.E. EULAR recommendations for the management of rheumatoid arthritis with synthetic and biological disease-modifying antirheumatic drugs: 2022 update. *Ann. Rheum. Dis.* **2023**, *82*, 3–18. [CrossRef] [PubMed]
85. Tanaka, Y.; Soen, S.; Hirata, S.; Okada, Y.; Fujiwara, S.; Tanaka, I.; Kitajima, Y.; Kubota, T.; Ebina, K.; Takashi, Y.; et al. The 2023 Guidelines for the management and treatment of glucocorticoid-induced osteoporosis. *J. Bone Miner. Metab.* **2024**, *42*, 143–154. [CrossRef]
86. Van Staa, T.P.; Leufkens, H.G.; Abenhaim, L.; Zhang, B.; Cooper, C. Use of oral corticosteroids and risk of fractures. *J. Bone Miner. Res.* **2000**, *15*, 993–1000. [CrossRef] [PubMed]
87. Amiche, M.A.; Abtahi, S.; Driessen, J.H.M.; Vestergaard, P.; de Vries, F.; Cadarette, S.M.; Burden, A.M. Impact of cumulative exposure to high-dose oral glucocorticoids on fracture risk in Denmark: A population-based case-control study. *Arch. Osteoporos.* **2018**, *13*, 30. [CrossRef]
88. Soen, S.; Kaku, M.; Okubo, N.; Onishi, Y.; Saito, K.; Kobayashi, M. Fracture risk associated with glucocorticoid-induced osteoporosis in Japan. *J. Bone Miner. Metab.* **2022**, *40*, 636–647. [CrossRef] [PubMed]
89. Nakajima, A.; Sakai, R.; Inoue, E.; Harigai, M. Prevalence of patients with rheumatoid arthritis and age-stratified trends in clinical characteristics and treatment, based on the National Database of Health Insurance Claims and Specific Health Checkups of Japan. *Int. J Rheum. Dis.* **2020**, *23*, 1676–1684. [CrossRef]
90. Yoshimura, N.; Muraki, S.; Oka, H.; Iidaka, T.; Kodama, R.; Kawaguchi, H.; Nakamura, K.; Tanaka, S.; Akune, T. Is osteoporosis a predictor for future sarcopenia or vice versa? Four-year observations between the second and third ROAD study surveys. *Osteoporos. Int.* **2017**, *28*, 189–199. [CrossRef]
91. Miyamoto, K.; Hirayama, A.; Sato, Y.; Ikeda, S.; Maruyama, M.; Soga, T.; Tomita, M.; Nakamura, M.; Matsumoto, M.; Yoshimura, N.; et al. A Metabolomic Profile Predictive of New Osteoporosis or Sarcopenia Development. *Metabolites* **2021**, *11*, 278. [CrossRef]
92. Hata, R.; Miyamoto, K.; Abe, Y.; Sasaki, T.; Oguma, Y.; Tajima, T.; Arai, Y.; Matsumoto, M.; Nakamura, M.; Kanaji, A.; et al. Osteoporosis and sarcopenia are associated with each other and reduced IGF1 levels are a risk for both diseases in the very old elderly. *Bone* **2023**, *166*, 116570. [CrossRef] [PubMed]
93. Bennett, J.L.; Pratt, A.G.; Dodds, R.; Sayer, A.A.; Isaacs, J.D. Rheumatoid sarcopenia: Loss of skeletal muscle strength and mass in rheumatoid arthritis. *Nat. Rev. Rheumatol.* **2023**, *19*, 239–251. [CrossRef] [PubMed]
94. Chiba, K.; Okazaki, N.; Kurogi, A.; Watanabe, T.; Mori, A.; Suzuki, N.; Adachi, K.; Era, M.; Yokota, K.; Inoue, T.; et al. Randomized controlled trial of daily teriparatide, weekly high-dose teriparatide, or bisphosphonate in patients with postmenopausal osteoporosis: The TERABIT study. *Bone* **2022**, *160*, 116416. [CrossRef] [PubMed]
95. Yue, J.; Griffith, J.F.; Xu, J.; Xiao, F.; Shi, L.; Wang, D.; Wong, P.C.H.; Li, E.K.; Li, M.; Li, T.K.; et al. Effect of treat-to-target strategies on bone erosion progression in early rheumatoid arthritis: An HR-pQCT study. *Semin. Arthritis Rheum.* **2018**, *48*, 374–383. [CrossRef]
96. Figueiredo, C.P.; Perez, M.O.; Sales, L.P.; Medeiros, A.C.; Caparbo, V.F.; Pereira, R.M.R. Bone erosion in the 2nd metacarpophalangeal head: Association with its bone mineral density by HR-pQCT in rheumatoid arthritis patients. *BMC Musculoskelet. Disord.* **2021**, *22*, 109. [CrossRef] [PubMed]

97. Ishikawa, K.; Tani, S.; Toyone, T.; Tsuchiya, K.; Towatari, T.; Oshita, Y.; Yamamura, R.; Wada, K.; Nagai, T.; Shirahata, T.; et al. The potential effect of romosozumab on perioperative management for instrumentation surgery. *JOR Spine* **2024**, *7*, e1356. [CrossRef] [PubMed]
98. Cortet, B.; Dennison, E.; Diez-Perez, A.; Locquet, M.; Muratore, M.; Nogués, X.; Ovejero Crespo, D.; Quarta, E.; Brandi, M.L. Radiofrequency Echographic Multi Spectrometry (REMS) for the diagnosis of osteoporosis in a European multicenter clinical context. *Bone* **2021**, *143*, 115786. [CrossRef]

Journal of
Clinical Medicine

MDPI

Review

Rheumatoid Factor: Diagnostic and Prognostic Performance and Therapeutic Implications in Rheumatoid Arthritis

Tasuku Togashi †, Ryuhei Ishihara †, Ryu Watanabe *, Mayu Shiomi, Yuya Yano, Yuhei Fujisawa, Masao Katsushima, Kazuo Fukumoto, Shinsuke Yamada and Motomu Hashimoto

Department of Clinical Immunology, Osaka Metropolitan University Graduate School of Medicine, Osaka 545-8585, Japan
* Correspondence: doctorwatanaberyu7@gmail.com; Tel.: +81-6-6645-3981
† These authors contributed equally to this work.

Abstract: Rheumatoid factor (RF) is the first autoantibody identified in rheumatoid arthritis (RA) which targets the fragment crystallizable (Fc) region of immunoglobulin (Ig) G. Although IgM isotype is predominant, other Ig isotypes, including IgG and IgA, also exist. While RF is not specific to RA, it remains a valuable serological test for diagnosing the disease, as evidenced by its inclusion in the 2010 classification criteria for RA based on elevated serum RF levels. RF is also associated with RA severity, including joint damage and extra-articular manifestations, serving as a poor prognostic factor and aiding in the identification of difficult-to-treat RA. Recent studies have demonstrated that high serum RF levels are associated with a reduced response to tumor necrosis factor (TNF) inhibitors. In contrast, anti-TNF antibodies lacking the Fc portion have shown stable efficacy in RA patients regardless of baseline RF levels. These findings reaffirm the clinical significance of RF measurement, 80 years after its initial discovery. This review explores the diagnostic and prognostic significance of RF and its impact on treatment selection in RA management.

Keywords: anti-citrullinated protein antibodies; rheumatoid arthritis; rheumatoid factor; tumor necrosis factor

1. Introduction

Rheumatoid arthritis (RA) is a systemic autoimmune disease characterized by chronic, progressive inflammation of synovial joints, often leading to irreversible structural damage to bone and cartilage [1]. This debilitating condition significantly impacts patients' quality of life and imposes a considerable economic burden on healthcare systems worldwide. Despite extensive research, the precise etiology of RA remains elusive. Several hypotheses, including genetic predisposition, environmental triggers, and dysregulated immune responses, have been proposed (Figure 1); however, none provide a comprehensive explanation for the disease's onset. Notably, evidence of arthritis-like changes has been identified in skeletal remains from prehistoric times, suggesting that RA is not a modern ailment but rather a condition that has coexisted with humanity for millennia [2].

Epidemiologically, RA affects approximately 0.46% of the global population, as indicated by a recent meta-analysis (95% confidence interval 0.39–0.54) [3]. This prevalence underscores the necessity for rheumatologists and general physicians alike to possess a robust understanding of the disease. Given its chronic and systemic nature, early and accurate diagnosis of RA is critical to initiating timely interventions that can mitigate disease progression and improve outcomes.

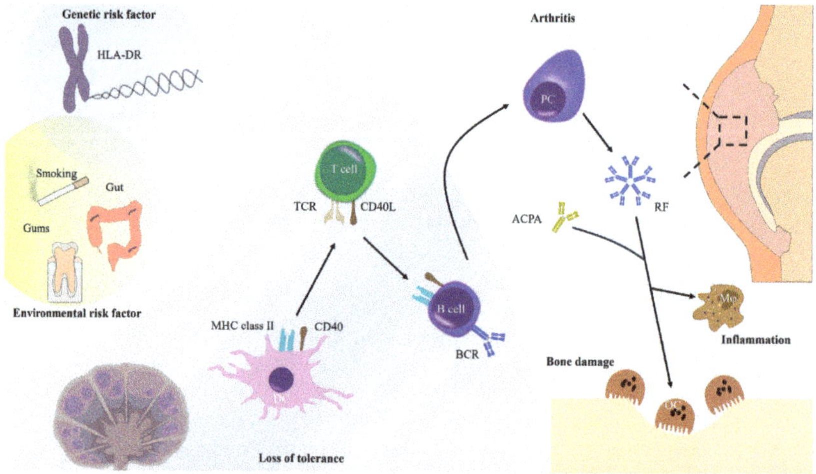

Figure 1. RF implicated in the pathogenesis of RA. The onset of rheumatoid arthritis (RA) is driven by a complex interplay of genetic and environmental factors. These factors lead to the generation of exogenous and endogenous antigens, which are subsequently presented by antigen-presenting cells (primarily dendritic cells) to CD4+ T cells. Upon activation, CD4+ T cells differentiate into self-antigen-specific subsets, including follicular helper T cells (Tfh) and peripheral helper T cells (Tph). These specialized CD4+ T cells facilitate B cell maturation and promote their differentiation into memory B cells and long-lived plasma cells. Plasma cells in inflamed synovial tissue produce significant quantities of rheumatoid factors (RF), predominantly Immunoglobulin M (IgM) type, and anti-citrullinated protein antibodies (ACPA). These autoantibodies form immune complexes with self-IgG in the synovium of RA patients. These immune complexes amplify complement activation, cytokine production by macrophages, and exacerbate joint damage by promoting osteoclast activation. Abbreviations: DC, dendritic cell; PC, plasma cells; Mφ, macrophage; OC, osteoclast; MHC, Major Histocompatibility Complex; TCR, T-cell receptor; BCR, B-cell receptor.

The diagnosis of RA is guided by several established classification criteria, among which the American College of Rheumatology/European League Against Rheumatism (ACR/EULAR) 2010 criteria are most widely used in clinical practice [4]. These criteria integrate clinical, serological, and imaging parameters to enhance diagnostic accuracy. In recent years, beyond these classification frameworks, there has been an increasing emphasis on early diagnosis and the incorporation of advanced imaging modalities, such as ultrasound and magnetic resonance imaging (MRI), which are pivotal in detecting subclinical synovitis [5,6].

Among the serological markers, rheumatoid factor (RF) and anti-citrullinated protein antibodies (ACPA) hold particular prominence. RF, a classical autoantibody discovered over eight decades ago, has been a cornerstone of RA diagnostics and research. Although its utility has been debated due to its presence in other autoimmune and inflammatory conditions, recent advancements have shed new light on its role, mechanisms, and potential implications in the pathophysiology and treatment of RA.

The evolving understanding of RF extends beyond its traditional use as a diagnostic tool. Emerging evidence suggests that RF plays a contributory role in disease mechanisms, including the formation of immune complexes and activation of complement pathways, which exacerbate joint damage. Furthermore, the prognostic value of RF in predicting disease severity and therapeutic response has gained increasing attention.

This review aims to provide a comprehensive exploration of the current evidence surrounding RF, with a focus on its clinical and biological significance in RA. We will discuss its historical context, diagnostic and prognostic performance, and therapeutic implications. By synthesizing recent advancements, we hope to elucidate the multifaceted roles of RF in RA and highlight potential directions for future research in this field.

2. Diagnostic Performance of RF

2.1. Detection Methods and Isotypes of RF

RF encompasses autoantibodies that recognize the fragment crystallizable region of immunoglobulin G (IgG) and were the first biomarkers identified in RA [7]. The discovery of RF dates back to 1940 when Waaler described a hemagglutinating factor in the serum of patients with RA [8]. Subsequently, in 1949, Pike coined the term "rheumatoid factor" to reflect its association with RA [9]. Since then, RF has remained a cornerstone in the study of autoimmune diseases, with its detection methods and clinical implications evolving significantly over the decades.

Various techniques have been developed for the measurement of RF, ranging from classical nephelometry and turbidimetry assays to more advanced methodologies. The former are isotype-nonspecific assays (Figure 2A) [10], while the advent of enzyme-linked immunosorbent assays (ELISA), fluorescence enzyme immunoassays (FEIA), chemiluminescence immunoassays (CLIA), and chemiluminescence microparticle immunoassays (CMIA) has allowed for isotype-specific RF detection, significantly advancing our understanding of its clinical relevance (Figure 2B) [11].

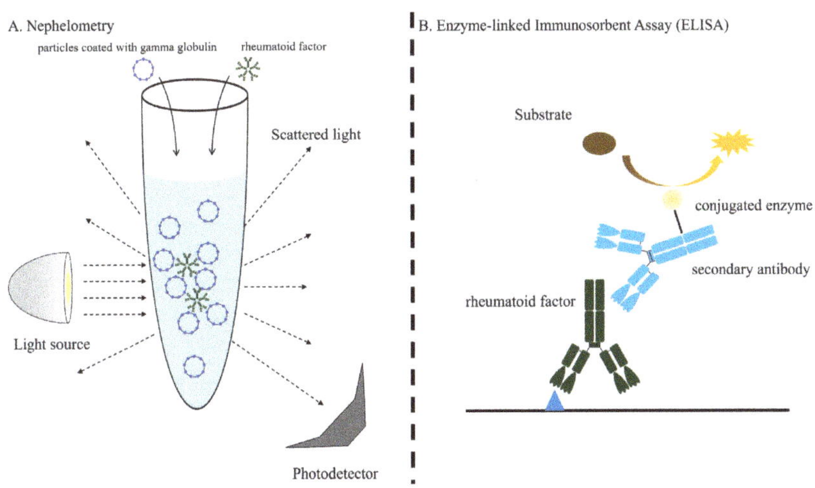

Figure 2. Methods for RF detection. (**A**) Nephelometry is based on the RF-induced aggregation of IgG-coupled particles. A laser beam is directed at the aggregates, and the intensity of the scattered light is quantified. The titer (IU/mL) is calculated from a standard curve, using serum aligned with the WHO's reference standard. The specific contribution of the various RF isotypes to the aggregation observed by nephelometry remains undetermined. (**B**) In the enzyme-linked immunosorbent assay (ELISA), the Fc portion of purified human IgG is immobilized on polystyrene microtiter plates and reacted with test serum. RF bound to the antigen is detected using an enzyme-conjugated secondary antibody specific to the immunoglobulin class, followed by the addition of an enzyme substrate.

The first World Health Organization (WHO) RF standard serum was established by pooling RA sera collected in 1963. In 1964, this pooled serum was divided into three batches, with the first batch designated as the international standard serum, W1066 [12]. The second batch was used to develop the first British standard serum, known as 64/002 [13]. Given their shared origin, W1066 and 64/002 are interchangeable as reference materials for RF measurement. The collaborative study involved 11 laboratories across 7 countries, all of which were required to utilize the sheep cell agglutination assay. Presently, most commercially available RF tests are standardized to W1066, with results expressed in international units (IU)/mL. However, at the time of the WHO standard W1066's publication in 1970 [14], isotype-specific assays had not yet been implemented. Results for IgA-RF and IgM-RF exhibit significant variability among commercially available assays, rendering them non-interchangeable for clinical and research applications [15,16].

Four subclasses of RF are detected by ELISA: IgM, IgG, IgA, and IgE [17], although IgE-RF measurements are rarely performed in recent years. Each isotype exhibits distinct associations with disease phenotypes and outcomes. IgG-RF and IgE-RF are particularly noteworthy for their links to vasculitic manifestations [18,19]. Additionally, IgE-RF levels are low in approximately half of patients with rheumatoid arthritis, whereas elevated concentrations are observed in individuals with rheumatoid vasculitis and Felty syndrome [19,20]. Conversely, patients positive for IgA-RF or IgM-RF often present with higher disease activity and greater radiological damage compared to seronegative patients [21–25]. Moreover, IgA-RF has been significantly associated with pulmonary lesions, while IgM-RF correlates strongly with the presence of rheumatoid nodules [26].

2.2. Sensitivity and Specificity of RF

The sensitivity and specificity of RF in diagnosing RA vary depending on disease stage, RF isotype, and detection method. The sensitivity of IgM-RF for RA is estimated to range from 41% to 66% in early RA and increases to 62% to 87% in established RA [27,28]. These figures underscore the dynamic nature of RF's diagnostic utility across the disease continuum. Moreover, the diagnostic performance of individual RF isotypes has been the focus of numerous studies, reflecting the complexity and heterogeneity of RF expression in RA patients.

A comprehensive systematic review and meta-analysis, involving 36 peer-reviewed studies and 7517 patients, provided insights into the sensitivity and specificity of various RF detection methods. Among the methods assessed, nephelometry and latex agglutination achieved the highest overall sensitivity (68.6%) across all isotypes. In contrast, isotype-specific assays such as ELISA and FEIA highlighted notable differences in sensitivity: IgM-RF exhibited the highest sensitivity (63.4%), followed by IgA-RF (49.1%) and IgG-RF (39.9%) [29]. Regarding specificity, IgA-RF demonstrated the highest specificity (91.4%), followed by IgM-RF (90%) and IgG-RF (78.9%). These results affirm IgM-RF as a robust marker for RA, with a diagnostic odds ratio of 21.7, compared to 16.0 for IgA-RF and 14.2 for IgG-RF, underscoring its clinical utility in identifying RA cases [29]. Furthermore, the presence of multiple RF isotypes enhances the likelihood of RA, highlighting the potential benefit of combined isotype detection in diagnostic and prognostic assessments [15,30].

Despite its diagnostic value, RF has limitations that complicate its interpretation. RF is positive in 5–25% of healthy individuals, and its prevalence increases with age, exceeding 25% in individuals older than 85 years [31]. Moreover, RF positivity has been reported to be more common among women and older individuals than men in the general population of the United States [32]. Additionally, in certain North American Indian tribes, the prevalence of RF positivity among healthy individuals reaches approximately 30%, highlighting population-specific variations in its distribution [33]. Even in studies focusing exclusively on patients with RA, RF positivity rates in the United States demonstrate racial and ethnic disparities, with lower prevalence reported in white individuals compared to Black, Hispanic, and Asian populations [34]. A more recent meta-analysis further revealed that among white individuals, men were significantly more likely to be seropositive than women. However, no significant association between sex and RF seropositivity was observed in Hispanic or Asian populations [35]. These findings suggest that proposing age- and sex-adjusted cutoff values for RF may hold clinical significance.

Additionally, RF is detected in various non-RA conditions, including other autoimmune diseases (e.g., Sjögren's syndrome and systemic lupus erythematosus), bacterial infections (e.g., infective endocarditis), viral infections (e.g., hepatitis C virus and Epstein–Barr virus), and cryoglobulinemia [28,36]. Environmental factors such as smoking have also been linked to RF production, independent of genetic predispositions like shared epitope alleles [37]. These findings highlight the importance of careful interpretation of RF results in clinical practice.

2.3. Distinct Binding Epitopes of RF in Healthy State and Autoimmunity

The mechanisms underlying RF production remain incompletely understood and appear to vary across conditions. RF can be produced during immunizations and secondary immune responses to infections, aiding in pathogen clearance [38–40]. In primary Sjögren's syndrome, RFs are linked to salivary gland mucosa-associated lymphoid tissue–type lymphomas, exhibiting high affinity and monoreactive binding to the IgG-Fc portion [41]. RFs may contribute to the activation and proliferation of B cells in chronic inflammatory sites via IgG immune complexes, increasing the risk of lymphoma development [41]. According to Wang et al., serum RFs in patients with primary Sjögren's syndrome exhibit clonal restriction and predominantly comprise a shared set of immunoglobulin M heavy chain variable region (IgVH) subfamilies, including 1–69, 3–15, 3–7, and 3–74. Furthermore, certain RF clonotypes have been detected in serum several years before the onset of mixed cryoglobulinemia (MC), and their levels decline following immunosuppressive therapy and MC remission, suggesting their potential role as early biomarkers and indicators of therapeutic response [41]. Recent studies have revealed significant differences in the RF repertoire between RA and other conditions. For instance, RF binding epitopes in healthy individuals and primary Sjögren's syndrome differ markedly from those in RA, suggesting distinct functional roles [42]. This distinction emphasizes the need for refined diagnostic assays that can differentiate between pathogenic and non-pathogenic RF.

Recent advancements in next-generation RF assays offer promising avenues for improving diagnostic accuracy [43]. These assays, which target RA-specific epitopes, have demonstrated potential in combination with ACPA to identify individuals at high risk of progressing to RA. Such tools hold promise for early diagnosis and intervention, particularly in preclinical or at-risk populations. Further studies are needed to validate these findings.

2.4. Comparison Between RF and ACPA

ACPA represent a more recently identified serological marker compared to RF and specifically target citrulline residues of filaggrin present in epithelial cells [44]. ACPA has been recognized for its early detection in the disease process, turning positive before IgM-RF during the preclinical phase of RA [44,45]. Extensive research has highlighted the critical role of ACPA in RA pathogenesis and its superior diagnostic performance. ACPA exhibits higher sensitivity and specificity than RF, particularly in the early stages of RA [46]. Furthermore, studies have demonstrated that double positivity for both RF and ACPA provides greater specificity than single-marker positivity, reinforcing the importance of simultaneous measurement of these antibodies for accurate diagnosis and disease classification [47].

Recent studies have identified glycosylation in the Fab region of ACPA as a distinctive feature associated with RA, suggesting its potential influence on autoantigen binding and the selection and activation threshold of B cells [48]. Beyond their role in disease progression, ACPAs have also exhibited therapeutic potential. Emerging evidence suggests that certain monoclonal ACPAs can attenuate arthritis and inflammation in murine models, underscoring their complex immunomodulatory properties [49]. Further research is needed to elucidate the precise mechanisms of ACPAs in RA pathogenesis and to explore their potential applications in targeted therapeutic strategies.

3. Prognostic Performance of RF

3.1. Disease Activity and Joint Destruction

Beyond its diagnostic utility, RF holds significant prognostic value in RA, offering insights into disease progression, severity, and treatment response. Studies consistently demonstrate that RF-positive patients at diagnosis are more likely to experience aggressive disease phenotypes characterized by greater joint damage, elevated inflammatory markers, and increased extra-articular manifestations compared to RF-negative individuals [50–55]. Notably, patients with high RF titers exhibit a faster progression to joint destruction, necessitating early and aggressive disease control [52,56–58]. These observations, supported by multiple studies, highlight RF's prognostic role in disease stratification and treatment planning [47,55,59].

It has recently been reported that the inflammation-inducing ability of RF is maximized in the presence of ACPA; IgM-RF forms a pentamer, which recognizes the Fc portion of ACPA and forms an immune complex, which stimulates macrophages and others to produce IL-6, TNFα, IL-1β etc. [60]. The combination of RF positivity with ACPA has been linked to higher rates of radiographic progression and poorer functional outcomes [61–65].

RF isotypes may further enhance its prognostic significance. Most of previous studies showed that among RF-positive patients, IgA-RF and IgM-RF are associated with severe disease courses [21–25]. However, recent meta-analysis demonstrated that the prognostic role of RF isotypes is not uniformly definitive, with inconsistent findings reported across studies [29]. While IgM-RF demonstrated modest associations with disease activity in 60% of cases, and IgA-RF showed predictive value for radiographic progression in approximately 50% of cases, results varied significantly due to differences in study designs and outcome definitions [29].

Conversely, a study has reported that the mean disease activity and quality of life in seronegative RA patients are comparable to those of seropositive RA patients, with similar proportions achieving disease remission [66]. Furthermore, certain findings suggest that seronegative RA patients may exhibit greater inflammatory activity than their seropositive counterparts, as assessed by ultrasound and radiography [67,68]. These observations challenge the conventional perception that seronegative RA represents a milder disease phenotype, leaving the debate regarding its relative severity unresolved.

3.2. Disease Progression

RF holds significant potential in predicting the onset of RA. RF levels are known to gradually increase over several years, up to 10 years, prior to the onset or diagnosis of RA [45]. Early studies have demonstrated that approximately 17% of IgM-RF-positive individuals presenting with joint pain eventually develop RA during the disease course [69]. More recently, a prospective cohort study conducted in Denmark reported that healthy individuals with elevated RF levels (>100 IU/mL) faced up to a 26-fold increased risk of developing RA, with a 10-year absolute risk as high as 32%. Even individuals with low-titer RF (25–50 IU/mL and 50.1–100 IU/mL) were found to have a 3.6-fold and 6.0-fold higher risk, respectively, of progressing to RA [70]. Notably, the sequential elevation of RF isotypes—beginning with IgM-RF, followed by IgA-RF and IgG-RF—suggests a temporal progression in isotype expression prior to the emergence of clinical manifestations [45,71,72].

These observations underscore the importance of longitudinal RF isotype monitoring as a tool for identifying individuals at risk of developing RA. Such monitoring could enable the implementation of early intervention strategies. Early detection not only improves diagnostic precision but also facilitates timely therapeutic interventions during the critical "window of opportunity", thereby potentially altering the disease trajectory [57,73–77].

3.3. Extra-Articular Manifestations

RA sometimes exhibit extra-articular manifestations [78–80], which are notably more prevalent in seropositive patients and those with a prolonged disease duration [81]. Among them, cardiovascular and pulmonary diseases represent the leading causes of mortality among RA patients [82]. RF assessment is essential to understand these systemic complications.

Previous studies have consistently shown that patients with RA face a significantly increased risk of coronary artery disease, congestive heart failure, and sudden cardiac death compared to the general population [24,83–88]. Additionally, Federico et al. reported that the presence of positive autoantibodies, including RF and ACPA, is associated with an elevated risk of future cardiovascular damage in patients with early-stage RA, within the first year of disease onset [89]. Furthermore, another study indicated that RF and antinuclear antibodies (ANA) are linked to an increased risk of cardiac disease and overall mortality, even in individuals without rheumatic disease [90]. Notably, disease activity and severity in RA are strongly correlated with cardiac dysfunction, and treatment for RA have been shown to improve cardiac outcomes [88,91–93]. Therefore, effective stratification of high-risk patients may play a crucial role in reducing cardiovascular events through the implementation of optimized immunomodulatory therapies.

Similarly, the presence of RF and ACPA has been demonstrated to correlate with a higher incidence and mortality of RA-associated interstitial lung disease (RA-ILD), a serious complication that carries substantial mortality risk [11,94–100]. Furthermore, high-titer RF seropositivity ($\geq$60 IU/mL) has been linked to mediastinal lymph node enlargement, CT-detected honeycombing, and reduced transplant-free survival, underscoring its prognostic value in RA-associated pulmonary complications [101]. The efficacy and safety of therapeutic agents, including conventional synthetic disease-modifying anti-rheumatic drugs (csDMARDs) and biologic DMARDs (bDMARDs), in the management of RA-ILD remain subjects of ongoing research and clinical uncertainty [102–104]. Nevertheless, growing evidence indicates that these treatments may contribute to slowing disease progression and improving the overall prognosis of RA-ILD [103,105–114]. Recent studies and meta-analyses have provided accumulating evidence that methotrexate exerts a suppressive effect on ILD [105,115]. The 2021 American College of Rheumatology Guideline for the Treatment of RA conditionally recommend methotrexate over alternative DMARDs for the management of inflammatory arthritis with moderate to severe disease activity in patients with mild, stable airway disease or pulmonary parenchymal disease [58]. Furthermore, in recent years, antifibrotic agents such as nintedanib have demonstrated the ability to slow the decline in forced vital capacity in patients with progressive fibrosing RA-ILD [116]. RA-ILD is a severe organ complication in which early detection is crucial for enhancing patient outcomes. RF titer may prove to be a valuable biomarker for identifying patients at increased risk of developing lung disease or facing mortality [101].

Rheumatoid vasculitis (RV) is a severe extra-articular complication of RA, characterized by inflammation of medium-sized arteries and capillaries. It is associated with a particularly poor prognosis, with high mortality rates attributed to vasculitic damage and the adverse effects of immunosuppressive therapy [117,118]. Several risk factors have been identified for RV, including long-standing RA, male sex, smoking, and the presence of rheumatoid nodules [119,120]. In a study of patients diagnosed with RV between 1980 and 1993, 68% had rheumatoid nodules, and most exhibited strong RF positivity [121]. Furthermore, multiple studies have consistently identified high RF titers as the most significant predictor of RV development [122,123]. Clinically, the prevalence of RV is estimated at 1–5% among RA cases, though autopsy studies suggest a much higher prevalence, ranging from 15 to 31% [124]. This discrepancy underscores the need for vigilant screening to improve early detection and prognosis, further highlighting the critical role of RF in identifying patients at risk for RV.

3.4. Difficult-to-Treat RA (D2T RA)

RF is also implicated in the disease mechanism of difficult-to-treat RA (D2T RA), a treatment-refractory subset characterized by inadequate therapeutic responses to ≥2 bDMARDs or targeted synthetic DMARDs with different mechanisms of action [125]. Previous studies have identified various patient-related factors associated with the development of D2T RA, such as young onset, multiple comorbidities, high disease activity, low-dose MTX use, and high-dose glucocorticoid use [126–131]. Among them, high RF titers have also been linked to the development of D2T RA [128,129,131], suggesting that high RF titers may serve as a biomarker for identifying patients who would benefit from early aggressive interventions or innovative therapeutic strategies [52,55].

Recent studies identified that RF titers are significantly correlated with serum type I interferon levels, which may contribute to therapeutic resistance in early RA [132,133]. Further investigations are warranted to elucidate the mechanisms by which RF contributes to D2T RA development and to explore its incorporation into personalized treatment paradigms.

3.5. RF in the 1987 ACR and 2010 ACR/EULAR Classification Criteria

The evolution of RA classification criteria reflects advancements in our understanding of the disease and the role of serological markers such as RF. The 1987 ACR classification criteria marked a pivotal moment by including RF as one of the key diagnostic parameters [134]. At that time, RF was primarily valued for its diagnostic utility, with its presence supporting a diagnosis of RA in conjunction with clinical symptoms such as joint swelling and morning stiffness. However, the criteria did not consider RF titers, limiting its prognostic utility.

The introduction of the 2010 ACR/EULAR classification criteria represented a significant paradigm shift, emphasizing earlier diagnosis and incorporating both RF and ACPA as critical serological markers [4]. RF's inclusion was prioritized based on its diagnostic and prognostic value, with higher titers contributing more points toward an RA diagnosis. This quantitative approach not only improved the sensitivity of the criteria but also highlighted the role of RF in identifying patients with more severe disease trajectories. Unlike the 1987 criteria, the 2010 framework acknowledged the additive value of combining RF with ACPA, which together enhance diagnostic specificity and prognostic accuracy.

Importantly, the 2010 criteria also shifted focus toward early RA, aiming to identify and treat patients before significant joint damage occurs. This early intervention model underscores the necessity of RF testing in stratifying patients based on disease severity and progression risk. The integration of RF into both sets of criteria illustrates its enduring relevance in RA classification, while ongoing research into RF isotypes and next-generation assays promises to refine its application further. Future updates to RA classification may benefit from incorporating insights into the differential roles of RF isotypes and their interactions with other biomarkers.

In light of these findings, the prognostic utility of RF in RA extends well beyond traditional diagnostic applications. By integrating RF analysis with other biomarkers and clinical parameters, clinicians can better stratify patients, predict disease trajectories, and tailor treatment plans. Future research should aim to further elucidate the mechanistic pathways linking RF to disease outcomes and explore novel therapeutic approaches targeting RF-mediated processes.

4. Therapeutic Implications of RF

The predictive value of RF extends to treatment response. RF-positive patients often exhibit differential responses to DMARDs, including both conventional synthetic and biologic agents. For instance, higher baseline RF titers have been associated with better responses to rituximab, a B-cell-targeting therapy [135], while potentially predicting reduced efficacy of tumor necrosis factor inhibitors [136–140]. This variability highlights the role of RF in guiding personalized treatment strategies and optimizing therapeutic outcomes.

4.1. Conventional DMARDs

According to the EULAR recommendations 2022 update for the management of RA, methotrexate (MTX) is recommended as the first-line therapeutic option for patients with RA [52]. MTX, approved by the FDA in 1988, remains the anchor drug and first-line therapy for RA due to its cost-effectiveness and favorable safety profile [141]. Numerous studies have demonstrated the efficacy of MTX as a first-line treatment regardless of the presence of RF or ACPA [142–144]. However, some studies suggest that RF positivity may correlate with MTX treatment failure and a higher likelihood of adverse events [145]. Although the precise mechanism underlying the relationship between RF positivity and MTX treatment failure remains unclear, research has shown that type I interferon (IFN) signaling pathway genes are significantly overexpressed in MTX non-responders [146]. Furthermore, the expression of IFN type I regulatory genes is markedly elevated in RA patients compared to healthy individuals and has been positively associated with RF [132,147]. These findings suggest that IFN-related pathways may play a critical role in the link between RF positivity and MTX treatment resistance. Despite these findings, MTX remains the cornerstone of RA management. However, clinical trials evaluating MTX monotherapy have reported that only approximately 40% of patients with early RA achieve a good response as defined by the ACR50 criteria, with even lower response rates observed with csDMARDs other than MTX [148–150]. High-titer RF has been identified as a poor prognostic indicator and its presence warrants a more proactive approach, including earlier use of bDMARDs [52].

4.2. Tumor Necrosis Factor Inhibitors

Tumor necrosis factor-alpha (TNFα) is a critical mediator that plays a central role in both inflammation and bone destruction in RA [151]. TNF inhibitors—such as infliximab (IFX), etanercept (ETA), adalimumab (ADA), golimumab (GOL), and certolizumab pegol (CZP)—are currently the most widely prescribed bDMARDs due to their proven high efficacy and favorable safety profile [152,153].

Previous studies have indicated that the presence of RF is associated with a diminished clinical response to TNF inhibitors [136–139,154–156]. However, more recent evidence suggests that CZP, in contrast to monoclonal antibodies such as IFX, ADA, GOL, and the receptor fusion protein ETA, demonstrates consistent efficacy regardless of RF levels [53,157–160]. The influence of RF on the pharmacokinetics of these therapies represents a critical aspect of our discussion. RFs are autoantibodies that specifically recognize the Fc region of IgG [161]. These RFs form immune complexes with IgG antibodies by binding to their Fc region. These immune complexes are then taken up by antigen-presenting cells (APCs), mainly macrophages, via Fc gamma receptors (FcγRs) for IgG (Figure 3A). Once taken up, these complexes are presumed to be transported to lysosomes, where they undergo enzymatic degradation as part of intracellular processing and clearance mechanisms [162,163]. CZP, however, lacks an Fc region and consequently avoids this pathway [164].

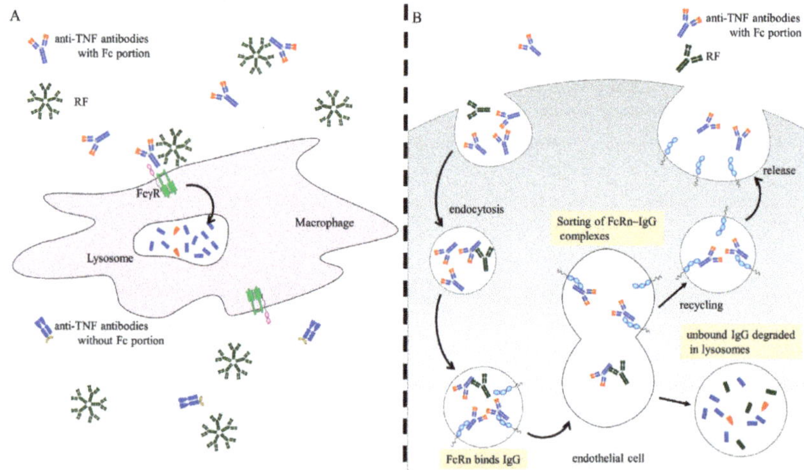

Figure 3. Mechanisms of attenuation of TNF antibody efficacy by RF. (**A**) The RF-IgG immune complex binds to the Fc receptors for IgG (FcγR) on the surface of antigen-presenting cells (APCs), leading to the internalization and subsequent lysosomal transport of the complex. Within the lysosomes, both the FcγR and the internalized antigen undergo proteolytic degradation. Anti-TNF antibodies lacking the Fc portion are hypothesized to evade this degradation pathway. (**B**) The neonatal Fc receptor for IgG (FcRn) is predominantly expressed on endothelial cells. These cells internalize serum IgG and engage FcRn within acidic endosomal compartments. FcRn subsequently recycles IgG back into circulation, thereby extending its serum half-life. In contrast, IgG that fails to bind FcRn is routed to lysosomes for degradation, bypassing intracellular sorting. Rheumatoid factor (RF) binds to the FcRn-binding sites of TNF antibodies and may interfere with their recycling process.

In addition, high-titer RF could impact IgG recycling mediated by the neonatal Fc receptor (FcRn). While TNF inhibitors containing an Fc region are incorporated into the endosome and recycled through binding to FcRn in endothelial cells, IgG that fail to bind to FcRn are degraded in lysosomes [165]. RF may interfere with this recycling process by binding to the FcRn-binding site on IgG [166] (Figure 3B).

Based on these mechanisms, the serum drug levels of TNF inhibitors containing the Fc region, such as IFX and ADA, are reduced or undetectable in patients with high-titer RF. In contrast, the serum drug levels of CZP remain stable regardless of RF titer [159]. Consequently, it has been reported that CZP demonstrates greater efficacy compared to TNF inhibitors with an Fc region in patients with high RF titers (166–204 IU/mL or higher) [53,157,160].

It is important to highlight the recently launched TNF inhibitor ozoralizumab, which is now available in Japan. This next-generation single-domain anti-TNF-α antibody has a unique structure comprising two anti-TNF-α nanobodies® and an anti-human serum albumin (HSA) nanobody®. With a molecular weight of 38 kDa—approximately one-fourth the size of conventional anti-TNF-α IgG antibodies—ozoralizumab represents a novel and advanced therapeutic option [167,168]. Notably, ozoralizumab lacks the Fc region in its structure, which may allow it to bypass the efficacy-reducing effects associated with RF.

4.3. Non-TNF Targeted Treatment

Treatment with TNF inhibitors have traditionally been the first-line therapy following an inadequate response to MTX. While TNF inhibitors significantly improve the quality of life for most RA patients, at least one-third of patients fail to respond to these drugs [169,170]. To provide alternative options, several newer antirheumatic therapies with distinct mechanisms of action are now available, including non-TNF biologics and Janus kinase (JAK) inhibitors [52,171]. These non-TNF biologics include a range of targeted therapies, including anti-B-cell agents such as rituximab (RTX), anti-T-cell co-stimulatory inhibitors such as abatacept, and interleukin-6 receptor inhibitors such as tocilizumab and sarilumab [172–174].

The importance of targeting B cells in the treatment of RA is clear, as evidenced by the efficacy of RTX, a B-cell depletion therapy. A meta-analysis of four randomized placebo-controlled trials (REFLEX, SERENE, DANCER, and IMAGE) revealed that RTX provides additional therapeutic benefits in seropositive RA, particularly in patients who have not responded to at least one TNF inhibitor [135]. Notably, RTX has demonstrated efficacy irrespective of the presence of RF [135]. Furthermore, in a large observational cohort study of RA patients treated with RTX, seropositive patients exhibited significantly lower Disease Activity Score 28 (DAS28) at 6 months compared to seronegative patients [135]. These findings offer critical insights for optimizing treatment strategies in RF-positive patients.

A recent study reported that serum IL-6 concentrations were significantly elevated in patients who failed to achieve remission with TNF inhibitors compared to those who did not. These findings suggest that such patients exhibit a high dependency on IL-6, making IL-6 signaling inhibition a rational and potentially effective therapeutic strategy [175]. While some studies suggest that RF positivity is associated with improved treatment outcomes in patients receiving IL-6 inhibitors, others report no significant correlation between RF positivity and treatment response [176–179]. Similarly, findings on the relationship between RF presence and treatment response to abatacept have been inconsistent [176,180–185], and data regarding RF's impact on the efficacy of JAK inhibitors remain limited [186–188]. However, there is no evidence to indicate that the presence of RF is linked to treatment discontinuation due to a lack of efficacy for these therapies. Consequently, the presence or absence of RF does not seem to restrict the clinical application of these therapies.

5. Conclusions

Over the decades, advancements in RF detection methods and a deeper understanding of its isotype-specific roles have significantly improved RA management. However, challenges such as diagnostic specificity, prognostic variability, and treatment resistance persist, highlighting the need for further research. Future efforts should focus on refining RF assays to enhance their diagnostic and prognostic precision, exploring the temporal dynamics of RF isotype progression, and integrating RF into personalized treatment paradigms.

Given the heterogeneity of RA, RF remains a key biomarker not only for its established diagnostic and prognostic value but also for its emerging role in guiding treatment stratification. RF, in combination with other biomarkers such as ACPA, may help identify patient subgroups more likely to benefit from specific therapeutic approaches. Moreover, high RF titers have been linked to treatment resistance, particularly with MTX and certain biologic therapies, underscoring the importance of personalized treatment strategies. Integrating RF status into precision medicine frameworks holds promise for optimizing therapeutic outcomes and advancing individualized RA management.

Author Contributions: T.T. and R.I. performed literature review. R.I. made Figures. T.T., R.I. and R.W. drafted the manuscript. M.H. read and finalized the manuscript. Other authors participated in the useful discussion. All authors have read and agreed to the published version of the manuscript.

Funding: This research received no external funding.

Institutional Review Board Statement: Not applicable.

Informed Consent Statement: Not applicable.

Data Availability Statement: Not applicable.

Conflicts of Interest: RW received a research grant from AbbVie and speaker's fee from AbbVie, Asahi Kasei, Chugai, Eli Lilly, GSK, and UCB Japan. MH received research grants and/or speaker fee from Abbvie, Asahi Kasei, Astellas, Brystol Meyers, Chugai, EA Pharma, Eisai, Daiichi Sankyo, Eli Lilly, Novartis Pharma, Taisho Toyama, Tanabe Mitsubishi, Towa Pharma, UCB Japan. These pharmaceutical companies had no role in the writing of the manuscript.

References

1. Smolen, J.S.; Aletaha, D.; Barton, A.; Burmester, G.R.; Emery, P.; Firestein, G.S.; Kavanaugh, A.; McInnes, I.B.; Solomon, D.H.; Strand, V.; et al. Rheumatoid arthritis. *Nat. Rev. Dis. Primers.* **2018**, *4*, 18001. [CrossRef] [PubMed]
2. Rothschild, B.M.; Turner, K.R.; DeLuca, M.A. Symmetrical erosive peripheral polyarthritis in the Late Archaic Period of Alabama. *Science* **1988**, *241*, 1498–1501. [CrossRef] [PubMed]
3. Almutairi, K.; Nossent, J.; Preen, D.; Keen, H.; Inderjeeth, C. The global prevalence of rheumatoid arthritis: A meta-analysis based on a systematic review. *Rheumatol. Int.* **2021**, *41*, 863–877. [CrossRef] [PubMed]
4. Aletaha, D.; Neogi, T.; Silman, A.J.; Funovits, J.; Felson, D.T.; Bingham, C.O., 3rd; Birnbaum, N.S.; Burmester, G.R.; Bykerk, V.P.; Cohen, M.D.; et al. 2010 rheumatoid arthritis classification criteria: An American College of Rheumatology/European League Against Rheumatism collaborative initiative. *Ann. Rheum. Dis.* **2010**, *69*, 1580–1588. [CrossRef]
5. Silvagni, E.; Zandonella Callegher, S.; Mauric, E.; Chiricolo, S.; Schreiber, N.; Tullio, A.; Zabotti, A.; Scirè, C.A.; Dejaco, C.; Sakellariou, G. Musculoskeletal ultrasound for treating rheumatoid arthritis to target—A systematic literature review. *Rheumatology* **2022**, *61*, 4590–4602. [CrossRef]
6. Hunt, L.; Eugénio, G.; Grainger, A.J. Magnetic resonance imaging in individuals at risk of rheumatoid arthritis. *Best Pract. Res. Clin. Rheumatol.* **2017**, *31*, 80–89. [CrossRef] [PubMed]
7. Steiner, G.; Toes, R.E.M. Autoantibodies in rheumatoid arthritis—Rheumatoid factor, anticitrullinated protein antibodies and beyond. *Curr. Opin. Rheumatol.* **2024**, *36*, 217–224. [CrossRef] [PubMed]
8. Waaler, E. On the occurrence of a factor in human serum activating the specific agglutintion of sheep blood corpuscles. *APMIS* **2007**, *115*, 422–438; discussion 439. [CrossRef]
9. Pike, R.M.; Sulkin, S.E.; Coggeshall, H.C. Serological reactions in rheumatoid arthritis; factors affecting the agglutination of sensitized sheep erythrocytes in rheumatid-arthritis serum. *J. Immunol.* **1949**, *63*, 441–446. [CrossRef]
10. Renaudineau, Y.; Jamin, C.; Saraux, A.; Youinou, P. Rheumatoid factor on a daily basis. *Autoimmunity* **2005**, *38*, 11–16. [CrossRef]
11. Brink, M.; Hansson, M.; Mathsson-Alm, L.; Wijayatunga, P.; Verheul, M.K.; Trouw, L.A.; Holmdahl, R.; Rönnelid, J.; Klareskog, L.; Rantapää-Dahlqvist, S. Rheumatoid factor isotypes in relation to antibodies against citrullinated peptides and carbamylated proteins before the onset of rheumatoid arthritis. *Arthritis Res. Ther.* **2016**, *18*, 43. [CrossRef]
12. WHO Reference Reagent Rheumatoid Arthritis Serum, Human NIBSC Code: W1066 Instructions for Use (Version 2.0, Dated 04/04/2008). Available online: https://nibsc.org/documents/ifu/W1066.pdf (accessed on 17 February 2025).
13. Non WHO Reference Material Rheumatoid Arthritis Serum, 1st British Standard NIBSC Code: 64/002 Instructions for Use (Version 6.0, Dated 04/04/2008). Available online: https://www.nibsc.org/documents/ifu/64-002.pdf (accessed on 17 February 2025).
14. Anderson, S.G.; Bentzon, M.W.; Houba, V.; Krag, P. International reference preparation of rheumatoid arthritis serum. *Bull. World Health Organ.* **1970**, *42*, 311–318. [PubMed]
15. Van Hoovels, L.; Vander Cruyssen, B.; Sieghart, D.; Bonroy, C.; Nagy, E.; Pullerits, R.; Čučnik, S.; Dahle, C.; Heijnen, I.; Bernasconi, L.; et al. IgA rheumatoid factor in rheumatoid arthritis. *Clin. Chem. Lab. Med.* **2022**, *60*, 1617–1626. [CrossRef]
16. Van Hoovels, L.; Vander Cruyssen, B.; Sieghart, D.; Bonroy, C.; Nagy, E.; Pullerits, R.; Čučnik, S.; Dahle, C.; Heijnen, I.; Bernasconi, L.; et al. Multicentre study to improve clinical interpretation of rheumatoid factor and anti-citrullinated protein/peptide antibodies test results. *RMD Open* **2022**, *8*, e002099. [CrossRef]
17. Gioud-Paquet, M.; Auvinet, M.; Raffin, T.; Girard, P.; Bouvier, M.; Lejeune, E.; Monier, J.C. IgM rheumatoid factor (RF), IgA RF, IgE RF, and IgG RF detected by ELISA in rheumatoid arthritis. *Ann. Rheum. Dis.* **1987**, *46*, 65–71. [CrossRef]
18. Mannik, M.; Nardella, F.A. IgG rheumatoid factors and self-association of these antibodies. *Clin. Rheum. Dis.* **1985**, *11*, 551–572. [CrossRef] [PubMed]
19. Mizushima, Y.; Shoji, Y.; Hoshi, K.; Kiyokawa, S. Detection and clinical significance of IgE rheumatoid factor. *J. Rheumatol.* **1984**, *11*, 22–26. [PubMed]
20. Merétey, K.; Falus, A.; Böhm, U.; Permin, H.; Wiik, A. IgE class immune complexes in Felty's syndrome: Characterisation of antibody activities in isolated complexes. *Ann. Rheum. Dis.* **1984**, *43*, 246–250. [CrossRef]
21. Arnason, J.A.; Jonsson, T.; Brekkan, A.; Sigurjonsson, K.; Valdimarsson, H. Relation between bone erosions and rheumatoid factor isotypes. *Ann. Rheum. Dis.* **1987**, *46*, 380–384. [CrossRef] [PubMed]

22. Eggelmeijer, F.; Otten, H.G.; de Rooy, H.H.; Daha, M.R.; Breedveld, F.C. Significance of rheumatoid factor isotypes in seronegative rheumatoid arthritis. *Rheumatol. Int.* **1990**, *10*, 43–46. [CrossRef] [PubMed]
23. Houssien, D.A.; Jonsson, T.; Davies, E.; Scott, D.L. Clinical significance of IgA rheumatoid factor subclasses in rheumatoid arthritis. *J. Rheumatol.* **1997**, *24*, 2119–2122. [PubMed]
24. Teitsson, I. IgA rheumatoid factor as predictor of disease activity. *Scand. J. Rheumatol. Suppl.* **1988**, *75*, 233–237. [CrossRef] [PubMed]
25. Winska Wiloch, H.; Thompson, K.; Young, A.; Corbett, M.; Shipley, M.; Hay, F. IgA and IgM rheumatoid factors as markers of later erosive changes in rheumatoid arthritis (RA). *Scand. J. Rheumatol. Suppl.* **1988**, *75*, 238–243. [CrossRef]
26. Ateş, A.; Kinikli, G.; Turgay, M.; Akay, G.; Tokgöz, G. Effects of rheumatoid factor isotypes on disease activity and severity in patients with rheumatoid arthritis: A comparative study. *Clin. Rheumatol.* **2007**, *26*, 538–545. [CrossRef]
27. Nishimura, K.; Sugiyama, D.; Kogata, Y.; Tsuji, G.; Nakazawa, T.; Kawano, S.; Saigo, K.; Morinobu, A.; Koshiba, M.; Kuntz, K.M.; et al. Meta-analysis: Diagnostic accuracy of anti-cyclic citrullinated peptide antibody and rheumatoid factor for rheumatoid arthritis. *Ann. Intern. Med.* **2007**, *146*, 797–808. [CrossRef]
28. Wu, C.Y.; Yang, H.Y.; Luo, S.F.; Lai, J.H. From Rheumatoid Factor to Anti-Citrullinated Protein Antibodies and Anti-Carbamylated Protein Antibodies for Diagnosis and Prognosis Prediction in Patients with Rheumatoid Arthritis. *Int. J. Mol. Sci.* **2021**, *22*, 686. [CrossRef] [PubMed]
29. Motta, F.; Bizzaro, N.; Giavarina, D.; Franceschini, F.; Infantino, M.; Palterer, B.; Sebastiani, G.D.; Selmi, C. Rheumatoid factor isotypes in rheumatoid arthritis diagnosis and prognosis: A systematic review and meta-analysis. *RMD Open* **2023**, *9*, e002817. [CrossRef] [PubMed]
30. Jaskowski, T.D.; Hill, H.R.; Russo, K.L.; Lakos, G.; Szekanecz, Z.; Teodorescu, M. Relationship between rheumatoid factor isotypes and IgG anti-cyclic citrullinated peptide antibodies. *J. Rheumatol.* **2010**, *37*, 1582–1588. [CrossRef] [PubMed]
31. van Schaardenburg, D.; Lagaay, A.M.; Otten, H.G.; Breedveld, F.C. The relation between class-specific serum rheumatoid factors and age in the general population. *Br. J. Rheumatol.* **1993**, *32*, 546–549. [CrossRef]
32. Dillon, C.F.; Weisman, M.H.; Miller, F.W. Population-based estimates of humoral autoimmunity from the U.S. National Health and Nutrition Examination Surveys, 1960–2014. *PLoS ONE* **2020**, *15*, e0226516. [CrossRef]
33. Newkirk, M.M. Rheumatoid factors: What do they tell us? *J. Rheumatol.* **2002**, *29*, 2034–2040.
34. Greenberg, J.D.; Spruill, T.M.; Shan, Y.; Reed, G.; Kremer, J.M.; Potter, J.; Yazici, Y.; Ogedegbe, G.; Harrold, L.R. Racial and ethnic disparities in disease activity in patients with rheumatoid arthritis. *Am. J. Med.* **2013**, *126*, 1089–1098. [CrossRef] [PubMed]
35. Hadwen, B.; Yu, R.; Cairns, E.; Barra, L. Presence of Autoantibodies in Males and Females with Rheumatoid Arthritis: A Systematic Review and Metaanalysis. *J. Rheumatol.* **2022**, *49*, 663–671. [CrossRef]
36. Ingegnoli, F.; Castelli, R.; Gualtierotti, R. Rheumatoid factors: Clinical applications. *Dis. Markers.* **2013**, *35*, 727–734. [CrossRef] [PubMed]
37. Ishikawa, Y.; Ikari, K.; Hashimoto, M.; Ohmura, K.; Tanaka, M.; Ito, H.; Taniguchi, A.; Yamanaka, H.; Mimori, T.; Terao, C. Shared epitope defines distinct associations of cigarette smoking with levels of anticitrullinated protein antibody and rheumatoid factor. *Ann. Rheum. Dis.* **2019**, *78*, 1480–1487. [CrossRef]
38. Slaughter, L.; Carson, D.A.; Jensen, F.C.; Holbrook, T.L.; Vaughan, J.H. In vitro effects of Epstein-Barr virus on peripheral blood mononuclear cells from patients with rheumatoid arthritis and normal subjects. *J. Exp. Med.* **1978**, *148*, 1429–1434. [CrossRef] [PubMed]
39. Van Snick, J.L.; Van Roost, E.; Markowetz, B.; Cambiaso, C.L.; Masson, P.L. Enhancement by IgM rheumatoid factor of in vitro ingestion by macrophages and in vivo clearance of aggregated IgG or antigen-antibody complexes. *Eur. J. Immunol.* **1978**, *8*, 279–285. [CrossRef]
40. Welch, M.J.; Fong, S.; Vaughan, J.; Carson, D. Increased frequency of rheumatoid factor precursor B lymphocytes after immunization of normal adults with tetanus toxoid. *Clin. Exp. Immunol.* **1983**, *51*, 299–304. [PubMed]
41. Wang, J.J.; Reed, J.H.; Colella, A.D.; Russell, A.J.; Murray-Brown, W.; Chataway, T.K.; Jackson, K.J.L.; Goodnow, C.C.; Gordon, T.P. Molecular Profiling and Clonal Tracking of Secreted Rheumatoid Factors in Primary Sjögren's Syndrome. *Arthritis Rheumatol.* **2018**, *70*, 1617–1625. [CrossRef] [PubMed]
42. Oskam, N.; Ooijevaar-De Heer, P.; Kos, D.; Jeremiasse, J.; van Boheemen, L.; Verstappen, G.M.; Kroese, F.G.M.; van Schaardenburg, D.; Wolbink, G.; Rispens, T. Rheumatoid factor autoantibody repertoire profiling reveals distinct binding epitopes in health and autoimmunity. *Ann. Rheum. Dis.* **2023**, *82*, 945–956. [CrossRef]
43. Oskam, N.; Ooijevaar-de Heer, P.; Kos, D.; van Boheemen, L.; van Schaardenburg, D.; Wolbink, G.; Rispens, T. Next-generation rheumatoid factor assay provides improved predictive power for the development of arthritis in patients at risk. *RMD Open* **2024**, *10*, e004172. [CrossRef] [PubMed]
44. Schellekens, G.A.; de Jong, B.A.; van den Hoogen, F.H.; van de Putte, L.B.; van Venrooij, W.J. Citrulline is an Essential Constituent of Antigenic Determinants Recognized by Rheumatoid Arthritis-specific Autoantibodies. 1998. *J. Immunol.* **2015**, *195*, 8–16. [PubMed]

45. Nielen, M.M.; van Schaardenburg, D.; Reesink, H.W.; van de Stadt, R.J.; van der Horst-Bruinsma, I.E.; de Koning, M.H.; Habibuw, M.R.; Vandenbroucke, J.P.; Dijkmans, B.A. Specific autoantibodies precede the symptoms of rheumatoid arthritis: A study of serial measurements in blood donors. *Arthritis Rheum.* **2004**, *50*, 380–386. [CrossRef] [PubMed]
46. Aggarwal, R.; Liao, K.; Nair, R.; Ringold, S.; Costenbader, K.H. Anti-citrullinated peptide antibody assays and their role in the diagnosis of rheumatoid arthritis. *Arthritis Rheum.* **2009**, *61*, 1472–1483. [CrossRef]
47. Steiner, G.; Van Hoovels, L.; Csige, D.; Gatto, M.; Iagnocco, A.; Szekanecz, Z. Should ACR/EULAR criteria be revised changing the RF and ACPA scores? *Autoimmun. Rev.* **2024**, *23*, 103421. [CrossRef] [PubMed]
48. Stork, E.M.; van Rijswijck, D.M.H.; van Schie, K.A.; Hoek, M.; Kissel, T.; Scherer, H.U.; Huizinga, T.W.J.; Heck, A.J.R.; Toes, R.E.M.; Bondt, A. Antigen-specific Fab profiling achieves molecular-resolution analysis of human autoantibody repertoires in rheumatoid arthritis. *Nat. Commun.* **2024**, *15*, 3114. [CrossRef] [PubMed]
49. Raposo, B.; Klareskog, L.; Robinson, W.H.; Malmström, V.; Grönwall, C. The peculiar features, diversity and impact of citrulline-reactive autoantibodies. *Nat. Rev. Rheumatol.* **2024**, *20*, 399–416. [CrossRef]
50. Albrecht, K.; Zink, A. Poor prognostic factors guiding treatment decisions in rheumatoid arthritis patients: A review of data from randomized clinical trials and cohort studies. *Arthritis Res. Ther.* **2017**, *19*, 68. [CrossRef] [PubMed]
51. Aletaha, D.; Alasti, F.; Smolen, J.S. Rheumatoid factor determines structural progression of rheumatoid arthritis dependent and independent of disease activity. *Ann. Rheum. Dis.* **2013**, *72*, 875–880. [CrossRef] [PubMed]
52. Smolen, J.S.; Landewé, R.B.M.; Bergstra, S.A.; Kerschbaumer, A.; Sepriano, A.; Aletaha, D.; Caporali, R.; Edwards, C.J.; Hyrich, K.L.; Pope, J.E.; et al. EULAR recommendations for the management of rheumatoid arthritis with synthetic and biological disease-modifying antirheumatic drugs: 2022 update. *Ann. Rheum. Dis.* **2023**, *82*, 3–18. [CrossRef]
53. Smolen, J.S.; Taylor, P.C.; Tanaka, Y.; Takeuchi, T.; Hashimoto, M.; Cara, C.; Lauwerys, B.; Tilt, N.; Ufuktepe, B.; Xavier, R.M.; et al. Impact of high rheumatoid factor levels on treatment outcomes with certolizumab pegol and adalimumab in patients with rheumatoid arthritis. *Rheumatology* **2024**, *63*, 3015–3024. [CrossRef]
54. Soubrier, M.; Barber Chamoux, N.; Tatar, Z.; Couderc, M.; Dubost, J.J.; Mathieu, S. Cardiovascular risk in rheumatoid arthritis. *Jt. Bone Spine* **2014**, *81*, 298–302. [CrossRef]
55. Vastesaeger, N.; Xu, S.; Aletaha, D.; St Clair, E.W.; Smolen, J.S. A pilot risk model for the prediction of rapid radiographic progression in rheumatoid arthritis. *Rheumatology* **2009**, *48*, 1114–1121. [CrossRef] [PubMed]
56. Balanean, A.; Brown-Bickerstaff, C.; Klink, A.; Patel, V.; Zheng, H.; N'Dri, L.; Wittstock, K.; Feinberg, B.; Chaballa, M.; Khaychuk, V.; et al. Real-world clinical outcomes and rationale for initiating abatacept as a first-line biologic for patients with anticitrullinated protein antibody- and rheumatoid factor-positive rheumatoid arthritis. *J. Comp. Eff. Res.* **2024**, *13*, e230144. [CrossRef] [PubMed]
57. Burgers, L.E.; Raza, K.; van der Helm-van Mil, A.H. Window of opportunity in rheumatoid arthritis—Definitions and supporting evidence: From old to new perspectives. *RMD Open* **2019**, *5*, e000870. [CrossRef] [PubMed]
58. Fraenkel, L.; Bathon, J.M.; England, B.R.; St Clair, E.W.; Arayssi, T.; Carandang, K.; Deane, K.D.; Genovese, M.; Huston, K.K.; Kerr, G.; et al. 2021 American College of Rheumatology Guideline for the Treatment of Rheumatoid Arthritis. *Arthritis Rheumatol.* **2021**, *73*, 1108–1123. [CrossRef] [PubMed]
59. Milchram, L.; Fischer, A.; Huber, J.; Soldo, R.; Sieghart, D.; Vierlinger, K.; Blüml, S.; Steiner, G.; Weinhäusel, A. Functional Analysis of Autoantibody Signatures in Rheumatoid Arthritis. *Molecules* **2022**, *27*, 1452. [CrossRef]
60. Pertsinidou, E.; Saevarsdottir, S.; Manivel, V.A.; Klareskog, L.; Alfredsson, L.; Mathsson-Alm, L.; Hansson, M.; Cornillet, M.; Serre, G.; Holmdahl, R.; et al. In early rheumatoid arthritis, anticitrullinated peptide antibodies associate with low number of affected joints and rheumatoid factor associates with systemic inflammation. *Ann. Rheum. Dis.* **2024**, *83*, 277–287. [CrossRef]
61. Guaracha-Basáñez, G.A.; Contreras-Yáñez, I.; Ortiz-Haro, A.B.; Pascual-Ramos, V. Differences in referral path, clinical and radiographic outcomes between seronegative and seropositive rheumatoid arthritis Mexican Mestizo patients: A cohort study. *PLoS ONE* **2024**, *19*, e0304953. [CrossRef]
62. Hetland, M.L.; Østergaard, M.; Stengaard-Pedersen, K.; Junker, P.; Ejbjerg, B.; Jacobsen, S.; Ellingsen, T.; Lindegaard, H.; Pødenphant, J.; Vestergaard, A.; et al. Anti-cyclic citrullinated peptide antibodies, 28-joint Disease Activity Score, and magnetic resonance imaging bone oedema at baseline predict 11 years' functional and radiographic outcome in early rheumatoid arthritis. *Scand. J. Rheumatol.* **2019**, *48*, 1–8. [CrossRef] [PubMed]
63. Lin, D.; Zhao, M.; Zhang, Y.; Xie, Y.; Cao, J.; Pan, Y. Seronegative rheumatic arthritis has milder inflammation and bone erosion in an ultrasound study of disease-modifying anti-rheumatic drugs (DMARDs)-naïve Chinese cohort. *Ann. Transl. Med.* **2022**, *10*, 661. [CrossRef] [PubMed]
64. Terao, C.; Yamakawa, N.; Yano, K.; Markusse, I.M.; Ikari, K.; Yoshida, S.; Furu, M.; Hashimoto, M.; Ito, H.; Fujii, T.; et al. Rheumatoid Factor Is Associated with the Distribution of Hand Joint Destruction in Rheumatoid Arthritis. *Arthritis Rheumatol.* **2015**, *67*, 3113–3123. [CrossRef] [PubMed]
65. van den Broek, M.; Dirven, L.; Klarenbeek, N.B.; Molenaar, T.H.; Han, K.H.; Kerstens, P.J.; Huizinga, T.W.; Dijkmans, B.A.; Allaart, C.F. The association of treatment response and joint damage with ACPA-status in recent-onset RA: A subanalysis of the 8-year follow-up of the BeSt study. *Ann. Rheum. Dis.* **2012**, *71*, 245–248. [CrossRef] [PubMed]

66. Mouterde, G.; Rincheval, N.; Lukas, C.; Daien, C.; Saraux, A.; Dieudé, P.; Morel, J.; Combe, B. Outcome of patients with early arthritis without rheumatoid factor and ACPA and predictors of rheumatoid arthritis in the ESPOIR cohort. *Arthritis Res. Ther.* **2019**, *21*, 140. [CrossRef]
67. Nordberg, L.B.; Lillegraven, S.; Lie, E.; Aga, A.B.; Olsen, I.C.; Hammer, H.B.; Uhlig, T.; Jonsson, M.K.; van der Heijde, D.; Kvien, T.K.; et al. Patients with seronegative RA have more inflammatory activity compared with patients with seropositive RA in an inception cohort of DMARD-naïve patients classified according to the 2010 ACR/EULAR criteria. *Ann. Rheum. Dis.* **2017**, *76*, 341–345. [CrossRef]
68. Geng, Y.; Zhou, W.; Zhang, Z.L. A comparative study on the diversity of clinical features between the sero-negative and sero-positive rheumatoid arthritis patients. *Rheumatol. Int.* **2012**, *32*, 3897–3901. [CrossRef] [PubMed]
69. de Bois, M.H.; Arndt, J.W.; Speyer, I.; Pauwels, E.K.; Breedveld, F.C. Technetium-99m labelled human immunoglobulin scintigraphy predicts rheumatoid arthritis in patients with arthralgia. *Scand. J. Rheumatol.* **1996**, *25*, 155–158. [CrossRef]
70. Nielsen, S.F.; Bojesen, S.E.; Schnohr, P.; Nordestgaard, B.G. Elevated rheumatoid factor and long term risk of rheumatoid arthritis: A prospective cohort study. *BMJ* **2012**, *345*, e5244. [CrossRef]
71. Deane, K.D.; Norris, J.M.; Holers, V.M. Preclinical rheumatoid arthritis: Identification, evaluation, and future directions for investigation. *Rheum. Dis. Clin. N. Am.* **2010**, *36*, 213–241. [CrossRef] [PubMed]
72. Kokkonen, H.; Mullazehi, M.; Berglin, E.; Hallmans, G.; Wadell, G.; Rönnelid, J.; Rantapää-Dahlqvist, S. Antibodies of IgG, IgA and IgM isotypes against cyclic citrullinated peptide precede the development of rheumatoid arthritis. *Arthritis Res. Ther.* **2011**, *13*, R13. [CrossRef]
73. Monti, S.; Montecucco, C.; Bugatti, S.; Caporali, R. Rheumatoid arthritis treatment: The earlier the better to prevent joint damage. *RMD Open* **2015**, *1*, e000057. [CrossRef] [PubMed]
74. González-Álvaro, I.; Ortiz, A.M.; Seoane, I.V.; García-Vicuña, R.; Martínez, C.; Gomariz, R.P. Biomarkers predicting a need for intensive treatment in patients with early arthritis. *Curr. Pharm. Des.* **2015**, *21*, 170–181. [CrossRef]
75. van Nies, J.A.; Krabben, A.; Schoones, J.W.; Huizinga, T.W.; Kloppenburg, M.; van der Helm-van Mil, A.H. What is the evidence for the presence of a therapeutic window of opportunity in rheumatoid arthritis? A systematic literature review. *Ann. Rheum. Dis.* **2014**, *73*, 861–870. [CrossRef] [PubMed]
76. Nagy, G.; van Vollenhoven, R.F. Sustained biologic-free and drug-free remission in rheumatoid arthritis, where are we now? *Arthritis Res. Ther.* **2015**, *17*, 181. [CrossRef] [PubMed]
77. van Nies, J.A.; Tsonaka, R.; Gaujoux-Viala, C.; Fautrel, B.; van der Helm-van Mil, A.H. Evaluating relationships between symptom duration and persistence of rheumatoid arthritis: Does a window of opportunity exist? Results on the Leiden early arthritis clinic and ESPOIR cohorts. *Ann. Rheum. Dis.* **2015**, *74*, 806–812. [CrossRef] [PubMed]
78. Cojocaru, M.; Cojocaru, I.M.; Silosi, I.; Vrabie, C.D.; Tanasescu, R. Extra-articular Manifestations in Rheumatoid Arthritis. *Maedica* **2010**, *5*, 286–291.
79. Conforti, A.; Di Cola, I.; Pavlych, V.; Ruscitti, P.; Berardicurti, O.; Ursini, F.; Giacomelli, R.; Cipriani, P. Beyond the joints, the extra-articular manifestations in rheumatoid arthritis. *Autoimmun. Rev.* **2021**, *20*, 102735. [CrossRef]
80. Radu, A.F.; Bungau, S.G. Management of Rheumatoid Arthritis: An Overview. *Cells* **2021**, *10*, 2857. [CrossRef] [PubMed]
81. Sahatciu-Meka, V.; Rexhepi, S.; Manxhuka-Kerliu, S.; Rexhepi, M. Extra-articular manifestations of seronegative and seropositive rheumatoid arthritis. *Bosn. J. Basic Med. Sci.* **2010**, *10*, 26–31. [CrossRef]
82. Figus, F.A.; Piga, M.; Azzolin, I.; McConnell, R.; Iagnocco, A. Rheumatoid arthritis: Extra-articular manifestations and comorbidities. *Autoimmun. Rev.* **2021**, *20*, 102776. [CrossRef]
83. Ahlers, M.J.; Lowery, B.D.; Farber-Eger, E.; Wang, T.J.; Bradham, W.; Ormseth, M.J.; Chung, C.P.; Stein, C.M.; Gupta, D.K. Heart Failure Risk Associated with Rheumatoid Arthritis-Related Chronic Inflammation. *J. Am. Heart Assoc.* **2020**, *9*, e014661. [CrossRef] [PubMed]
84. Corrao, S.; Messina, S.; Pistone, G.; Calvo, L.; Scaglione, R.; Licata, G. Heart involvement in rheumatoid arthritis: Systematic review and meta-analysis. *Int. J. Cardiol.* **2013**, *167*, 2031–2038. [CrossRef] [PubMed]
85. Holmström, M.; Koivuniemi, R.; Korpi, K.; Kaasalainen, T.; Laine, M.; Kuuliala, A.; Leirisalo-Repo, M.; Kupari, M.; Kivistö, S. Cardiac magnetic resonance imaging reveals frequent myocardial involvement and dysfunction in active rheumatoid arthritis. *Clin. Exp. Rheumatol.* **2016**, *34*, 416–423. [PubMed]
86. Khalid, Y.; Dasu, N.; Shah, A.; Brown, K.; Kaell, A.; Levine, A.; Dasu, K.; Raminfard, A. Incidence of congestive heart failure in rheumatoid arthritis: A review of literature and meta-regression analysis. *ESC Heart Fail.* **2020**, *7*, 3745–3753. [CrossRef] [PubMed]
87. Mantini, C.; Maffei, E.; Toia, P.; Ricci, F.; Seitun, S.; Clemente, A.; Malagò, R.; Runza, G.; La Grutta, L.; Midiri, M.; et al. Influence of image reconstruction parameters on cardiovascular risk reclassification by Computed Tomography Coronary Artery Calcium Score. *Eur. J. Radiol.* **2018**, *101*, 1–7. [CrossRef] [PubMed]

88. Plein, S.; Erhayiem, B.; Fent, G.; Horton, S.; Dumitru, R.B.; Andrews, J.; Greenwood, J.P.; Emery, P.; Hensor, E.M.; Baxter, P.; et al. Cardiovascular effects of biological versus conventional synthetic disease-modifying antirheumatic drug therapy in treatment-naïve, early rheumatoid arthritis. *Ann. Rheum. Dis.* **2020**, *79*, 1414–1422. [CrossRef] [PubMed]
89. Federico, J.A.; Syväranta, S.A.; Tuohinen, S.S.; Holmström, M.M.; Peltomaa, R.L.; Koivuniemi, R.P.; Kestilä, M.H.; Kaasalainen, T.T.; Peltonen, J.I.; Leirisalo-Repo, M.T.K.; et al. Myocardial T1 mapping by cardiac magnetic resonance imaging shows early myocardial changes in treatment-naive patients with active rheumatoid arthritis and positive autoantibodies. *Clin. Exp. Rheumatol.* **2024**, *42*, 1368–1376. [CrossRef]
90. Liang, K.P.; Kremers, H.M.; Crowson, C.S.; Snyder, M.R.; Therneau, T.M.; Roger, V.L.; Gabriel, S.E. Autoantibodies and the risk of cardiovascular events. *J. Rheumatol.* **2009**, *36*, 2462–2469. [CrossRef] [PubMed]
91. Hanvivadhanakul, P.; Buakhamsri, A. Disease activity is associated with LV dysfunction in rheumatoid arthritis patients without clinical cardiovascular disease. *Adv. Rheumatol.* **2019**, *59*, 56. [CrossRef]
92. Løgstrup, B.B.; Deibjerg, L.K.; Hedemann-Andersen, A.; Ellingsen, T. Left ventricular function in treatment-naive early rheumatoid arthritis. *Am. J. Cardiovasc. Dis.* **2014**, *4*, 79–86. [CrossRef]
93. Çakmak, E.; Fındıkçıoğlu, U.; Tezcan, M.E. Disease severity affects myocardial functions in patients with treatment-naive early rheumatoid arthritis. *Int. J. Rheum. Dis.* **2021**, *24*, 494–501. [CrossRef]
94. Koduri, G.M.; Podlasek, A.; Pattapola, S.; Zhang, J.; Laila, D.; Nandagudi, A.; Dubey, S.; Kelly, C. Four-factor risk score for the prediction of interstitial lung disease in rheumatoid arthritis. *Rheumatol. Int.* **2023**, *43*, 1515–1523. [CrossRef] [PubMed]
95. Lingampalli, N.; Sokolove, J.; Lahey, L.J.; Edison, J.D.; Gilliland, W.R.; Holers, V.M.; Deane, K.D.; Robinson, W.H. Combination of anti-citrullinated protein antibodies and rheumatoid factor is associated with increased systemic inflammatory mediators and more rapid progression from preclinical to clinical rheumatoid arthritis. *Clin. Immunol.* **2018**, *195*, 119–126. [CrossRef]
96. Natalini, J.G.; Baker, J.F.; Singh, N.; Mahajan, T.D.; Roul, P.; Thiele, G.M.; Sauer, B.C.; Johnson, C.R.; Kawut, S.M.; Mikuls, T.R.; et al. Autoantibody Seropositivity and Risk for Interstitial Lung Disease in a Prospective Male-Predominant Rheumatoid Arthritis Cohort of U.S. Veterans. *Ann. Am. Thorac. Soc.* **2021**, *18*, 598–605. [CrossRef] [PubMed]
97. Xie, S.; Li, S.; Chen, B.; Zhu, Q.; Xu, L.; Li, F. Serum anti-citrullinated protein antibodies and rheumatoid factor increase the risk of rheumatoid arthritis-related interstitial lung disease: A meta-analysis. *Clin. Rheumatol.* **2021**, *40*, 4533–4543. [CrossRef] [PubMed]
98. Xue, J.; Hu, W.; Wu, S.; Wang, J.; Chi, S.; Liu, X. Development of a Risk Nomogram Model for Identifying Interstitial Lung Disease in Patients with Rheumatoid Arthritis. *Front. Immunol.* **2022**, *13*, 823669. [CrossRef]
99. Zhang, M.; Yin, J.; Zhang, X. Factors associated with interstitial lung disease in patients with rheumatoid arthritis: A systematic review and meta-analysis. *PLoS ONE* **2023**, *18*, e0286191. [CrossRef] [PubMed]
100. Ajeganova, S.; Humphreys, J.H.; Verheul, M.K.; van Steenbergen, H.W.; van Nies, J.A.; Hafström, I.; Svensson, B.; Huizinga, T.W.; Trouw, L.A.; Verstappen, S.M.; et al. Anticitrullinated protein antibodies and rheumatoid factor are associated with increased mortality but with different causes of death in patients with rheumatoid arthritis: A longitudinal study in three European cohorts. *Ann. Rheum. Dis.* **2016**, *75*, 1924–1932. [CrossRef] [PubMed]
101. Tyker, A.; Ventura, I.B.; Lee, C.T.; Strykowski, R.; Garcia, N.; Guzy, R.; Jablonski, R.; Vij, R.; Strek, M.E.; Chung, J.H.; et al. High-titer rheumatoid factor seropositivity predicts mediastinal lymphadenopathy and mortality in rheumatoid arthritis-related interstitial lung disease. *Sci. Rep.* **2021**, *11*, 22821. [CrossRef]
102. Fragoulis, G.E.; Nikiphorou, E.; Larsen, J.; Korsten, P.; Conway, R. Methotrexate-Associated Pneumonitis and Rheumatoid Arthritis-Interstitial Lung Disease: Current Concepts for the Diagnosis and Treatment. *Front. Med.* **2019**, *6*, 238. [CrossRef]
103. Baker, M.C.; Liu, Y.; Lu, R.; Lin, J.; Melehani, J.; Robinson, W.H. Incidence of Interstitial Lung Disease in Patients with Rheumatoid Arthritis Treated with Biologic and Targeted Synthetic Disease-Modifying Antirheumatic Drugs. *JAMA Network Open* **2023**, *6*, e233640. [CrossRef]
104. Bendstrup, E.; Møller, J.; Kronborg-White, S.; Prior, T.S.; Hyldgaard, C. Interstitial Lung Disease in Rheumatoid Arthritis Remains a Challenge for Clinicians. *J. Clin. Med.* **2019**, *8*, 2038. [CrossRef] [PubMed]
105. Kiely, P.; Busby, A.D.; Nikiphorou, E.; Sullivan, K.; Walsh, D.A.; Creamer, P.; Dixey, J.; Young, A. Is incident rheumatoid arthritis interstitial lung disease associated with methotrexate treatment? Results from a multivariate analysis in the ERAS and ERAN inception cohorts. *BMJ Open* **2019**, *9*, e028466. [CrossRef]
106. Fragoulis, G.E.; Conway, R.; Nikiphorou, E. Methotrexate and interstitial lung disease: Controversies and questions. A narrative review of the literature. *Rheumatology* **2019**, *58*, 1900–1906. [CrossRef] [PubMed]
107. Dawson, J.K.; Quah, E.; Earnshaw, B.; Amoasii, C.; Mudawi, T.; Spencer, L.G. Does methotrexate cause progressive fibrotic interstitial lung disease? A systematic review. *Rheumatol. Int.* **2021**, *41*, 1055–1064. [CrossRef]
108. Druce, K.L.; Iqbal, K.; Watson, K.D.; Symmons, D.P.M.; Hyrich, K.L.; Kelly, C. Mortality in patients with interstitial lung disease treated with rituximab or TNFi as a first biologic. *RMD Open* **2017**, *3*, e000473. [CrossRef] [PubMed]
109. Md Yusof, M.Y.; Kabia, A.; Darby, M.; Lettieri, G.; Beirne, P.; Vital, E.M.; Dass, S.; Emery, P. Effect of rituximab on the progression of rheumatoid arthritis-related interstitial lung disease: 10 years' experience at a single centre. *Rheumatology* **2017**, *56*, 1348–1357. [CrossRef] [PubMed]

110. Cassone, G.; Manfredi, A.; Atzeni, F.; Venerito, V.; Vacchi, C.; Picerno, V.; Furini, F.; Erre, G.L.; Tomietto, P.; Fedele, A.L.; et al. Safety of Abatacept in Italian Patients with Rheumatoid Arthritis and Interstitial Lung Disease: A Multicenter Retrospective Study. *J. Clin. Med.* **2020**, *9*, 277. [CrossRef] [PubMed]
111. Fernández-Díaz, C.; Loricera, J.; Castañeda, S.; López-Mejías, R.; Ojeda-García, C.; Olivé, A.; Rodríguez-Muguruza, S.; Carreira, P.E.; Pérez-Sandoval, T.; Retuerto, M.; et al. Abatacept in patients with rheumatoid arthritis and interstitial lung disease: A national multicenter study of 63 patients. *Semin. Arthritis Rheum.* **2018**, *48*, 22–27. [CrossRef] [PubMed]
112. Mena-Vázquez, N.; Godoy-Navarrete, F.J.; Manrique-Arija, S.; Aguilar-Hurtado, M.C.; Romero-Barco, C.M.; Ureña-Garnica, I.; Espildora, F.; Añón-Oñate, I.; Pérez-Albaladejo, L.; Gomez-Cano, C.; et al. Non-anti-TNF biologic agents are associated with slower worsening of interstitial lung disease secondary to rheumatoid arthritis. *Clin. Rheumatol.* **2021**, *40*, 133–142. [CrossRef]
113. Manfredi, A.; Cassone, G.; Furini, F.; Gremese, E.; Venerito, V.; Atzeni, F.; Arrigoni, E.; Della Casa, G.; Cerri, S.; Govoni, M.; et al. Tocilizumab therapy in rheumatoid arthritis with interstitial lung disease: A multicentre retrospective study. *Intern. Med. J.* **2020**, *50*, 1085–1090. [CrossRef] [PubMed]
114. Narváez, J.; Aguilar-Coll, M.; Roig-Kim, M.; Maymó-Paituvi, P.; Palacios-Olid, J.; Nolla, J.M.; D, L.L. Janus kinase inhibitors in rheumatoid arthritis-associated interstitial lung disease: A systematic review and meta-analysis. *Autoimmun. Rev.* **2024**, *23*, 103636. [CrossRef] [PubMed]
115. Rojas-Serrano, J.; González-Velásquez, E.; Mejía, M.; Sánchez-Rodríguez, A.; Carrillo, G. Interstitial lung disease related to rheumatoid arthritis: Evolution after treatment. *Reumatol. Clin.* **2012**, *8*, 68–71. [CrossRef] [PubMed]
116. Matteson, E.L.; Aringer, M.; Burmester, G.R.; Mueller, H.; Moros, L.; Kolb, M. Effect of nintedanib in patients with progressive pulmonary fibrosis associated with rheumatoid arthritis: Data from the INBUILD trial. *Clin. Rheumatol.* **2023**, *42*, 2311–2319. [CrossRef]
117. Turesson, C.; O'Fallon, W.M.; Crowson, C.S.; Gabriel, S.E.; Matteson, E.L. Occurrence of extraarticular disease manifestations is associated with excess mortality in a community based cohort of patients with rheumatoid arthritis. *J. Rheumatol.* **2002**, *29*, 62–67.
118. Makol, A.; Crowson, C.S.; Wetter, D.A.; Sokumbi, O.; Matteson, E.L.; Warrington, K.J. Vasculitis associated with rheumatoid arthritis: A case-control study. *Rheumatology* **2014**, *53*, 890–899. [CrossRef]
119. Turesson, C.; Matteson, E.L. Vasculitis in rheumatoid arthritis. *Curr. Opin. Rheumatol.* **2009**, *21*, 35–40. [CrossRef]
120. Turesson, C.; O'Fallon, W.M.; Crowson, C.S.; Gabriel, S.E.; Matteson, E.L. Extra-articular disease manifestations in rheumatoid arthritis: Incidence trends and risk factors over 46 years. *Ann. Rheum. Dis.* **2003**, *62*, 722–727. [CrossRef] [PubMed]
121. Voskuyl, A.E.; Zwinderman, A.H.; Westedt, M.L.; Vandenbroucke, J.P.; Breedveld, F.C.; Hazes, J.M. Factors associated with the development of vasculitis in rheumatoid arthritis: Results of a case-control study. *Ann. Rheum. Dis.* **1996**, *55*, 190–192. [CrossRef] [PubMed]
122. Vollertsen, R.S.; Conn, D.L.; Ballard, D.J.; Ilstrup, D.M.; Kazmar, R.E.; Silverfield, J.C. Rheumatoid vasculitis: Survival and associated risk factors. *Medicine (Baltimore)* **1986**, *65*, 365–375. [CrossRef]
123. Geirsson, A.J.; Sturfelt, G.; Truedsson, L. Clinical and serological features of severe vasculitis in rheumatoid arthritis: Prognostic implications. *Ann. Rheum. Dis.* **1987**, *46*, 727–733. [CrossRef] [PubMed]
124. Genta, M.S.; Genta, R.M.; Gabay, C. Systemic rheumatoid vasculitis: A review. *Semin. Arthritis Rheum.* **2006**, *36*, 88–98. [CrossRef] [PubMed]
125. Nagy, G.; Roodenrijs, N.M.T.; Welsing, P.M.; Kedves, M.; Hamar, A.; van der Goes, M.C.; Kent, A.; Bakkers, M.; Blaas, E.; Senolt, L.; et al. EULAR definition of difficult-to-treat rheumatoid arthritis. *Ann. Rheum. Dis.* **2021**, *80*, 31–35. [CrossRef]
126. Leon, L.; Madrid-Garcia, A.; Lopez-Viejo, P.; González-Álvaro, I.; Novella-Navarro, M.; Freites Nuñez, D.; Rosales, Z.; Fernandez-Gutierrez, B.; Abasolo, L. Difficult-to-treat rheumatoid arthritis (D2T RA): Clinical issues at early stages of disease. *RMD Open* **2023**, *9*, e002842. [CrossRef] [PubMed]
127. Roodenrijs, N.M.T.; van der Goes, M.C.; Welsing, P.M.J.; Tekstra, J.; Lafeber, F.; Jacobs, J.W.G.; van Laar, J.M. Difficult-to-treat rheumatoid arthritis: Contributing factors and burden of disease. *Rheumatology* **2021**, *60*, 3778–3788. [CrossRef]
128. Watanabe, R.; Ebina, K.; Gon, T.; Okano, T.; Murata, K.; Murakami, K.; Maeda, Y.; Jinno, S.; Shirasugi, I.; Son, Y.; et al. Predictive factors and treatment outcomes associated with difficult-to-treat rheumatoid arthritis conditions: The ANSWER cohort study. *Rheumatology* **2024**, *63*, 2418–2426. [CrossRef] [PubMed]
129. Watanabe, R.; Hashimoto, M.; Murata, K.; Murakami, K.; Tanaka, M.; Ohmura, K.; Ito, H.; Matsuda, S. Prevalence and predictive factors of difficult-to-treat rheumatoid arthritis: The KURAMA cohort. *Immunol. Med.* **2022**, *45*, 35–44. [CrossRef]
130. Watanabe, R.; Okano, T.; Gon, T.; Yoshida, N.; Fukumoto, K.; Yamada, S.; Hashimoto, M. Difficult-to-treat rheumatoid arthritis: Current concept and unsolved problems. *Front. Med.* **2022**, *9*, 1049875. [CrossRef] [PubMed]
131. Hofman, Z.L.M.; Roodenrijs, N.M.T.; Nikiphorou, E.; Kent, A.L.; Nagy, G.; Welsing, P.M.J.; van Laar, J.M. Difficult-to-treat rheumatoid arthritis: What have we learned and what do we still need to learn? *Rheumatology* **2025**, *64*, 65–73. [CrossRef] [PubMed]

132. Cooles, F.A.H.; Tarn, J.; Lendrem, D.W.; Naamane, N.; Lin, C.M.; Millar, B.; Maney, N.J.; Anderson, A.E.; Thalayasingam, N.; Diboll, J.; et al. Interferon-α-mediated therapeutic resistance in early rheumatoid arthritis implicates epigenetic reprogramming. *Ann. Rheum. Dis.* **2022**, *81*, 1214–1223. [CrossRef] [PubMed]
133. Iwasaki, T.; Watanabe, R.; Ito, H.; Fujii, T.; Okuma, K.; Oku, T.; Hirayama, Y.; Ohmura, K.; Murata, K.; Murakami, K.; et al. Dynamics of Type I and Type II Interferon Signature Determines Responsiveness to Anti-TNF Therapy in Rheumatoid Arthritis. *Front. Immunol.* **2022**, *13*, 901437. [CrossRef] [PubMed]
134. Arnett, F.C.; Edworthy, S.M.; Bloch, D.A.; McShane, D.J.; Fries, J.F.; Cooper, N.S.; Healey, L.A.; Kaplan, S.R.; Liang, M.H.; Luthra, H.S.; et al. The American Rheumatism Association 1987 revised criteria for the classification of rheumatoid arthritis. *Arthritis Rheum.* **1988**, *31*, 315–324. [CrossRef]
135. Chatzidionysiou, K.; Lie, E.; Nasonov, E.; Lukina, G.; Hetland, M.L.; Tarp, U.; Gabay, C.; van Riel, P.L.; Nordström, D.C.; Gomez-Reino, J.; et al. Highest clinical effectiveness of rituximab in autoantibody-positive patients with rheumatoid arthritis and in those for whom no more than one previous TNF antagonist has failed: Pooled data from 10 European registries. *Ann. Rheum. Dis.* **2011**, *70*, 1575–1580. [CrossRef]
136. Potter, C.; Hyrich, K.L.; Tracey, A.; Lunt, M.; Plant, D.; Symmons, D.P.; Thomson, W.; Worthington, J.; Emery, P.; Morgan, A.W.; et al. Association of rheumatoid factor and anti-cyclic citrullinated peptide positivity, but not carriage of shared epitope or PTPN22 susceptibility variants, with anti-tumour necrosis factor response in rheumatoid arthritis. *Ann. Rheum. Dis.* **2009**, *68*, 69–74. [CrossRef] [PubMed]
137. De Rycke, L.; Verhelst, X.; Kruithof, E.; Van den Bosch, F.; Hoffman, I.E.; Veys, E.M.; De Keyser, F. Rheumatoid factor, but not anti-cyclic citrullinated peptide antibodies, is modulated by infliximab treatment in rheumatoid arthritis. *Ann. Rheum. Dis.* **2005**, *64*, 299–302. [CrossRef] [PubMed]
138. Blaschke, S.; Rinke, K.; Maring, M.; Flad, T.; Patschan, S.; Jahn, O.; Mueller, C.A.; Mueller, G.A.; Dihazi, H. Haptoglobin-α1, -α2, vitamin D-binding protein and apolipoprotein C-III as predictors of etanercept drug response in rheumatoid arthritis. *Arthritis Res. Ther.* **2015**, *17*, 45. [CrossRef] [PubMed]
139. Bobbio-Pallavicini, F.; Caporali, R.; Alpini, C.; Avalle, S.; Epis, O.M.; Klersy, C.; Montecucco, C. High IgA rheumatoid factor levels are associated with poor clinical response to tumour necrosis factor alpha inhibitors in rheumatoid arthritis. *Ann. Rheum. Dis.* **2007**, *66*, 302–307. [CrossRef] [PubMed]
140. Sebastiani, M.; Manfredi, A.; Iannone, F.; Gremese, E.; Bortoluzzi, A.; Favalli, E.; Bazzani, C.; Salaffi, F.; Fusaro, E.; Foti, R.; et al. Factors Predicting Early Failure of Etanercept in Rheumatoid Arthritis: An Analysis from the Gruppo Italiano di Studio sulla Early Arthritis (Italian Group for the Study of Early Arthritis) Registry. *Arch. Rheumatol.* **2020**, *35*, 163–169. [CrossRef] [PubMed]
141. Zhao, Z.; Hua, Z.; Luo, X.; Li, Y.; Yu, L.; Li, M.; Lu, C.; Zhao, T.; Liu, Y. Application and pharmacological mechanism of methotrexate in rheumatoid arthritis. *Biomed. Pharmacother.* **2022**, *150*, 113074. [CrossRef] [PubMed]
142. Hider, S.L.; Silman, A.J.; Thomson, W.; Lunt, M.; Bunn, D.; Symmons, D.P. Can clinical factors at presentation be used to predict outcome of treatment with methotrexate in patients with early inflammatory polyarthritis? *Ann. Rheum. Dis.* **2009**, *68*, 57–62. [CrossRef] [PubMed]
143. Saevarsdottir, S.; Wallin, H.; Seddighzadeh, M.; Ernestam, S.; Geborek, P.; Petersson, I.F.; Bratt, J.; van Vollenhoven, R.F. Predictors of response to methotrexate in early DMARD naive rheumatoid arthritis: Results from the initial open-label phase of the SWEFOT trial. *Ann. Rheum. Dis.* **2011**, *70*, 469–475. [CrossRef] [PubMed]
144. Dekkers, J.S.; Bergstra, S.A.; Chopra, A.; Tikly, M.; Fonseca, J.E.; Salomon-Escoto, K.; Huizinga, T.W.J.; van der Woude, D. Autoantibody status is not associated with early treatment response to first-line methotrexate in patients with early rheumatoid arthritis. *Rheumatology* **2019**, *58*, 149–153. [CrossRef]
145. Bluett, J.; Sergeant, J.C.; MacGregor, A.J.; Chipping, J.R.; Marshall, T.; Symmons, D.P.M.; Verstappen, S.M.M. Risk factors for oral methotrexate failure in patients with inflammatory polyarthritis: Results from a UK prospective cohort study. *Arthritis Res. Ther.* **2018**, *20*, 50. [CrossRef]
146. Plant, D.; Maciejewski, M.; Smith, S.; Nair, N.; Hyrich, K.; Ziemek, D.; Barton, A.; Verstappen, S. Profiling of Gene Expression Biomarkers as a Classifier of Methotrexate Nonresponse in Patients with Rheumatoid Arthritis. *Arthritis Rheumatol.* **2019**, *71*, 678–684. [CrossRef] [PubMed]
147. van der Pouw Kraan, T.C.; Wijbrandts, C.A.; van Baarsen, L.G.; Voskuyl, A.E.; Rustenburg, F.; Baggen, J.M.; Ibrahim, S.M.; Fero, M.; Dijkmans, B.A.; Tak, P.P.; et al. Rheumatoid arthritis subtypes identified by genomic profiling of peripheral blood cells: Assignment of a type I interferon signature in a subpopulation of patients. *Ann. Rheum. Dis.* **2007**, *66*, 1008–1014. [CrossRef] [PubMed]
148. Emery, P.; Breedveld, F.C.; Lemmel, E.M.; Kaltwasser, J.P.; Dawes, P.T.; Gömör, B.; Van Den Bosch, F.; Nordström, D.; Bjorneboe, O.; Dahl, R.; et al. A comparison of the efficacy and safety of leflunomide and methotrexate for the treatment of rheumatoid arthritis. *Rheumatology* **2000**, *39*, 655–665. [CrossRef] [PubMed]
149. Lie, E.; Uhlig, T.; van der Heijde, D.; Rødevand, E.; Kalstad, S.; Kaufmann, C.; Mikkelsen, K.; Kvien, T.K. Effectiveness of sulfasalazine and methotrexate in 1102 DMARD-naive patients with early RA. *Rheumatology* **2012**, *51*, 670–678. [CrossRef]

150. Hazlewood, G.S.; Barnabe, C.; Tomlinson, G.; Marshall, D.; Devoe, D.; Bombardier, C. Methotrexate monotherapy and methotrexate combination therapy with traditional and biologic disease modifying antirheumatic drugs for rheumatoid arthritis: Abridged Cochrane systematic review and network meta-analysis. *BMJ* **2016**, *353*, i1777. [CrossRef] [PubMed]
151. McInnes, I.B.; Buckley, C.D.; Isaacs, J.D. Cytokines in rheumatoid arthritis—Shaping the immunological landscape. *Nat. Rev. Rheumatol.* **2016**, *12*, 63–68. [CrossRef] [PubMed]
152. Kievit, W.; Fransen, J.; Adang, E.M.; den Broeder, A.A.; Bernelot Moens, H.J.; Visser, H.; van de Laar, M.A.; van Riel, P.L. Long-term effectiveness and safety of TNF-blocking agents in daily clinical practice: Results from the Dutch Rheumatoid Arthritis Monitoring register. *Rheumatology* **2011**, *50*, 196–203. [CrossRef] [PubMed]
153. Ochi, S.; Saito, K.; Mizoguchi, F.; Kato, S.; Tanaka, Y. Insensitivity versus poor response to tumour necrosis factor inhibitors in rheumatoid arthritis: A retrospective cohort study. *Arthritis Res. Ther.* **2020**, *22*, 41. [CrossRef] [PubMed]
154. Mancarella, L.; Bobbio-Pallavicini, F.; Ceccarelli, F.; Falappone, P.C.; Ferrante, A.; Malesci, D.; Massara, A.; Nacci, F.; Secchi, M.E.; Manganelli, S.; et al. Good clinical response, remission, and predictors of remission in rheumatoid arthritis patients treated with tumor necrosis factor-alpha blockers: The GISEA study. *J. Rheumatol.* **2007**, *34*, 1670–1673. [PubMed]
155. Santos-Moreno, P.; Sánchez, G.; Castro, C. Rheumatoid factor as predictor of response to treatment with anti-TNF alpha drugs in patients with rheumatoid arthritis: Results of a cohort study. *Medicine* **2019**, *98*, e14181. [CrossRef]
156. Hambardzumyan, K.; Hermanrud, C.; Marits, P.; Vivar, N.; Ernestam, S.; Wallman, J.K.; van Vollenhoven, R.F.; Fogdell-Hahn, A.; Saevarsdottir, S. Association of female sex and positive rheumatoid factor with low serum infliximab and anti-drug antibodies, related to treatment failure in early rheumatoid arthritis: Results from the SWEFOT trial population. *Scand. J. Rheumatol.* **2019**, *48*, 362–366. [CrossRef]
157. Nakayama, Y.; Watanabe, R.; Murakami, K.; Murata, K.; Tanaka, M.; Ito, H.; Yamamoto, W.; Ebina, K.; Hata, K.; Hiramatsu, Y.; et al. Differential efficacy of TNF inhibitors with or without the immunoglobulin fragment crystallizable (Fc) portion in rheumatoid arthritis: The ANSWER cohort study. *Rheumatol. Int.* **2022**, *42*, 1227–1234. [CrossRef] [PubMed]
158. Tanaka, Y.; Takeuchi, T.; Haaland, D.; Hall, S.; Inanc, N.; Li, Z.; Xavier, R.M.; Cara, C.; Tilt, N.; Taylor, P.C. Efficacy of certolizumab pegol across baseline rheumatoid factor subgroups in patients with rheumatoid arthritis: Post-hoc analysis of clinical trials. *Int. J. Rheum. Dis.* **2023**, *26*, 1248–1259. [CrossRef]
159. Martínez-Feito, A.; Plasencia-Rodríguez, C.; Novella-Navarro, M.; Gehin, J.E.; Hernández-Breijo, B.; Brenis, C.M.; Villalba-Yllán, A.; Fernández, E.; Monjo-Henry, I.; Pascual-Salcedo, D.; et al. Influence of rheumatoid factor on serum drug levels of TNF inhibitors with different structures in rheumatoid arthritis. *Clin. Exp. Rheumatol.* **2024**, *42*, 999–1005. [CrossRef]
160. López-Medina, C.; Calvo-Gutiérrez, J.; Ábalos-Aguilera, M.C.; Cepas, F.; Plasencia-Rodríguez, C.; Martínez-Feito, A.; Balsa, A.; Faré-García, R.; Juan-Mas, A.; Ruiz-Esquide, V.; et al. Exploring the influence of baseline rheumatoid factor levels on TNF inhibitor retention rate in patients with rheumatoid arthritis: A multicentre and retrospective study. *RMD Open* **2024**, *10*, e003975. [CrossRef] [PubMed]
161. van Delft, M.A.M.; Huizinga, T.W.J. An overview of autoantibodies in rheumatoid arthritis. *J. Autoimmun.* **2020**, *110*, 102392. [CrossRef] [PubMed]
162. Takai, T. Roles of Fc receptors in autoimmunity. *Nat. Rev. Immunol.* **2002**, *2*, 580–592. [CrossRef] [PubMed]
163. Junker, F.; Gordon, J.; Qureshi, O. Fc Gamma Receptors and Their Role in Antigen Uptake, Presentation, and T Cell Activation. *Front. Immunol.* **2020**, *11*, 1393. [CrossRef] [PubMed]
164. Mease, P.J. Certolizumab pegol in the treatment of rheumatoid arthritis: A comprehensive review of its clinical efficacy and safety. *Rheumatology* **2011**, *50*, 261–270. [CrossRef] [PubMed]
165. Ward, E.S.; Ober, R.J. Targeting FcRn to Generate Antibody-Based Therapeutics. *Trends Pharmacol. Sci.* **2018**, *39*, 892–904. [CrossRef]
166. Roopenian, D.C.; Akilesh, S. FcRn: The neonatal Fc receptor comes of age. *Nat. Rev. Immunol.* **2007**, *7*, 715–725. [CrossRef] [PubMed]
167. Oyama, S.; Ebina, K.; Etani, Y.; Hirao, M.; Kyuuma, M.; Fujii, Y.; Iwata, K.; Ogawa, B.; Hasegawa, T.; Kawano, S.; et al. A novel anti-TNF-α drug ozoralizumab rapidly distributes to inflamed joint tissues in a mouse model of collagen induced arthritis. *Sci. Rep.* **2022**, *12*, 18102. [CrossRef]
168. Takeuchi, T.; Kawanishi, M.; Nakanishi, M.; Yamasaki, H.; Tanaka, Y. Phase II/III Results of a Trial of Anti-Tumor Necrosis Factor Multivalent NANOBODY Compound Ozoralizumab in Patients with Rheumatoid Arthritis. *Arthritis Rheumatol.* **2022**, *74*, 1776–1785. [CrossRef] [PubMed]
169. Taylor, P.C.; Matucci Cerinic, M.; Alten, R.; Avouac, J.; Westhovens, R. Managing inadequate response to initial anti-TNF therapy in rheumatoid arthritis: Optimising treatment outcomes. *Ther. Adv. Musculoskelet. Dis.* **2022**, *14*, 1759720X221114101. [CrossRef]
170. Rubbert-Roth, A.; Szabó, M.Z.; Kedves, M.; Nagy, G.; Atzeni, F.; Sarzi-Puttini, P. Failure of anti-TNF treatment in patients with rheumatoid arthritis: The pros and cons of the early use of alternative biological agents. *Autoimmun. Rev.* **2019**, *18*, 102398. [CrossRef]

171. Shams, S.; Martinez, J.M.; Dawson, J.R.D.; Flores, J.; Gabriel, M.; Garcia, G.; Guevara, A.; Murray, K.; Pacifici, N.; Vargas, M.V.; et al. The Therapeutic Landscape of Rheumatoid Arthritis: Current State and Future Directions. *Front. Pharmacol.* **2021**, *12*, 680043. [CrossRef]
172. Mohamed Ahamada, M.; Wu, X. Analysis of efficacy and safety of abatacept for rheumatoid arthritis: Systematic review and meta-analysis. *Clin. Exp. Rheumatol.* **2023**, *41*, 1882–1900. [CrossRef] [PubMed]
173. Wang, M.; Chen, L.; He, J.; Xia, W.; Ye, Z.; She, J. Structural insights into IL-6 signaling inhibition by therapeutic antibodies. *Cell Rep.* **2024**, *43*, 113819. [CrossRef]
174. Tavakolpour, S.; Alesaeidi, S.; Darvishi, M.; GhasemiAdl, M.; Darabi-Monadi, S.; Akhlaghdoust, M.; Elikaei Behjati, S.; Jafarieh, A. A comprehensive review of rituximab therapy in rheumatoid arthritis patients. *Clin. Rheumatol.* **2019**, *38*, 2977–2994. [CrossRef]
175. Miyazaki, Y.; Nakano, K.; Nakayamada, S.; Kubo, S.; Iwata, S.; Hanami, K.; Fukuyo, S.; Miyagawa, I.; Yamaguchi, A.; Kawabe, A.; et al. Serum TNFα levels at 24 h after certolizumab pegol predict effectiveness at week 12 in patients with rheumatoid arthritis from TSUBAME study. *Arthritis Res. Ther.* **2021**, *23*, 154. [CrossRef] [PubMed]
176. Maneiro, R.J.; Salgado, E.; Carmona, L.; Gomez-Reino, J.J. Rheumatoid factor as predictor of response to abatacept, rituximab and tocilizumab in rheumatoid arthritis: Systematic review and meta-analysis. *Semin. Arthritis Rheum.* **2013**, *43*, 9–17. [CrossRef] [PubMed]
177. Kawashiri, S.Y.; Kawakami, A.; Iwamoto, N.; Fujikawa, K.; Aramaki, T.; Tamai, M.; Yamasaki, S.; Nakamura, H.; Origuchi, T.; Ueki, Y.; et al. In rheumatoid arthritis patients treated with tocilizumab, the rate of clinical disease activity index (CDAI) remission at 24 weeks is superior in those with higher titers of IgM-rheumatoid factor at baseline. *Mod. Rheumatol.* **2011**, *21*, 370–374. [CrossRef]
178. Burmester, G.R.; Feist, E.; Kellner, H.; Braun, J.; Iking-Konert, C.; Rubbert-Roth, A. Effectiveness and safety of the interleukin 6-receptor antagonist tocilizumab after 4 and 24 weeks in patients with active rheumatoid arthritis: The first phase IIIb real-life study (TAMARA). *Ann. Rheum. Dis.* **2011**, *70*, 755–759. [CrossRef]
179. Emery, P.; van Hoogstraten, H.; Mangan, E.K.; van Adelsberg, J.; Fan, C.; Kivitz, A.; Pinheiro, G.d.R.C.; Huizinga, T.W. 229. Clinical responses of sarilumab based on rheumatoid factor and anti-cyclic citrullinated peptide antibody status in patients with rheumatoid arthritis. *Rheumatology* **2017**, *56*, kex062.230. [CrossRef]
180. Gottenberg, J.E.; Ravaud, P.; Cantagrel, A.; Combe, B.; Flipo, R.M.; Schaeverbeke, T.; Houvenagel, E.; Gaudin, P.; Loeuille, D.; Rist, S.; et al. Positivity for anti-cyclic citrullinated peptide is associated with a better response to abatacept: Data from the 'Orencia and Rheumatoid Arthritis' registry. *Ann. Rheum. Dis.* **2012**, *71*, 1815–1819. [CrossRef] [PubMed]
181. Gottenberg, J.E.; Courvoisier, D.S.; Hernandez, M.V.; Iannone, F.; Lie, E.; Canhão, H.; Pavelka, K.; Hetland, M.L.; Turesson, C.; Mariette, X.; et al. Brief Report: Association of Rheumatoid Factor and Anti-Citrullinated Protein Antibody Positivity with Better Effectiveness of Abatacept: Results from the Pan-European Registry Analysis. *Arthritis Rheumatol.* **2016**, *68*, 1346–1352. [CrossRef] [PubMed]
182. Alten, R.; Mariette, X.; Lorenz, H.M.; Nüßlein, H.; Galeazzi, M.; Navarro, F.; Chartier, M.; Heitzmann, J.; Poncet, C.; Rauch, C.; et al. Predictors of abatacept retention over 2 years in patients with rheumatoid arthritis: Results from the real-world ACTION study. *Clin. Rheumatol.* **2019**, *38*, 1413–1424. [CrossRef] [PubMed]
183. Bozec, A.; Luo, Y.; Engdahl, C.; Figueiredo, C.; Bang, H.; Schett, G. Abatacept blocks anti-citrullinated protein antibody and rheumatoid factor mediated cytokine production in human macrophages in IDO-dependent manner. *Arthritis Res. Ther.* **2018**, *20*, 24. [CrossRef]
184. Lend, K.; Lampa, J.; Padyukov, L.; Hetland, M.L.; Heiberg, M.S.; Nordström, D.C.; Nurmohamed, M.T.; Rudin, A.; Østergaard, M.; Haavardsholm, E.A.; et al. Association of rheumatoid factor, anti-citrullinated protein antibodies and shared epitope with clinical response to initial treatment in patients with early rheumatoid arthritis: Data from a randomised controlled trial. *Ann. Rheum. Dis.* **2024**, *83*, 1657–1665. [CrossRef] [PubMed]
185. Okazaki, S.; Watanabe, R.; Harigae, H.; Fujii, H. Better Retention of Abatacept Is Associated with High Rheumatoid Factor: A Five-Year Follow-Up Study of Patients with Rheumatoid Arthritis. *Tohoku J. Exp. Med.* **2020**, *250*, 153–159. [CrossRef] [PubMed]
186. Martinez-Molina, C.; Gich, I.; Diaz-Torné, C.; Park, H.S.; Feliu, A.; Vidal, S.; Corominas, H. Patient-related factors influencing the effectiveness and safety of Janus Kinase inhibitors in rheumatoid arthritis: A real-world study. *Sci. Rep.* **2024**, *14*, 172. [CrossRef]
187. Bird, P.; Hall, S.; Nash, P.; Connell, C.A.; Kwok, K.; Witcombe, D.; Thirunavukkarasu, K. Treatment outcomes in patients with seropositive versus seronegative rheumatoid arthritis in Phase III randomised clinical trials of tofacitinib. *RMD Open* **2019**, *5*, e000742. [CrossRef] [PubMed]
188. Pope, J.E.; Keystone, E.; Jamal, S.; Wang, L.; Fallon, L.; Woolcott, J.; Lazariciu, I.; Chapman, D.; Haraoui, B. Persistence of Tofacitinib in the Treatment of Rheumatoid Arthritis in Open-Label, Long-Term Extension Studies up to 9.5 Years. *ACR Open Rheumatol.* **2019**, *1*, 73–82. [CrossRef]

Journal of
Clinical Medicine

MDPI

Review

Immunosuppressants/Immunomodulators and Malignancy

Norishige Iizuka [1], Yoshihiko Hoshida [2,*], Atsuko Tsujii Miyamoto [3,4], Hotaka Shigyo [4], Akira Nishigaichi [4], Gensuke Okamura [5] and Shiro Ohshima [4]

1 Department of Pathology, Kishiwada City Hospital, Kishiwada 596-8501, Osaka, Japan; iizuka.n@gmail.com
2 Department of Pathology, NHO Osaka Minami Medical Center, Kawachinagano 586-8521, Osaka, Japan
3 Department of Respiratory Medicine and Clinical Immunology, Graduate School of Medicine, The University of Osaka, Suita 565-0871, Osaka, Japan; a.tsujii@imed3.med.osaka-u.ac.jp
4 Department of Rheumatology and Allergology, NHO Osaka Minami Medical Center, Kawachinagano 586-8521, Osaka, Japan; hokaka306@gmail.com (H.S.); nishigaichi.akira.za@mail.hosp.go.jp (A.N.); ohshima.shiro.tr@mail.hosp.go.jp (S.O.)
5 Department of Orthopedics, NHO Osaka Minami Medical Center, Kawachinagano 586-8521, Osaka, Japan; gensuke.okamura@gmail.com
* Correspondence: hoshida65317@gmail.com; Tel.: +81-721-53-5761; Fax: +81-721-53-8904

Abstract: Individuals with immunosuppressive conditions are at a higher risk of developing malignancies than those in the general population. Immunosuppression weakens tumor immunity, hinders the detection of pro-oncogenic cells, and activates oncogenic viruses. Malignancies arising in immunosuppressed patients tend to be aggressive, have a high incidence of virus-associated cancers, and are reversible in some cases. Notably, immunosuppressive agents influence the frequency and type of malignancies, as well as their clinicopathological features. Organ transplant recipients receive long-term immunosuppressants to prevent acute rejection. Post-transplant malignancies vary depending on the type of drug administered before the onset of these diseases. Patients with rheumatoid arthritis (RA) are treated with long-term immunosuppressive medications, such as methotrexate (MTX). MTX is widely recognized as being associated with a specific type of lymphoproliferative disorder (LPD), known as MTX-associated LPD. Our recent report indicated that the clinicopathological features of rheumatoid arthritis-associated lymphoproliferative disorder (RA-LPD) also vary based on the other anti-RA agents used, such as tacrolimus and tumor necrosis factor inhibitors. Therefore, the clinicopathological characteristics of post-transplant LPD and RA-LPD evolve alongside the changes in the immunosuppressants/immunomodulators administered. Understanding the various characteristics and time trends of immunosuppressive neoplasms, particularly LPDs, in relation to different immunosuppressant/immunomodulator medications is highly valuable in clinical practice.

Keywords: post-transplant malignancy; post-transplant lymphoproliferative disorders; rheumatoid arthritis-associated lymphoproliferative disorders; rheumatoid arthritis-associated malignancy; methotrexate; immunosuppressive agents; anti-rheumatic agents

1. Introduction

Malignant neoplasms in patients with immunosuppressive conditions exhibit distinct characteristics compared to those in immunocompetent individuals [1–4]. This difference arises from the restoration of tumor immunity in the host following the reestablishment of defenses against tumors and oncogenic viral antigens [5]. A noteworthy aspect is the reversible nature of immunosuppressive neoplasms; spontaneous regression can occur after the administration, reduction, and alteration of the immunosuppressive agent [6]. This phenomenon has been observed in patients with various cancer types, including skin cancer, malignant melanoma (MM), Kaposi's sarcoma (KS), lymphoproliferative disorder (LPD), hepatocellular carcinoma, and Merkel cell carcinoma [7–11].

The frequency and clinicopathological features of immunosuppressive neoplasms vary according to the specific immunosuppressive state [1–4]. Immunosuppressive conditions are categorized into inborn errors of immunity (congenital) and acquired forms; the latter is further divided into groups, including patients with acquired immunodeficiency syndrome (AIDS) and iatrogenic cases. The iatrogenic group includes solid organ transplant recipients and individuals with autoimmune diseases such as rheumatoid arthritis (RA), who are treated long-term with immunosuppressive agents [4,12]. Immunosuppressive agents have also enhanced the efficacy of organ transplantation over the years [13]. The introduction of powerful immunosuppressive agents may be associated with reduced survival rates as a result of the increased frequency and progression of malignant neoplasms [14–16]. Notably, the choice and dosage of immunosuppressive agent may influence the incidence and type of malignancy observed [1,2,4,17–19].

For patients with RA, the development of neoplasia, especially LPD, is associated not only with the immunosuppressive conditions induced by the anti-RA agents but also with the immune dysregulation inherent in RA itself [20]. For over half a century, patients with RA have been recognized as vulnerable to LPDs because of their hyperimmune state [21,22]. Epidemiological studies have indicated that the incidence of LPDs is two to four times higher in patients with RA before the introduction of methotrexate (MTX) as an immunosuppressive agent [23,24]. Baecklund et al. observed a correlation between LPD incidence and RA disease activity, emphasizing that diffuse large B-cell lymphoma (DLBCL) is more likely to develop in patients with RA [25,26]. Consequently, RA-LPDs, which arise from the immune dysregulation associated with RA, may be classified as disease-associated LPDs. Meanwhile, LPDs in RA patients receiving MTX have garnered significant attention since Elliman's report in 1991 [27]. The 2001 World Health Organization (WHO) classification highlighted the immunosuppressive effects of MTX and was the first to define the terminology for MTX-associated LPD (MTX-LPD) [28]. In this context, RA-associated LPD (RA-LPD), linked to the immunosuppressive state caused by RA therapy, especially MTX, should be recognized as a therapy-related LPD. Thus, RA-LPD encompasses both disease- and therapy-related LPDs.

Over the past 30 years, significant advancements in the understanding of RA pathogenesis have ushered in a new era of treatment [29–32]. Previously, RA management primarily involved the use of prednisolone (PSL) and non-steroidal anti-inflammatory drugs (NSAIDs). The emergence of conventional synthetic disease-modifying anti-rheumatic drugs (csDMARDs) in the 1990s, such as salazosulfapyridine (SASP), led to the introduction of MTX and tacrolimus (TAC) as immunosuppressive agents [33]. MTX at a low dose causes immunosuppression by disrupting pyrimidine and purine synthesis and increasing adenosine levels, while TAC causes immunosuppression by blocking calcineurin. This was followed by a series of biologic DMARDs (bDMARDs), including anti-tumor necrosis factor (TNF)-α biologics such as infliximab (IFX), etanercept (ETN), adalimumab (ADA), golimumab (GLM), and certolizumab (CZP), and non-anti-TNF-α biologics, including tocilizumab (TCZ), which targets the interleukin (IL)-6 receptor, and abatacept (ABT), which uses CTLA4-Ig. Subsequently, targeted synthetic DMARDs (tsDMARDs) based on Janus kinase (JAK) inhibitors (JAKi), such as tofacitinib (TOF), upadacitinib (UPA), and baricitinib (BAR) were developed [29–32].

Recently, our group reported that the clinicopathological characteristics of RA-LPD vary based on the type and frequency of the anti-RA agent used, and that these characteristics change over time, resembling the effects of post-transplant malignancies [34]. This article mainly describes the malignancies that develop under immunosuppressive and immune dysregulated conditions, highlighting how the immunosuppressants/immunomodulators affect the post-transplantation-LPD (PT-LPD) and RA-LPD.

2. Immunosuppressive Agents and Organ Transplantation

2.1. Post-Solid Organ Transplantation Malignancy and Immunosuppressive Agents (Figure 1)

Patients who receive solid organ transplants develop malignant tumors at a rate that is two to four times higher than in the general population [1,5,17]. Malignant neoplasms in transplant recipients tend to display a more aggressive clinical course, with a rising prevalence of infection-related cancers such as human papillomavirus (HPV)-associated skin cancer and Epstein–Barr virus (EBV)-related lymphoma than in the general population.

According to a cohort report of 175,732 transplants in the United States from 1987 to 2008, the standard incidence ratios (SIRs) for developing malignancies in transplant recipients were significantly elevated for most infection-related malignancies compared to the general population, including non-Hodgkin lymphoma (NHL) (SIR: 7.54), Kaposi sarcoma (SIR: 61.46), and cancers of the liver (SIR: 11.56), anus (SIR: 5.84), and vulva (SIR: 7.60). Among infection-unrelated malignancies, SIRs were significantly elevated for lung (SIR: 1.97), kidney (SIR: 4.65), skin (non-melanoma, non-epithelial) (SIR: 13.85), lip (SIR: 16.78), and intrahepatic bile duct cancers (SIR: 5.76). In contrast, the risk of breast cancer (SIR: 0.85) and, to a lesser extent, prostate cancer (SIR: 0.92) decreased [1].

The type of cancer varies based on the transplanted organ and the immunosuppressive agents used [1,2,4,17–19].

Immunosuppressive therapy is vital for preventing organ transplantation rejection. Historically, immunosuppressive agents have been improved to decrease rejection rates and enhance the retention of the transplanted organs. In the 1960s, the use of maintenance immunosuppressive agents in organ transplantation began with azathioprine (AZ). In the 1980s, calcineurin inhibitors (CNI) such as cyclosporine A (CyA) and TAC were introduced, followed by mycophenolate mofetil (MPA) and mycophenolate (MMF). In the 2000s, everolimus (EVL) and sirolimus (SRL) emerged as a mammalian target of rapamycin (mTOR) inhibitors [35]. Considering these factors, the history of post-transplant malignancies can be classified into three eras based on the type of immunosuppressant used for the maintenance therapy [36]; these are outlined below.

2.1.1. Azathioprine (AZ) Era

Since AZ was approved by the Food and Drug Administration (FDA) in 1963, the AZ era began in the 1960s and lasted until the 1970s. AZ is widely used as a maintenance immunosuppressant in transplantation medicine. It suppresses the immune system by inhibiting purine, DNA and RNA synthesis, and T-cell proliferation [36]. Additionally, AZ has been reported to be carcinogenic in cases where the DNA in the epidermal cells is mutated due to ultraviolet exposure, as it directly inhibits the DNA repair mechanisms [37,38].

An epidemiological study of the AZ era reported on 693 cases of malignant tumors in the Denver Transplant Tumor Registry (DTTR) prior to August 1978, before the introduction of CyA. The most common types of malignant tumor were skin and lip cancer (40.0%), followed by LPD (19.2%), cervical cancer (7.1%), lung cancer (5.2%), colorectal cancer (3.0%), and KS (2.9%) [39]. A 2016 meta-analysis also showed that transplant patients who received AZ had a higher incidence of squamous cell carcinoma of the skin than those who did not (odds ratio (OR) = 1.56; 95% confidence interval (CI): 1.11–2.18) [40].

2.1.2. Calcineurin Inhibitor (CNI) Era

The 1980s and the 1990s were the era of CNIs. In 1983, CyA was approved by the FDA for immunosuppression in transplantation, and TAC was approved in 1994. These medications are now widely used in transplantation. CyA binds to cyclophilin A, whereas TAC binds to the intracellular protein FKBP12. In both of these CNIs, their binding forms a complex consisting of Ca^{2+}, calmodulin, and calcineurin, which inhibits the phosphatase activity of calcineurin. This inhibition prevents the dephosphorylation and nuclear translocation of NFATs, thereby inhibiting the production of IL-2. As a result, CNIs inhibit T- cell activation and proliferation, contributing to immunosuppression [35,36].

CNIs also act as carcinogens by increasing transforming growth factor (TGF)-β1 [41,42], a potent inhibitor of IL-2-stimulated T-cell proliferation, and by stimulating the tumor angiogenesis factor vascular endothelial growth factor (VEGF) [41]. Additionally, the elevated IL-6 levels in EBV-infected B-cells promote the activation, proliferation, and possibly the immortalization of these cells [43,44].

The frequency of malignant tumors was higher in the CyA group than in the AZ group [18]. Penn reported that, among 773 CyA monotherapy regimen transplants in the CTTR until March 1995, the most common types of malignant tumor were skin and lip cancer (25.1%), followed by lymphoma (22.5%), KS (8.4%), kidney cancer (6.5%), cervical cancer (1.6%), and vulvar/perineum cancer (0.6%) [45]. Compared with the AZ therapy, the incidence of lymphoma, KS, and renal cancer increased, whereas the incidence of squamous cell carcinoma (SCC), cervical cancer, and vulvar cancer decreased [46]. A report from Japan published in the same era also showed that the CyA group had a lower frequency of SCC, no KS, and a higher frequency of kidney and thyroid cancers than the non-CyA group, which consisted mainly of AZ-treated patients [18]. Compared with TAC and CyA, OPTN/UNOS data indicated that TAC significantly reduced the incidence of all non-skin cancers, non-lymphoma solid tumors, and non-MM skin cancers compared with CyA [36,47].

2.1.3. Mammalian Target of Rapamycin (mTOR) Inhibitor Era

Since the start of the new millennium, new immunosuppressants have become available for use in transplantation. SRL was approved by the FDA in 1999, marking the beginning of the era of mTOR inhibitors in 2000, followed by the approval of EVL in 2010. Both are representative mTOR agents [48]. The immunosuppressive activity of the mTOR inhibitors is based on their binding to immunophilin (FKBP12), which downregulates p70S6 kinase activity and blocks the IL-2 stimulation of lymphocyte proliferation [49].

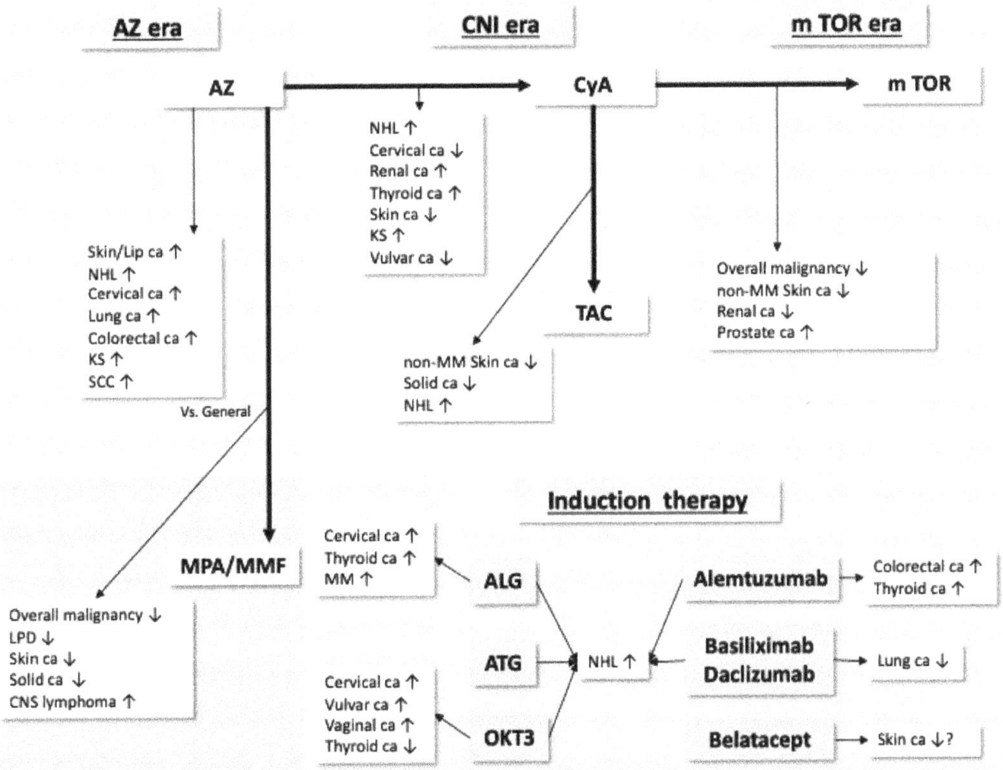

Figure 1. Changing patterns of post-transplant malignancy according to immunosuppressive agent [2,14,15,18,36,39,40,45–47,50–62]. The type of cancer depends on the immunosuppressive agents used before the development of the malignancies. As immunosuppressive therapies have advanced, the patterns of malignant tumors in transplant patients have changed, as shown in this figure. Abbreviations: AZ: azathioprine, ca: carcinoma, NHL: non-Hodgkin lymphoma, KS: Kaposi's sarcoma, SCC: squamous cell carcinoma, MPA: mycophenolate mofetil, MMF: mycophenolate, LPD: lymphoproliferative disorders, CNS: central nervous system, CNI: calcineurin inhibitors, CyA: cyclosporine A, TAC: tacrolimus, MM: malignant melanoma, mTOR: mammalian target of rapamycin, ALG: anti-lymphocyte globulin, ATG: anti-thymocyte globulin.

mTOR demonstrates anti-tumor effects by inhibiting cell proliferation through the PI3 kinase [63] and p70S6 kinase pathways as a result of the deletion of PTEN. It induces growth arrest by upregulating E-cadherin, enhancing the expression of cell cycle inhibitors (e.g., p27kip1) [64], decreasing IL-10 secretion, preventing the constitutive activation of signal transducer and activator of transcription (STAT)1 and STAT3 [65], and disrupting VEGF production, which hinders the VEGF-induced stimulation of vascular endothelial cells [49,66].

Although the risk of post-transplant MM has increased significantly over the last decade, a meta-analysis revealed that the overall incidence of all malignancies and non-MM skin cancers has decreased [2,50–53]. Another study reported a decline in renal cancer, alongside an increased incidence of prostate cancer, when compared with CyA [2,53,54].

2.1.4. Mycophenolic Acid (MPA)/Mycophenolate Mofetil (MMF)

Mycophenolic acid (MPA) and mycophenolate mofetil (MMF) were approved for kidney transplantation in 1995 and are currently widely used as alternatives to AZ. Both agents are combined with CNIs or mTOR inhibitors for maintenance therapy. They exert immunosuppressive effects as purine synthesis inhibitors that target inosine monophosphate dehydrogenase (IMD) [14,67], reducing the incidence of malignant tumors by inhibiting IMD proliferation, which is increased in tumor cells. However, sufficient immunosuppression is also thought to decrease the need for potent immunosuppressive agents [68].

Compared with other immunosuppressive treatments, MMF significantly reduces the incidence of PT-LPD, total cancer, skin cancer, and solid tumors [14,36,55]. However, as discussed later, MMF administration increases the incidence of CNS lymphoma [56,57].

2.1.5. Immunosuppressants for Transplant Induction Therapy

Transplant induction therapy is a short-term medication used during transplant induction or in cases of acute rejection. Immunosuppressive agents for this therapy are classified as polyclonal antibodies (anti-lymphocyte globulin (ALG)) and monoclonal antibodies. The former includes thymoglobulin (RATG, FDA approved in 1999) and anti-thymocyte globulin (ATG, approved in 1998), while the latter encompasses OKT3 (anti-CD3 antibodies, approved in 1985), alemtuzumab (anti-CD52, approved in 2014), basiliximab (anti-CD25, IL-2α receptor, approved in 1998), daclimuzab (anti-CD25, IL-2α receptor, approved in 1997, discontinued in 2009), and belatacept (anti-CD80/86, approved in 2011) [58,69–76].

All antibody induction therapies, including ALG, ATG, OKT3, alemtuzumab, basiliximab, and daclizumab, increase the frequency of PT-LPD [15,58–60]. In addition to lymphoma, ALG therapy elevates the incidence of colorectal cancer, thyroid cancer, and MM [58,59]. OKT3 therapy increases the incidence of cervical, vaginal, and vulvar cancers [59,61] and decreases the incidence of thyroid cancer [58]. The anti-IL-2α receptor treatments, namely, basiliximab and daclizumab, reduce lung cancer incidence. Alemtuzumab is linked to a higher incidence of colorectal and thyroid cancers [58]. Belatacept has been reported to lower the risk of skin cancer [62]; however, recent studies have reported contradictory results [77].

2.2. *Post-Transplantation Lymphoproliferative Disorders (PT-LPD) and Immunosuppressive Agents (Figure 1)*

Post-transplantation lymphoproliferative disorders (PT-LPDs) are the second most common malignant neoplasms that arise following organ or bone marrow transplantation, comprising clinically and morphologically diverse lymphoid proliferative disorders [4]. PT-LPDs are histologically classified into four groups: non-destructive PT-LPDs, which includes reactive plasmacytic hyperplasia; polymorphic PT-LPDs, monomorphic PT-LPDs, and other types, including plasmacytoma-like PT-LPDs. PT-LPDs are mainly associated with EBV and tend to have an aggressive clinical course. While PT-LPDs mainly involve B-cells, T-cells, and natural killer (NK) cells, Hodgkin lymphoma (HL) can also occur [78–80]. A noteworthy aspect is the reversible nature of PT-LPDs, as first reported by Starzl et al. [6]. Non-destructive LPDs and the majority of polymorphic PT-LPDs regress spontaneously after the discontinuation of immunosuppressive agents [81].

In this section, we discuss the types of immunosuppressants and the clinicopathological characteristics of PT-LPDs.

2.3. *Central Nervous System (CNS) Lymphoma*

Central nervous system (CNS) involvement frequently occurs in immunosuppressive LPD cases. Various immunodeficiency conditions and immunosuppressive drugs affect the frequency of CNS-LPD. Before the advent of combination antiretroviral therapy (cART), primary CNS lymphomas were more prevalent among HIV-positive patients. Since the introduction of cART, the frequency of non-Hodgkin lymphoma (NHL) has decreased by 50% [82]. CNS-LPD is a common post-transplant malignancy among patients receiving Aza, MMF, and belatacept regimens [56,57,83–85]. However, it has become rare since the introduction of CyA [18]. Conversely, it has also been suggested that CyA treatment may suppress CNS-LPD.

2.4. Time Trends According to Changes in Immunosuppressants

Since 1983, CyA has been widely used for transplantation instead of AZ. In addition to the decreased frequency of CNS lymphoma, changes in the characteristics of PT-LPD have been observed. PT-LPDs in patients receiving the CyA regimen occur earlier after transplantation, with increased rates of widespread lymph node involvement, gastrointestinal tract issues, and a higher regression rate following the reduction or cessation of immunosuppressive therapy when compared to those receiving AZ [46]. There were better prognoses in the CyA era than in the AZ era [80].

In 1994, TAC was introduced into transplant medicine and became widely used in the field. Regarding LPD, although reports suggest that its administration increases the incidence of LPD [15,43,86,87], no differences were found between the two groups in terms of LPD incidence or clinicopathological features compared to the TAC and CyA groups [14]. At the outset of TAC's introduction, concerns emerged that it could elevate the incidence of PT-LPD, particularly in pediatric liver transplantation [88–91]. According to a report from Pittsburgh, the incidence of PT-LPD was the same for CyA and TAC; however, the incidence of PT-LPD in pediatric liver transplantation tended to be higher for TAC than for CyA ($p = 0.06$) [86]. Nevertheless, in 2013 Narkewicz et al. examined the incidence of PT-LPD in pediatric liver transplantation over a 12-year period (1995–2007) and reported a decrease in PT-LPD incidence. This decrease was attributed to weight loss resulting from immunosuppressant dosing and the monitoring of EBV DNA levels in the blood [89].

A 2011 report from Sweden indicated a statistically significant decrease in the NHL risk among non-kidney transplant recipients from 2000 to 2008 compared to those from 1990 to 1999 [88]. Tsai et al. observed a shift in the histological type and the time to onset of PT-LPD, as documented over time using the UNOS OPTN database from 1999 to 2013. They identified that while the proportion of polymorphic LPD (P-LPD) decreased, the proportion of monomorphic LPD (M-LPD) increased, with an extended time to onset. This change was attributed to the increased use of TAC and a possible increase in the transplant patients' survival rates [92].

The EBV positivity rate also appears to have changed over time. Nelson noted that the proportion of EBV-negative PT-LPD was 2% until 1991 but rose to 23% during the 1990s [93]. EBV-negative PT-LPD has distinct genetic features compared to EBV-positive PT-LPD and is genetically similar to de novo lymphoma [94]. Luskin also indicated that the percentage of EBV-negative PT-LPD increased from 10% in 1990–1995 to 48% in 2008–2013 [95]. Leblond reported that the median time between organ transplantation and tumor diagnosis for EBV-negative PT-LPD was 1800 days, compared to 180 days for EBV-positive LPD; thus, EBV-negative PT-LPD may be a late complication of organ transplantation, induced by the different regimens of immunosuppressive agents [96].

3. Anti-RA Agents and Malignancy

3.1. Malignancy in Patients with RA and Anti-RA Agents

RA is an autoimmune disorder marked by persistent inflammation in the joints and synovium, leading to joint damage and the loss of function, along with the production of autoantibodies, including rheumatoid factor (RF) and anti-citrullinated protein antibody

(ACPA) [97,98]. The incidence of malignant tumors in patients with RA has been reported to be either higher or lower than that in the general population, making this point epidemiologically controversial [33,99–101]. However, the frequency of immune dysregulation and the use of anti-RA agents in patients with RA differ from those in the general population for each type of malignancy.

Patients with RA have a higher risk of developing lymphoma and lung cancer but a lower risk of developing colorectal and breast cancers than the general population [33,102–104]. Additionally, a recent report from France highlighted a significant increase in the incidence of bladder cancer, cervical cancer, prostate cancer, MM, DLBCL, multiple myeloma, and HL. In contrast, the incidence of pancreatic, breast, and endometrial cancers is low [105]. Other studies have indicated a high incidence of leukemia, particularly acute myeloid leukemia (AML) [106], and non-MM skin cancer [107,108]. Conversely, other studies have reported a low incidence of liver [33] and prostate cancers [109].

The pathogenesis of neoplasia in patients with RA may arise from the immune dysregulated state inherent to RA or from an immunosuppressive state induced by antirheumatic agents [20]. It is well established that the hyperimmune state in RA contributes to the increased frequency of LPD [21,22], and that these LPDs can be classified as disease-associated LPDs. Furthermore, the increased frequency of lung cancer has been linked to a hyperimmune state associated with interstitial lung disease and smoking. Moreover, the influence of anti-rheumatic agents on malignant tumor development should not be overlooked.

Anti-RA agents have advanced significantly over the past 30 years, providing substantial benefits to RA patients [29–31]. Traditionally, anti-inflammatory PSLs and analgesic NSAIDs have been used to alleviate the pain associated with RA. Additionally, SASP was approved by the FDA in 1950 as an immunomodulator, followed by the introduction of cDMARDs, with MTX, leflunomide (LEF), and TAC being approved as immunosuppressants in 1988, 1998, and 2005, respectively. Subsequently, bcDMARDs for RA were introduced, including the soluble TNFi ETN (approved in 1998); TNFi monoclonal antibodies such as IFX (approved in 1999); ADA (approved in 2002); GLM (approved in 2009); CZP (approved in 2009); rituximab (RTX) (approved in 1998), which targets the anti-CD20 antibody; ABT (approved in 2005), which utilizes CTLA4-Ig; and TCZ (approved in 2010), which targets the IL-6 receptor. Furthermore, TOF (approved in 2012), upadacitinib (UPA) (approved in 2019), and baricitinib (BAR) (approved in 2022) which are small-molecule compounds classified as JAKis, have also been employed as tsDMARDs [29–32,110].

3.1.1. Non-Steroidal Anti-Inflammatory Drugs (NSAIDs)

Traditionally, anti-inflammatory PSLs and analgesic NSAIDs have been used to alleviate the pain associated with RA [29]. The selective inhibition of cyclooxygenase-2 by NSAIDs suppresses the production of prostaglandins, thereby preventing the incidence of colorectal, breast, lung, and prostate cancers [111–113]. Recent reports from Japan indicate that the incidence of colorectal cancer significantly decreased in the 2000s; however, this notable difference disappeared in the early 2010s [114]. These phenomena are believed to result from the reduced frequency of NSAID use among patients with RA due to the advancements in RA treatment drugs, as suggested [33]. The lower risk of developing colorectal and breast cancers is thought to be due to the use of NSAIDs [99,112,115].

3.1.2. Conventional Synthetic DMARD (csDMARD)

Methotrexate (MTX)

MTX is now recognized as an anchor drug for RA [29–33]. Methotrexate is a folate analog that inhibits dihydrofolate reductase, thereby hindering DNA synthesis and inducing cell death. The anti-inflammatory effects of MTX may involve mechanisms beyond dihydrofolate reductase inhibition. Specifically, these include suppressing cell proliferation by inhibiting purine metabolism, increasing the rate of T-cell apoptosis by inhibiting T-cell activation, enhancing endogenous adenosine release, inhibiting the production of cytokines and intercellular adhesion molecules, and blocking IL-1β receptor binding [116].

The tumorigenic effect of MTX may arise from an immunosuppressive state that reduces tumor immunity. Feng et al. [117] suggested that the unique impact of MTX, which induces EBV replication while promoting immunosuppression, could explain its association with the development of EBV-LPD in RA patients. Regarding the direct carcinogenicity of MTX, it has been reported to exhibit chromosomal cytogenetic effects [20]; however, no further findings have been reported.

The statistical evidence surrounding the overall risk of malignancies, including LPD, in patients with RA treated with MTX remains controversial. Although the incidence of non-MM skin cancer is reportedly increased, many studies have not reported that LPD risk is associated with MTX treatment [26,118,119]. Conversely, some studies have indicated a significant increase in LPD incidence with MTX treatment [33,120,121]. Owing to its characteristic clinicopathological findings, such as the regression of the LPD after MTX cessation, it was designated MTX-LPD in the 2001 WHO classification [28]. These findings support an association between MTX and the development of LPD, which is categorized as a treatment-related LPD. The LPD is discussed in the next section.

Tacrolimus (TAC)

The immunosuppressive effects and carcinogenic properties of TAC were discussed in the section on PT-LPD [36]. Several studies have reported a significant association between TAC administration and the occurrence of malignancies in patients with rheumatoid arthritis [33,122].

Other csDMARD

SASP and LEF do not appear to be associated with cancer risk [116].

3.1.3. Biologic DMARDs (bDMARDs)

Tumor Necrosis Factor Inhibitors (TNFis)

TNF-α was initially identified as a factor that induces tumor necrosis and was subsequently shown to act as a carcinogenic promoter in chronic inflammation. TNF-α activates downstream signaling pathways, including NF-κB, leading to inflammation and the induction of cancer-associated chemokines, cytokines, growth factors, and angiogenesis. Additionally, TNF-α binds to TNF receptor 1, forming the TNFR-associated death domain/Fas-associated death domain complex, which activates caspase-8 and induces apoptosis in cells. Tumor necrosis factor inhibitors (TNFis) not only exhibit anti-inflammatory and anti-tumor effects but also promote tumor growth by inhibiting apoptosis [123].

Most previous studies have reported no significant increase in the incidence of malignancies overall following TNFi treatment [119,124–136]. However, meta-analyses conducted soon after the introduction of TNFis indicated an increased incidence of these events [137]. In contrast, other studies have indicated a decrease in incidence [133,138]. Several studies have reported an increase in LPDs [119,137,139], as well as in instances of non-MM skin cancer [128,135,140], MM [141], and urinary tract cancer [138], but not in other solid tumors. The relationship between LPD and TNFi treatment is discussed in the following section.

Rituximab (RTX)

RTX is a CD20 antibody that depletes circulating mature B lymphocytes [142]. This reduction in antigen presentation by the B-cells leads to T-cell activation. A prolonged period of rituximab-induced B-cell depletion may compromise the immune system, including tumor immuno-surveillance [143]. Since 2000, RTX has been used in combination with CHOP therapy for the treatment of DLBCL. However, a report from California, USA, investigated the occurrence of secondary cancers before and after combination therapy with RTX and DLBCL and revealed that the incidence of AML and thyroid cancer increased after RTX introduction [144]. Furthermore, several studies have shown that the overall incidence of malignant tumors was increased [145].

Patients with RA treated with RTX face an increased overall risk of malignancy, particularly lung, bladder, urinary tract, otopharyngeal, and head and neck cancers, as well as HL and MM, while demonstrating a decreased risk of breast and endometrial cancers compared with the general population [101,136]. However, Huss reported that RTX was not related to the overall incidence of malignancy [136].

Abatacept (ABT)

ABT is a fusion protein composed of the extracellular domain of human CTLA-4, which selectively modulates the co-stimulation of T lymphocytes by inhibiting their activation through binding to CD80/CD86, thereby preventing interaction with the CD28 expressed on T-cells [29].

ABT therapy is associated with an overall increased risk of malignancies in patients with RA [101,136,146]. Compared to the general population, the incidence of lung, bladder, and urinary tract cancers is higher [101,136]. However, other studies have not found a significant difference in the comparison of patients with RA treated with other DMARDs [147–151]. Nonetheless, ABT treatment was associated with a slightly elevated risk of non-melanotic skin cancer and malignant melanoma compared to other DMARDs [146–149,152]. The increased incidence of melanoma is consistent with the widespread use of the CTLA-4 inhibitor ipilimumab for MM treatment [153].

Tocilizumab (TCZ)

Tocilizumab (TCZ) blocks IL-6-mediated signaling by preventing IL-6 from binding to both the transmembrane and soluble forms of the IL-6 receptor. IL-6 plays a crucial role in regulating immunity and inflammation [154] by activating the JAK2 and STAT3 signaling pathways. The activation of the JAK2/STAT3 signaling pathway contributes to tumorigenesis. It promotes the formation of an inflammatory microenvironment in tumors and is closely associated with the development and progression of various cancers. Therefore, IL-6 inhibitors are being studied for their potential application as key molecules in cancer therapy that target the IL-6/JAK2/STAT3 signaling pathway [155].

Compared to the general population, TCZ therapy does not appear to be associated with an increased overall risk of malignancies in patients with RA [101,137,156]. However, the incidence of lung, bladder, and cervical cancers has increased, whereas that of breast cancer has decreased [101,157].

3.1.4. Targeted Synthetic DMARDs (tsDAMRDs)

Janus Kinase Inhibitors (JAKis)

JAKs are tyrosine kinases that play a role in cytokine receptor signaling. JAK regulates the transcription of several genes associated with inflammatory, immune, and cancerous conditions [32]. The excessive activation of JAK and its associated JAK/STAT signaling promotes cancer hallmarks such as proliferation, survival, and angiogenesis, in both the tumor and its surrounding environment, through the activation of STAT3, IL-6, IL-11, IL-22, IL-23, and interferon-γ (IFN-γ) [158]. Inhibiting JAK may provide an alternative cancer treatment [159]; a JAKi has been approved as an anticancer therapy for myelofibrosis [160]. However, JAKs also prevent tumor progression by activating CD8-positive

T-cells and natural killer cells, raising the crucial question of whether JAKis increase the risk of malignancy.

TOF primarily targets ATP-binding sites, specifically JAK1 and JAK3, disrupting cytokines such as IL-2, IL-6, type 1 IFNs, and IFN-γ [161]. BAR selectively binds to the ATP-binding sites of JAK1 and JAK2, whereas UPA selectively binds to JAK1 [32]. Although many reports suggest that there is no significant increase in the incidence of malignancies with TOF, UPA, and BAR [162–168], others have documented a noticeable increase in the frequency of malignancies compared to that in patients treated with TNFis [169–173], thereby the FDA and European Medicine Agency (EMA) emitted warnings in 2021 and 2023, respectively [174]. This is particularly evident in patients aged $\geq$ 50 years, who are at risk of cardiovascular disease [169]. The incidence of non-MM skin cancer and lung cancer is reportedly higher in patients receiving JAKis than in those treated with TNFis [163,169,175].

3.2. *Time Trends of Malignancy in Patients with RA*

Comparisons between two meta-analyses conducted in Canada in 2008 and the United States in 2015 can be utilized to understand the time trends of malignancy in patients with RA [99,102]. The 2008 meta-analysis conducted in Canada did not confirm an increased overall risk of malignant tumors in patients treated with DMARDs. In contrast, the 2015 report indicated that the overall incidence of malignant tumors, particularly lymphomas, was higher in patients than in the general population. However, no differences were observed in the incidence of malignant melanoma, cervical cancer, or prostate cancer between the two groups.

According to the Japanese IORRA cohort [103], the period from 2000 to 2013 was divided into three phases: the pre-biological agent period (the early 2000s, 2000–2004), the biological agent period (the late 2000s, 2005–2009), and the late biological agent period (the early 2010s, 2010–2013). Changes in malignant tumors over time have been reported. The report indicated that the frequencies of all malignant tumors and lymphomas remained unchanged. However, while the incidence of breast cancer was not significantly different between patients with RA and the general population in the 2000s, it decreased significantly in the early 2010s. Furthermore, although the incidence of lung cancer was considerably higher in the early 2000s, this disparity decreased from the late 2000s to the early 2010s. These results suggest that while malignant tumors and lung cancer are experiencing a downward trend compared to the general population, the incidence of colorectal cancer is increasing. Although the incidence of malignant lymphoma is decreasing, it remains significantly higher than in the general population.

Factors contributing to the decrease in lung cancer patients with rheumatoid arthritis include a reduction in the smoking population, decreased chronic inflammation due to interstitial pneumonia, and the influence of a downward trend in CRP levels [176]. The decline in lymphoma, particularly DLBCL, may be attributed to the reduced disease activity associated with improved treatment. This advancement has resulted in a decrease in the incidence of disease-related LPD. Furthermore, a heightened awareness of MTX-LPD and the widespread use of MTX alternatives may contribute to the occurrence of treatment-related LPD.

4. Rheumatoid Arthritis Associated Lymphoproliferative Disorders (RA-LPDs) and Anti-RA Agents (Figure 2)

RA-LPD has distinct characteristics that differentiate it from general lymphomas. It occurs in approximately 1 in 2000 patients with RA, and its frequency is two to four times higher than that in the general population [23,24,114]. According to our database, the male-to-female ratio was 1:2.24, indicating a predominance in females, with a median age at disease onset of 70 years. The median duration from RA onset to LPD onset was 12 years, and the median time from the first administration of MTX to LPD onset was just over five years. The EBV-encoded small RNA-1 (EBER-1) positivity rate was notably high at 51.8%, and C-reactive protein (CRP) and lactate dehydrogenase (LDH) levels were elevated at the onset of LPD [34].

All histological types of malignant lymphomas are present in RA-LPD; however, immunodeficiency-associated LPD can also occur. The most common histological type is DLBCL, followed by HL, mucosa-associated lymphoid tissue lymphoma (MALToma), P-LPD, follicular lymphoma (FL), angioimmunoblastic lymphoma (AITL), HL-like lesions, and EBV-positive mucocutaneous ulcer (EBV-MCU). Compared to sporadic LPD, RA-LPD is characterized by the presence of immunodeficiency lymphomas, such as P-LPD, HL-like lesions, and EBV-MCU, along with an increased proportion of HL, P-LPD, and AITL. Conversely, MALToma, FL, and T-cell phenotypes, such as peripheral T-cell lymphoma (PTCL), anaplastic large cell lymphoma (ALCL), and adult T-cell leukemia/lymphoma (ATLL), are less prevalent [34].

In our database, RA-LPD regressed in 81.6% of cases within 2 weeks to 3 months after the discontinuation of MTX. In 32.1% of the regressions, re-growth occurred at a median of 1 year (1–92 months). The 5-year remission maintenance rate (5y-PregFS) after regression following MTX discontinuation was 63.8%. In contrast to PT-LPD, the proportion of cases achieving CR owing to treatment effects was high. The tumor death rate was 16.3%, and the 5-year survival rate was 86.3%, indicating that the prognosis is better than that for sporadic LPD [34].

4.1. Pre-MTX Era Conventional Therapy and RA-LPD

Before MTX use, patients with RA were treated with medications such as SASP, BCL, sodium aurothiomalate, and PSL. This group can be considered to have disease-related LPD affected by the disease activity of RA without the influence of anti-RA drugs, and an increased frequency of DLBCL has been reported [25,26]. In our database, this naïve group showed a lower frequency of EBER-1 positivity than the other groups. Extranodal origins, particularly from the breast, stomach, and orbit, as well as the B-cell phenotype, including MALToma and FL, may characterize the original nature of RA-LPD. Similar to PT-LPD [34], indolent lymphomas such as FL and MALToma may not be immunosuppressive LPDs in RA-LPD.

4.1.1. Conventional Synthetic DMARD (csDMARD) and RA-LPD

MTX is now recognized as a cost-effective cornerstone of RA therapy [28–31]. The MTX group is prominent, and numerous recent studies have highlighted its clinicopathological features [4,28,34,120,177–188]. This is also detailed in the WHO classification [4,28,82]. In our database, a comparison of the MTX monotherapy group with the naïve group elucidated the pathology of pure MTX-LPD. The MTX monotherapy group had a higher proportion of primary oral lesions and a lower proportion of primary orbital or gastric lesions and MALTomas than the naïve group. In the MTX monotherapy group, the incidence of oral primary lesions increased, whereas that of orbital or gastric primary lesions and MALTomas decreased.

Regarding TAC, a comparison between the MTX plus TAC combination and MTX monotherapy groups revealed a significant increase in the proportion of primary lesions and ALCL in the pharyngeal and parotid glands, along with a decrease in the proportion of primary lesions in the lungs [34]. TAC also affects lymphoma formation in RA-LPD. We allowed overlap with our other drugs and compared 78 of the 518 patients with RA to

78 patients receiving TAC and 440 patients without TAC. Consequently, an increase in EBER-1 positivity, P-LPD subtype, and advanced age at LPD onset were identified as independent poor prognostic factors in patients treated with TAC therapy [123]. Patients receiving TAC medications for RA may require a detailed follow-up to assess LPD development.

4.1.2. Biologic DMARDs (bDMARDs) and RA-LPD

A TNFi does not increase the incidence of LPD, as described above in the relationship between TNFi administration and the development of LPD [125–135]. Although the FDA expressed concern about LPD development in the early stages of TNFi administration [119,139,189], following several studies reporting cases of LPD, particularly within the first few months of TNFi treatment [190], no similar reports have yet been published.

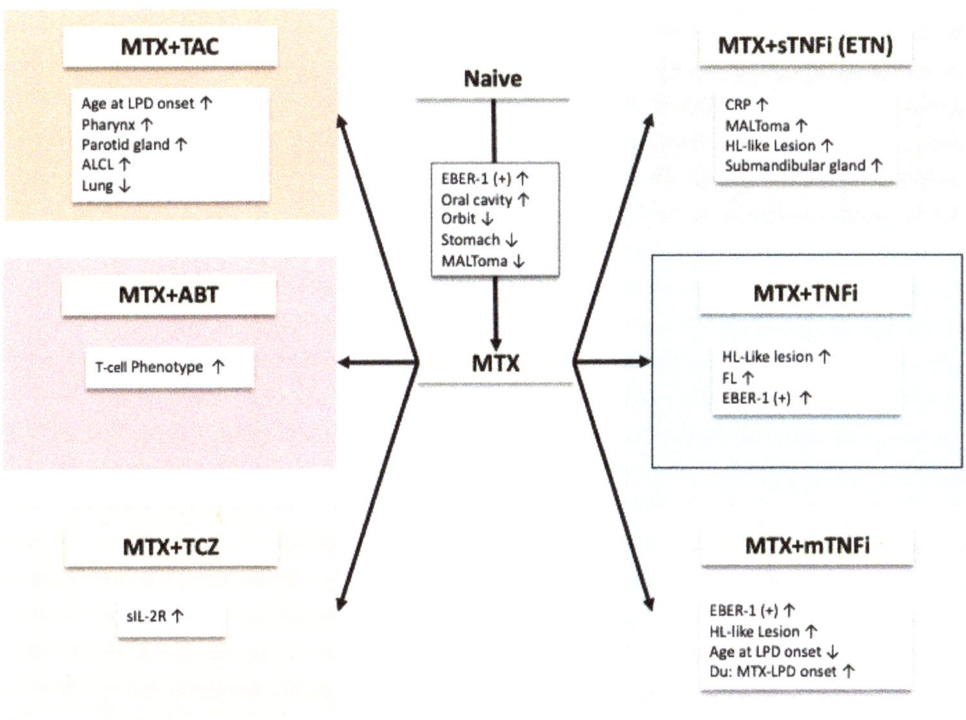

Figure 2. Changing patterns of rheumatoid arthritis-associated lymphoproliferative disorders according to anti-rheumatic agent [34,191] The clinicopathological features of rheumatoid arthritis-associated lymphoproliferative disorder (RA-LPD) also differ based on the anti-RA agent used, including methotrexate, tacrolimus, and tumor necrosis factor inhibitors, among others, as illustrated in this figure. Abbreviations: MTX: methotrexate, TAC: tacrolimus, LPD: lymphoproliferative disorder, ALCL: anaplastic large cell lymphoma, ABT: abatacept, TCZ: tocilizumab, sIL-2R: soluble interleukin-2 receptor, EBER-1: Epstein–Barr virus-encoded small RNA-1, MALToma: mucosa-associated lymphoid tissue lymphoma, ref.: reference, sTNFi: soluble tumor necrosis factor inhibitor, ETN: etanercept, CRP: C-reactive protein, HL-like lesion: Hodgkin lymphoma-like lesion, TNFi: tumor necrosis factor inhibitor, FL: follicular lymphoma, mTNFi: monoclonal tumor necrosis factor inhibitor, MTX-LPD: methotrexate-associated lymphoid tissue lymphoma, Du: duration.

The incidence and histologic subtypes of the LPDs depend on each anti-RA agent, including TNFis, and have recently garnered more interest [192]. Although previous studies have not shown any correlation with the histological subtypes of LPDs [130,186,193], our database allowed us to statistically demonstrate the effect of TNFi administration on LPD. The MTX plus TNFi combination groups were compared with the MTX monotherapy group. In the MTX plus TNFi groups, there was an increase in EBER-1-positive cases, a higher proportion of HL-like lesions, and a decrease in the proportion of FL than in the MTX monotherapy group [34].

TNF is a trimeric protein produced by various cells and exists in both soluble and membrane-bound forms [194]. Compared with sTNFis, mTNFis have a significant impact on Crohn's disease, uveitis, and psoriasis, and are associated with an increased risk of infectious complications, including opportunistic infections and tuberculosis [195–198]. TNFis were categorized into two groups: the soluble TNFi (sTNFi) group, specifically etanercept (ETN), and the monoclonal antibody TNFi (mTNFi) group. The mTNFis and sTNFis (ETN) function through different mechanisms, dependent on their unique ability to bind soluble and transmembrane TNFs and their capacity to induce apoptosis [194]. In vitro, mTNFi inhibits IFN-γ production, but sTNFi does not [199], which may suggest a difference in their susceptibility to bacterial and viral infections.

Interestingly, the clinicopathological features of RA-LPD varied between the MTX plus mTNFi and MTX plus sTNFi (ETN) groups [191]. In the MTX and sTNFi (ETN) group, CRP levels at LPD onset were higher than those in the MTX monotherapy group, and the rates of HL-like lesions, MALToma, and primary submandibular lesions increased. Additionally, the proportion of HL-like lesions was higher in the MTX group than in the mTNFi and MTX alone groups. However, the age of LPD onset increased, LDH levels decreased, the duration between the first MTX dose and the onset of LPD shortened, and the frequency of EBER-1 positive cases increased.

Patients with DLBCL treated with RTX plus CHOP therapy have an increased risk of HL compared to the general population [144]. As previously described, patients with RA who receive RTX have a high incidence of HL and MM [101]. Regarding ABT, the MTX plus ABT group showed a higher occurrence of T-LPD than the MTX-only group in our database.

TCZ is an IL-6 antagonist. IL-6 plays a role in DLBCL pathogenesis, particularly in the activated B-cell type, via the STAT3 signaling pathway [155]. Blockade of the IL-6 signaling cascade by TCZ may lower the risk of re-growth after spontaneous regression (SR), resulting in a favorable prognosis. RTX is a chimeric monoclonal antibody that targets the CD20 molecules expressed on the surface of B-cells. The MTX plus TCZ group exhibited elevated sIL-2R levels. TCZ increases the frequency of bladder and cervical cancers while decreasing the incidence of endometrial cancer [101].

4.1.3. Targeted Synthetic DMARDs (tsDMARDs) and RA-LPD

Concerning JAKis, while numerous reports have suggested that there is no significant rise in the incidence of malignancies associated with JAKis [162–169], Mariette et al. noted that the age- and sex-adjusted SIR of lymphoma was 2.62 (95%CI: 1.58–4.09) [200]. This has been observed in patients treated with JAKis for the myelofibrosis associated with aggressive lymphoma [201]. Furthermore, patients with RA treated with JAKis were more often positive for ACPA and RF [200]. Harada et al. indicated that the lymphoma occurring in patients with RA undergoing treatment with JAKis was aggressive B-cell lymphoma [188].

4.2. EBV Status and RA-LPD

RA-LPD exhibited a higher EBER-1 positivity rate (18.4%) than sporadic LPD (51.8%). Moreover, MTX monotherapy (50.3%), MTX plus TAC (59.4%), and MTX plus TNFi (65.2%) demonstrated higher EBER-1 positivity rates than those in the naïve group. Additionally, the combined MTX plus TNFi treatment group had a higher EBER-1 positivity rate than the MTX monotherapy group [34]. Furthermore, among TNFi, mTNFis showed a higher EBER-1 positivity (65.4%) than sTNFis (ETN) (47.9%) [191]. Patients treated with mTNFis are more susceptible to EBV infection, which may result in a higher proportion of EBER-1-positive patients compared to those treated with sTNFis (ETN). In patients with RA, blood EBV antibody titers have been reported to be higher than those in the general population [202]. Moreover, it has been noted that the administration does not increase EBV antibody titers in the blood [203]. This discrepancy may arise from geographic differences in EBV positivity, highlighting the need for further studies.

4.3. Time Trends of RA-LPD According to Changes in Anti-Rheumatic Agents

Our large-scale study assessed the statistical differences in the characteristics of RA-LPD over time [34]. Concerning anti-RA agents administered before LPD onset, naïve cases were less frequent in the 2010s-LPD group than in the 2000s-LPD group. Conversely, MTX, TAC, TNFis, and ABT were used more frequently in the 2010s-LPD group than in the 2000s-LPD group. The estimated cumulative and weekly MTX doses in the 2010s-LPD group were higher than those in the 2000s-LPD group.

The age at RA-LPD onset was higher in the 2010s-LPD group than in the 2000s-LPD group. Immunosuppressive markers, including P-LPD and EBER-1, were increased during the later stages. The incidence of NK/T-cell lymphoma and MALToma was significantly lower in the later period [34]. In contrast, when comparing our previous and most recent publication, the prognosis for RA-LPD was worse than that for sporadic LPD in the 2007 report [179], but it reversed and improved in the 2024 report [34]. In the former case, the proportion of DLBCL was significantly higher, whereas in the latter, the significant difference disappeared.

Furthermore, the report stated that the incidence of bladder cancer, cervical cancer, prostate cancer, MM, DLBCL, multiple myeloma, and HL have increased significantly. In contrast, the incidence of pancreatic, breast, and endometrial cancers is low [101].

5. Discussion

This review describes the effects of various immunosuppressants and immunomodulators administered before the onset of malignancies, particularly PT-LPD and RA-LPD, as well as their changing patterns over time. Recent advances in immunosuppressants and immunomodulators have significantly improved the quality of life (QOL) of organ transplant recipients and patients with RA, leading to better long-term survival while also addressing the need to prevent malignant tumor development. As immunosuppressants and immunomodulators continue to evolve, further research is necessary to identify the optimal therapy and dosage that balances the maintenance of the transplanted organ's function and the QOL of RA patients with a reduction in the risk of malignancy. The weaknesses of this review article include the content of the published reports, such as past studies, limited statistical analysis, small sample sizes, restricted geographic areas, insufficient verification, and low risk factors. However, essential trends that might otherwise be concealed in a large-scale meta-analysis can be identified. We believe that addressing these minor factors is important.

Overall, building evidence regarding the influence of drugs is challenging. Furthermore, determining which drug is responsible for an effect is particularly difficult when multiple drugs are administered to a single patient, considering the pharmacological synergy of all the drugs involved. The dataset from the British Society for Rheumatology Biological Registry of Rheumatoid Arthritis (BSRBR-RA) used in this study indicated that over 50% of patients who started their first TNFi later switched to alternative agents [125,204]. Prior reports examining the relationship between RA drugs, especially TNFis, and RA-LPD pathology failed to yield significant results because of inconsistencies in the group definitions and the extent of the information studied [130,189,194]. There was also potential bias in the follow-up methods, observation periods, data collection techniques, and number of cases evaluated.

In our database, 35% of patients with RA-LPD received multiple drugs, either simultaneously or at different time points. Nonetheless, significant results were obtained owing to the large number of cases, the accumulation of detailed information on the cases, and the division of patients into non-overlapping 1:1 groups, coupled with the statistical analysis of a vast quantity of data [34]. It would be intriguing to see the outcomes of earlier reports that utilized the same classification methods but did not produce significant results.

6. Conclusions

The trends in malignancies arising in patients treated with immunosuppressive/ immunomodulatory agents are continually evolving. With advancements in medicine, understanding the various characteristics and temporal changes in immunosuppressive malignant tumors, particularly LPD, is beneficial for daily clinical practice and may lead to significant medical breakthroughs, such as the development of new drugs and improved monitoring methods for cancer treatment. Immunosuppressive malignancies including LPDs are continuously changing their characteristics due to the effect of the immunosuppressive/immunomodulatory agents.

Author Contributions: A.N. and Y.H. performed the literature review and drafted the manuscript. Other authors contributed to the productive discussion. All authors have read and agreed to the published version of the manuscript.

Funding: This publication was supported by JSPS KAKENHI Grant Numbers 17K08734 and 20K07384 to YH and a Grant-in-Aid for Clinical Research from the National Hospital Organization Grant Numbers H28-NHO(TAKYO)-2, H31-NHO(TAKYO)-2 and R4-NHO(TAKYO)-1 to YH.

Acknowledgments: We are thankful to Dan Chi from Osaka Minami Medical Center for her administrative assistance and to Misato Igarashi from Osaka Minami Medical Center for serving as the librarian.

Conflicts of Interest: The authors declare no conflicts of interest.

References

1. Engels, E.A.; Pfeiffer, R.M.; Fraumeni, J.F., Jr.; Kasiske, B.L.; Israni, A.K.; Snyder, J.J.; Wolfe, R.A.; Goodrich, N.P.; Bayakly, A.R.; Clarke, C.A.; et al. Spectrum of cancer risk among US solid organ transplant recipients. *JAMA* **2011**, *306*, 1891–1901. [CrossRef] [PubMed]
2. Bhat, M.; Mara, K.; Dierkhising, R.; Watt, K.D.S. Immunosuppression, race, and donor-related risk factors affect de novo cancer incidence across solid organ transplant recipients. *Mayo Clin. Proc.* **2018**, *93*, 1236–1246. [CrossRef] [PubMed]
3. Grulich, A.E.; van Leeuwen, M.T.; Falster, M.O.; Vajdic, C.M. Incidence of cancers in people with HIV/AIDS compared with immunosuppressed transplant recipients: A meta-analysis. *Lancet* **2007**, *370*, 59–67. [CrossRef] [PubMed]
4. Swerdlow, S.H.; Campo, E.; Harris, N.L.; Jaffe, E.S.; Pileri, S.A.; Stein, H.; Thiele, J.; Arber, D.A.; Hasserjian, R.P.; Le Beau, M.M.; et al. *WHO Classification of Tumours of Haematopoietic and Lymphoid Tissues*, 4th ed.; IARC: Lyon, France, 2017; pp. 443–464.
5. Doycheva, L.; Amer, S.; Watt, K.D. De novo malignancies after transplantation: Risk and surveillance strategies. *Med. Clin. N. Am.* **2016**, *100*, 551–567. [CrossRef] [PubMed]

6. Starzl, T.E.; Nalesnik, M.A.; Porter, K.A.; Ho, M.; Iwatsuki, S.; Griffith, B.P.; Rosenthal, J.T.; Hakala, T.R.; Shaw, B.W., Jr.; Hardesty, R.L.; et al. Reversibility of lymphomas and lymphoproliferative lesions developing under cyclosporin-steroid therapy. *Lancet* **1984**, *1*, 583–587. [CrossRef] [PubMed]
7. Otley, C.C.; Coldiron, B.M.; Stasko, T.; Goldman, G.D. Decreased skin cancer after cessation of therapy with transplant-associated immunosuppressants. *Arch. Dermatol.* **2001**, *137*, 459–463. [PubMed]
8. Penn, I. Kaposi's sarcoma in immunosuppressed patients. *J. Clin. Lab. Immunol.* **1983**, *12*, 1–10. [PubMed]
9. Friedlaender, M.M.; Rubinger, D.; Rosenbaum, E.; Amir, G.; Siguencia, E. Temporary regression of Merkel cell carcinoma metastases after cessation of cyclosporine. *Transplantation* **2002**, *73*, 1849–1850. [CrossRef] [PubMed]
10. Elder, G.J.; Hersey, P.; Branley, P. Remission of transplanted melanoma—Clinical course and tumour cell characterisation. *Clin. Transplant.* **1997**, *11*, 565–568. [CrossRef] [PubMed]
11. Chuang, F.R.; Hsieh, H.; Hsu, K.T.; Huang, H.F. Increasing transplant cancer patient survival by conversion of immunosuppressive agents. *Transplant. Proc.* **1996**, *28*, 1346–1347. [PubMed]
12. de Jong, D.; Chan, J.K.C.; Coupland, S.E.; Naresh, K.N.; Siebert, R. Lymphoid proliferations and lymphomatous associated with immune deficiency and dysregulation: Introduction. In *WHO Classification of Tumours Editorial Board. Haematolymphoid Tumoures*, 5th ed.; The WHO Classification of Tumours Editorial Board, Ed.; IARC: Lyon, France, 2024; pp. 549–554.
13. Wang, J.H.; Pfeiffer, R.M.; Musgrove, D.; Castenson, D.; Fredrickson, M.; Miller, J.; Gonsalves, L.; Hsieh, M.C.; Lynch, C.F.; Zeng, Y.; et al. Cancer mortality among solid organ transplant recipients in the United States during 1987–2018. *Transplantation* **2023**, *107*, 2433–2442. [CrossRef] [PubMed]
14. Cherikh, W.S.; Kauffman, H.M.; McBride, M.A.; Maghirang, J.; Swinnen, L.J.; Hanto, D.W. Association of the type of induction immunosuppression with posttransplant lymphoproliferative disorder, graft survival, and patient survival after primary kidney transplantation. *Transplantation* **2003**, *76*, 1289–1293. [CrossRef] [PubMed]
15. Caillard, S.; Dharnidharka, V.; Agodoa, L.; Bohen, E.; Abbott, K. Posttransplant lymphoproliferative disorders after renal transplantation in the United States in era of modern immunosuppression. *Transplantation* **2005**, *80*, 1233–1243. [CrossRef] [PubMed]
16. Howard, R.J.; Patton, P.R.; Reed, A.I.; Hemming, A.W.; Van der Werf, W.J.; Pfaff, W.W.; Srinivas, T.R.; Scornik, J.C. The changing causes of graft loss and death after kidney transplantation. *Transplantation* **2002**, *73*, 1923–1928. [CrossRef] [PubMed]
17. Rossi, A.P.; Klein, C.L. Posttransplant malignancy. *Surg. Clin. N. Am.* **2019**, *99*, 49–64. [CrossRef] [PubMed]
18. Hoshida, Y.; Tsukuma, H.; Yasunaga, Y.; Xu, N.; Fujita, M.Q.; Satoh, T.; Ichikawa, Y.; Kurihara, K.; Imanishi, M.; Matsuno, T.; et al. Cancer risk after renal transplantation in Japan. *Int. J. Cancer* **1997**, *71*, 517–520. [CrossRef]
19. Opelz, G.; Naujokat, C.; Daniel, V.; Terness, P.; Döhler, B. Disassociation between risk of graft loss and risk of non-Hodgkin lymphoma with induction agents in renal transplant recipients. *Transplantation* **2006**, *81*, 1227–1233. [CrossRef] [PubMed]
20. Georgescu, L.; Quinn, G.C.; Schwartzman, S.; Paget, S.A. Lymphoma in patients with rheumatoid arthritis: Association with the disease state or methotrexate treatment. *Semin. Arthritis Rheum.* **1997**, *26*, 794–804. [CrossRef] [PubMed]
21. Lea, A.J. An association between the rheumatic disease and the reticulosis. *Ann. Rheum. Dis.* **1964**, *23*, 480–484. [CrossRef] [PubMed]
22. Miller, D.G. The association of immune disease and malignant lymphoma. *Ann. Intern. Med.* **1967**, *66*, 507–521. [CrossRef] [PubMed]
23. Isomäki, H.A.; Hakulinen, T.; Joutsenlahti, U. Excess risk of lymphomas, leukemia and myeloma in patients with rheumatoid arthritis. *J. Chronic Dis.* **1978**, *31*, 691–696. [CrossRef] [PubMed]
24. Thomas, E.; Brewster, D.H.; Black, R.J.; Macfarlane, G.J. Risk of malignancy among patients with rheumatic conditions. *Int. J. Cancer* **2000**, *88*, 497–502. [CrossRef] [PubMed]
25. Baecklund, E.; Iliadou, A.; Askling, J.; Ekbom, A.; Backlin, C.; Granath, F.; Catrina, A.I.; Rosenquist, R.; Feltelius, N.; Sundström, C. Association of chronic inflammation, not its treatment, with increased lymphoma risk in rheumatoid arthritis. *Arthritis Rheum.* **2006**, *54*, 692–701. [CrossRef] [PubMed]
26. Baecklund, E.; Sundström, C.; Ekbom, A.; Catrina, A.I.; Biberfeld, P.; Feltelius, N.; Klareskog, L. Lymphoma subtypes in patients with rheumatoid arthritis. Increased proportion of diffuse large B cell lymphoma. *Arthritis Rheum.* **2003**, *48*, 1543–1550. [CrossRef] [PubMed]
27. Ellman, M.H.; Hurwitz, H.; Thomas, C.; Kozloff, M. Lymphoma developing in a patient with rheumatoid arthritis taking low dose weekly methotrexate. *J. Rheumatol.* **1991**, *18*, 1741–1743. [PubMed]
28. Harris, N.L.; Swerdlow, S.H. Methotrexate-associated lymphoproliferative disorders. In *Pathology and Genetics. Tumors of Hematopoietic and Lymphoid Tissues. WHO Classification of Tumours of Haematopoietic and Lymphoid Tissues*, 3rd ed.; Jaffe, E.S., Harris, N.L., Stein, H., Vardiman, J.W., Eds.; IARC: Lyon, France, 2001; pp. 270–271.
29. Meier, F.M.P.; Frerix, M.; Hermann, W.; Müller-Ladner, U. Current immunotherapy in rheumatoid arthritis. *Immunotherapy* **2013**, *5*, 955–974. [CrossRef] [PubMed]

30. Kerrigan, S.A.; McInnes, I.B. Reflections on 'older' drugs: Learning new lessons in rheumatology. *Nat. Rev. Rheumatol.* **2020**, *16*, 179–183. [CrossRef] [PubMed]
31. Burmester, G.R.; Pope, J.E. Novel treatment strategies in rheumatoid arthritis. *Lancet* **2017**, *389*, 2338–2348. [CrossRef] [PubMed]
32. Shawky, A.M.; Almalki, F.A.; Abdalla, A.N.; Abdelazeem, A.H.; Gouda, A.M. A comprehensive overview of globally approved JAK inhibitors. *Pharmaceutics* **2022**, *14*, 1001. [CrossRef] [PubMed]
33. Hashimoto, A.; Chiba, N.; Tsuno, H.; Komiya, A.; Furukawa, H.; Matsui, T.; Nishino, J.; Tohma, S. Incidence of malignancy and the risk of lymphoma in Japanese patients with rheumatoid arthritis compared to the general population. *J. Rheumatol.* **2015**, *42*, 564–571. [CrossRef] [PubMed]
34. Hoshida, Y.; Tsujii, A.; Ohshima, S.; Saeki, Y.; Yagita, M.; Miyamura, T.; Katayama, M.; Kawasaki, T.; Hiramatsu, Y.; Oshima, H.; et al. Effect of recent antirheumatic drug on features of rheumatoid arthritis-associated lymphoproliferative disorders. *Arthritis Rheumatol.* **2024**, *76*, 869–881. [CrossRef] [PubMed]
35. Khan, M.A.; Hanna, A.; Sridhara, S.; Chaudhari, H.; Me, H.M.; Attieh, R.M.; Abu Jawdeh, B.G. Maintenance immunosuppression in kidney transplantation: A review of the current status and future directions. *J. Clin. Med.* **2025**, *14*, 1821. [CrossRef] [PubMed]
36. Kauffman, H.M.; Cherikh, W.S.; McBride, M.A.; Cheng, Y.; Hanto, D.W. Post-transplant de novo malignancies in renal transplant recipients: The past and present. *Transpl. Int.* **2006**, *19*, 607–620. [CrossRef] [PubMed]
37. Perrett, C.M.; Walker, S.L.; O'Donovan, P.; Warwick, J.; Harwood, C.A.; Karran, P.; McGregor, J.M. Azathioprine treatment photosensitizes human skin to ultraviolet A radiation. *Br. J. Dermatol.* **2008**, *159*, 198–204. [CrossRef] [PubMed]
38. Taylor, A.E.; Shuster, S. Skin cancer after renal transplantation: The causal role of azathioprine. *Acta Derm. Venereol.* **1992**, *7*, 115–119. [CrossRef]
39. Penn, I. Tumor incidence in human allograft recipients. *Transplant. Proc.* **1979**, *11*, 1047–1051. [PubMed]
40. Jiyad, Z.; Olsen, C.M.; Burke, M.T.; Isbel, N.M.; Green, A.C. Azathioprine and risk of skin cancer in organ transplant recipients: Systematic review and meta-analysis. *Am. J. Transplant.* **2016**, *16*, 3490–3503. [CrossRef] [PubMed]
41. Hojo, M.; Morimoto, T.; Maluccio, M.; Asano, T.; Morimoto, K.; Lagman, M.; Shimbo, T.; Suthanthiran, M. Cyclosporine induces cancer progression by a cell-autonomous mechanism. *Nature* **1999**, *397*, 530–534. [CrossRef] [PubMed]
42. Kehrl, J.H.; Wakefield, L.M.; Roberts, A.B.; Jakowlew, S.; Alvarez-Mon, M.; Derynck, R.; Sporn, M.B.; Fauci, A.S. Production of transforming growth factor beta by human T lymphocytes and its potential role in the regulation of T cell growth. *J. Exp. Med.* **1986**, *163*, 1037–1050. [CrossRef] [PubMed]
43. Tanner, J.E.; Menezes, J. Interleukin-6 and Epstein-Barr virus induction by cyclosporine A: Potential role in lymphoproliferative disease. *Blood* **1994**, *84*, 3956–3964. [CrossRef] [PubMed]
44. Walz, G.; Zanker, B.; Melton, L.B.; Suthanthiran, M.; Strom, T.B. Possible association of the immunosuppressive and B cell lymphoma-promoting properties of cyclosporine. *Transplantation* **1990**, *49*, 191–194. [CrossRef] [PubMed]
45. Penn, I. Cancers in cyclosporine-treated vs azathioprine treated patients. *Transplant. Proc.* **1996**, *28*, 876–878. [PubMed]
46. Penn, I. The changing pattern of posttransplant malignancies. *Transplant. Proc.* **1991**, *23*, 1101–1103. [PubMed]
47. Opelz, G.; Döhler, B. Lymphomas after solid organ transplantation: A collaborative transplant study report. *Am. J. Transplant.* **2004**, *4*, 222–230. [CrossRef] [PubMed]
48. Aala, A.; Brennan, D.C. Transformation in Immunosuppression: Are We Ready for it? *J. Am. Soc. Nephrol.* **2018**, *29*, 1791–1792. [CrossRef] [PubMed]
49. Luan, F.L.; Hojo, M.; Maluccio, M.; Yamaji, K.; Suthanthiran, M. Rapamycin blocks tumor progression: Unlinking immunosuppression from antitumor efficacy. *Transplantation* **2002**, *73*, 1565–1572. [CrossRef] [PubMed]
50. Fattouh, K.; Ducroux, E.; Decullier, E.; Kanitakis, J.; Morelon, E.; Boissonnat, P.; Sebbag, L.; Jullien, D.; Euvrard, S. Increasing incidence of melanoma after solid organ transplantation: A retrospective epidemiological study. *Transpl. Int.* **2017**, *30*, 1172–1180. [CrossRef] [PubMed]
51. Euvrard, S.; Morelon, E.; Rostaing, L.; Goffin, E.; Brocard, A.; Tromme, I.; Broeders, N.; del Marmol, V.; Chatelet, V.; Dompmartin, A.; et al. Sirolimus and secondary skin-cancer prevention in kidney transplantation. *N. Engl. J. Med.* **2012**, *367*, 329–339. [CrossRef] [PubMed]
52. Knoll, G.A.; Kokolo, M.B.; Mallick, R.; Beck, A.; Buenaventura, C.D.; Ducharme, R.; Barsoum, R.; Bernasconi, C.; Blydt-Hansen, T.D.; Ekberg, H.; et al. Effect of sirolimus on malignancy and survival after kidney transplantation: Systematic review and meta-analysis of individual patient data. *BMJ* **2014**, *349*, g6679. [CrossRef] [PubMed]
53. Yanik, E.L.; Siddiqui, K.; Engels, E.A. Sirolimus effects on cancer incidence after kidney transplantation: A meta-analysis. *Cancer Med.* **2015**, *4*, 1448–1459. [CrossRef] [PubMed]
54. Kauffman, H.M.; Cherikh, W.S.; Cheng, Y.; Hanto, D.W.; Kahan, B.D. Maintenance immunosuppression with target-of-rapamycin inhibitors is associated with a reduced incidence of de novo malignancies. *Transplantation* **2005**, *80*, 883–889. [CrossRef] [PubMed]
55. Robson, R.; Cecka, J.M.; Opelz, G.; Budde, M.; Sacks, S. Prospective registry-based observational cohort study of the long-term risk of malignancies in renal transplant patients treated with mycophenolate mofetil. *Am. J. Transplant.* **2005**, *5*, 2954–2960. [CrossRef] [PubMed]

56. Evens, A.M.; Choquet, S.; Kroll-Desrosiers, A.R.; Jagadeesh, D.; Smith, S.M.; Morschhauser, F.; Leblond, V.; Roy, R.; Barton, B.; Gordon, L.I.; et al. Primary CNS posttransplant lymphoproliferative disease (PTLD): An international report of 84 cases in the modern era. *Am. J. Transplant.* **2013**, *13*, 1512–1522. [CrossRef] [PubMed]
57. Crane, G.M.; Powell, H.; Kostadinov, R.; Rocafort, P.T.; Rifkin, D.E.; Burger, P.C.; Ambinder, R.F.; Swinnen, L.J.; Borowitz, M.J.; Duffield, A.S. Primary CNS lymphoproliferative disease, mycophenolate and calcineurin inhibitor usage. *Oncotarget* **2015**, *6*, 33849–33866. [CrossRef] [PubMed]
58. Hall, E.C.; Engels, E.A.; Pfeiffer, R.M.; Segev, D.L. Association of antibody induction immunosuppression with cancer after kidney transplantation. *Transplantation* **2015**, *99*, 1051–1057. [CrossRef] [PubMed]
59. Hibberd, A.D.; Trevillian, P.R.; Wlodarzcyk, J.H.; Gillies, A.H.; Stein, A.M.; Sheil, A.G.; Disney, A.P. Cancer risk associated with ATG/OKT3 in renal transplantation. *Transplant. Proc.* **1999**, *31*, 1271–1272. [CrossRef] [PubMed]
60. Swinnen, L.J.; Costanzo-Nordin, M.R.; Fisher, S.G.; O'Sullivan, E.J.; Johnson, M.R.; Heroux, A.L.; Dizikes, G.J.; Pifarre, R.; Fisher, R.I. Increased incidence of lymphoproliferative disorder after immunosuppression with the monoclonal antibody OKT3 in cardiac- transplant recipients. *N. Engl. J. Med.* **1990**, *323*, 1723–1728. [CrossRef] [PubMed]
61. Malvezzi, P.; Jouve, T.; Rostaing, L. Induction by anti-thymocyte globulins in kidney transplantation: A review of the literature and current usage. *J. Nephropathol.* **2015**, *4*, 10–115.
62. Wang, M.; Mittal, A.; Colegio, O.R. Belatacept reduces skin cancer risk in kidney transplant recipients. *J. Am. Acad. Dermatol.* **2020**, *82*, 996–998. [CrossRef] [PubMed]
63. Guba, M.; von Breitenbuch, P.; Steinbauer, M.; Koehl, G.; Flegel, S.; Hornung, M.; Bruns, C.J.; Zuelke, C.; Farkas, S.; Anthuber, M.; et al. Rapamycin inhibits primary and metastatic tumor growth by antiangiogenesis: Involvement of vascular endothelial growth factor. *Nat. Med.* **2002**, *8*, 128–135. [CrossRef] [PubMed]
64. Nourse, J.; Firpo, E.; Flanagan, W.M.; Coats, S.; Polyak, K.; Lee, M.H.; Massague, J.; Crabtree, G.R.; Roberts, J.M. Interleukin-2-mediated elimination of the p27Kip1 cyclin-dependent kinase inhibitor prevented by rapamycin. *Nature* **1994**, *372*, 570–573. [CrossRef] [PubMed]
65. Chen, H.; Lee, J.M.; Zong, Y.; Borowitz, M.; Ng, M.H.; Ambinder, R.F.; Hayward, S.D. Linkage between STAT regulation and Epstein-Barr virus gene expression in tumors. *J. Virol.* **2001**, *75*, 2929–2937. [CrossRef] [PubMed]
66. Koehl, G.E.; Andrassy, J.; Guba, M.; Richter, S.; Kroemer, A.; Scherer, M.N.; Steinbauer, M.; Graeb, C.; Schlitt, H.J.; Jauch, K.W.; et al. Rapamycin protects allografts from rejection while simultaneously attacking tumors in immunosuppressed mice. *Transplantation* **2004**, *77*, 1319–1326. [CrossRef] [PubMed]
67. Guba, M.; Graeb, C.; Jauch, K.W.; Geissler, E.K. Pro- and anti-cancer effects of immunosuppressive agents used in organ transplantation. *Transplantation* **2004**, *77*, 1777–1782. [CrossRef] [PubMed]
68. Buell, J.F.; Gross, T.G.; Woodle, E.S. Malignancy after transplantation. *Transplantation* **2005**, *80*, S254–S264. [CrossRef] [PubMed]
69. van der Zwan, M.; Baan, C.C.; van Gelder, T.; Hesselink, D.A. Review of the clinical pharmacokinetics and pharmacodynamics of Alemtuzumab and its use in kidney transplantation. *Clin. Pharmacokinet.* **2018**, *57*, 191–207. [CrossRef] [PubMed]
70. Shemshadi, M.; Hoseini, R.; Zareh, R.; Otukesh, H. Use of Basiliximab with the standard immunosuppressive protocol in pediatric renal transplantation:a double-blind randomized clinical trial. *Int. J. Organ. Transplant. Med.* **2020**, *11*, 8–14. [PubMed]
71. Iglesias, M.; Brennan, D.C.; Larsen, C.P.; Raimondi, G. Targeting inflammation and immune activation to improve CTLA4-Ig-based modulation of transplant rejection. *Front. Immunol.* **2022**, *13*, 926648. [CrossRef] [PubMed]
72. Smith, S.L. Ten years of Orthoclone OKT3 (muromonab-CD3): A review. *J. Transpl. Coord.* **1996**, *6*, 109–119. [PubMed]
73. Alloway, R.R.; Woodle, E.S.; Abramowicz, D.; Segev, D.L.; Castan, R.; Ilsley, J.N.; Jeschke, K.; Somerville, K.T.; Brennan, D.C. Rabbit anti-thymocyte globulin for the prevention of acute rejection in kidney transplantation. *Am. J. Transplant.* **2019**, *19*, 2252–2261. [CrossRef] [PubMed]
74. Mahmud, N.; Klipa, D.; Ahsan, N. Antibody immunosuppressive therapy in solid-organ transplant: Part, I. *MAbs* **2010**, *2*, 148–156. [CrossRef] [PubMed]
75. Bustami, R.T.; Ojo, A.O.; Wolfe, R.A.; Merion, R.M.; Bennett, W.M.; McDiarmid, S.V.; Leichtman, A.B.; Held, P.J.; Port, F.K. Immunosuppression and the risk of post-transplant malignancy among cadaveric first kidney transplant recipients. *Am. J. Transplant.* **2004**, *4*, 87–93. [CrossRef] [PubMed]
76. Kim, A.P.; Baker, D.E. Daclizumab. *Hosp. Pharm.* **2016**, *51*, 928–939. [CrossRef] [PubMed]
77. Jew, O.S.; Liu, W.W.; Stamey, C.; Kheterpal, M.; Myers, S.A.; Ellis, M.J.; Byrns, J.; Wheless, L.; Whitley, M.J. De novo belatacept does not reduce the rate of skin cancer in renal transplant recipients compared to standard therapy. *J. Am. Acad. Dermatol.* **2024**, *91*, 720–722. [CrossRef] [PubMed]
78. Nalesnik, M.A.; Jaffe, R.; Starzl, T.E.; Demetris, A.J.; Porter, K.; Burnham, J.A.; Makowka, L.; Ho, M.; Locker, J. The pathology of posttransplant lymphoproliferative disorders occurring in the setting of cyclosporine A-prednisone immunosuppression. *Am. J. Pathol.* **1988**, *133*, 173–192. [PubMed]
79. Hoshida, Y.; Aozasa, K. Malignancies in organ transplant recipients. *Pathol. Int.* **2004**, *54*, 649–658. [CrossRef] [PubMed]

80. Hoshida, Y.; Li, T.; Dong, Z.; Tomita, Y.; Yamauchi, A.; Hanai, J.; Aozasa, K. Lymphoproliferative disorders in renal transplant patients in Japan. *Int. J. Cancer* **2001**, *91*, 869–875. [CrossRef] [PubMed]
81. Ghobrial, I.M.; Habermann, T.M.; Maurer, M.J.; Geyer, S.M.; Ristow, K.M.; Larson, T.S.; Walker, R.C.; Ansell, S.M.; Macon, W.R.; Gores, G.G.; et al. Prognostic analysis for survival in adult solid organ transplant recipients with post-transplantation lymphoproliferative disorders. *J. Clin. Oncol.* **2005**, *23*, 7574–7582. [CrossRef] [PubMed]
82. Naresh, K.N.; Bhaget, G.; Bower, M.; Chadburn, A.; Chan, J.K.C.; Dierickx, D.; Gratzinger, D.; Michelow, P.; Natkunam, Y.; Sato, Y.; et al. Lymphomas arising in immune deficiency/dysregulation. In *WHO Classification of Tumours Editorial Board. Haematolymphoid Tumoures*, 5th ed.; The WHO Classification of Tumours Editorial Board, Ed.; IARC: Lyon, France, 2024; pp. 568–572.
83. Hoover, R.; Fraumeni, J.F., Jr. Risk of cancer in renal-transplant recipients. *Lancet* **1973**, *2*, 55–57. [CrossRef] [PubMed]
84. Grinyó, J.; Charpentier, B.; Pestana, J.M.; Vanrenterghem, Y.; Vincenti, F.; Reyes-Acevedo, R.; Apanovitch, A.M.; Gujrathi, S.; Agarwal, M.; Thomas, D.; et al. An integrated safety profile analysis of belatacept in kidney transplant recipients. *Transplantation* **2010**, *90*, 1521–1527. [CrossRef] [PubMed]
85. Vincenti, F.; Charpentier, B.; Vanrenterghem, Y.; Rostaing, L.; Bresnahan, B.; Darji, P.; Massari, P.; Mondragon-Ramirez, G.A.; Agarwal, M.; Di Russo, G.; et al. A phase III study of belatacept-based immunosuppression regimens versus cyclosporine in renal transplant recipients (BENEFIT study). *Am. J. Transplant.* **2010**, *10*, 535–546. [CrossRef] [PubMed]
86. Jain, A.; Nalesnik, M.; Reyes, J.; Pokharna, R.; Mazariegos, G.; Green, M.; Eghtesad, B.; Marsh, W.; Cacciarelli, T.; Fontes, P.; et al. Posttransplant lymphoproliferative disorders in liver transplantation: A 20-year experience. *Ann. Surg.* **2002**, *236*, 429–436. [CrossRef] [PubMed]
87. Fernberg, P.; Edgren, G.; Adami, J.; Ingvar, A.; Bellocco, R.; Tufveson, G.; Höglund, P.; Kinch, A.; Simard, J.F.; Baecklund, E.; et al. Time trends in risk and risk determinants of non-Hodgkin lymphoma in solid organ transplant recipients. *Am. J. Transplant.* **2011**, *11*, 2472–2482. [CrossRef] [PubMed]
88. Cox, K.L.; Lawrence-Miyasaki, L.S.; Garcia-Kennedy, R.; Lennette, E.T.; Martinez, O.M.; Krams, S.M.; Berquist, W.E.; So, S.K.; Esquivel, C.O. An increased incidence of Epstein-Barr virus infection and lymphoproliferative disorder in young children on FK506 after liver transplantation. *Transplantation* **1995**, *59*, 524–529. [CrossRef] [PubMed]
89. Narkewicz, M.R.; Green, M.; Dunn, S.; Millis, M.; McDiarmid, S.; Mazariegos, G.; Anand, R.; Yin, W. Studies of Pediatric Liver Transplantation Research Group. Decreasing incidence of symptomatic Epstein-Barr virus disease and posttransplant lymphoproliferative disorder in pediatric liver transplant recipients: Report of the studies of pediatric liver transplantation experience. *Liver Transpl.* **2013**, *19*, 730–740. [PubMed]
90. Holmes, R.D.; Sokol, R.J. Epstein-Barr virus and post-transplant lymphoproliferative disease. *Pediatr. Transplant.* **2002**, *6*, 456–464. [CrossRef] [PubMed]
91. Reding, R.; Wallemacq, P.E.; Lamy, M.E.; Rahier, J.; Sempoux, C.; Debande, B.; Jamart, J.; Barker, A.; Sokal, E.; De Ville de Goyet, J.; et al. Conversion from cyclosporine to FK506 for salvage of immunocompromised pediatric liver allografts. Efficacy, toxicity, and dose regimen in 23 children. *Transplantation* **1994**, *57*, 93–100. [CrossRef] [PubMed]
92. Tsai, D.E.; Bagley, S.; Reshef, R.; Shaked, A.; Bloom, R.D.; Ahya, V.; Goldberg, L.; Chung, A.; Debonera, F.; Schuster, S.J.; et al. The changing face of adult posttrasplant lymphoproliferative disorders: Changes in history between 1999 and 2013. *Am. J. Hematol.* **2018**, *93*, 874–881. [CrossRef] [PubMed]
93. Nelson, B.P.; Nalesnik, M.A.; Bahler, D.W.; Locker, J.; Fung, J.J.; Swerdlow, S.H. Epstein-Barr virus-negative post-transplant lymphoproliferative disorders: A distinct entity? *Am. J. Surg. Pathol.* **2000**, *24*, 375–385. [CrossRef] [PubMed]
94. Ferreiro, J.F.; Morscio, J.; Dierickx, D.; Vandenberghe, P.; Gheysens, O.; Verhoef, G.; Zamani, M.; Tousseyn, T.; Wlodarska, I. EBV-Positive and EBV-Negative Posttransplant Diffuse Large B Cell Lymphomas Have Distinct Genomic and Transcriptomic Features. *Am. J. Transplant.* **2016**, *16*, 414–425. [CrossRef] [PubMed]
95. Luskin, M.R.; Heil, D.S.; Tan, K.S.; Choi, S.; Stadtmauer, E.A.; Schuster, S.J.; Porter, D.L.; Vonderheide, R.H.; Bagg, A.; Heitjan, D.F.; et al. The Impact of EBV Status on Characteristics and Outcomes of Posttransplantation Lymphoproliferative Disorder. *Am. J. Transplant.* **2015**, *15*, 2665–2673. [CrossRef] [PubMed]
96. Leblond, V.; Davi, F.; Charlotte, F.; Dorent, R.; Bitker, M.O.; Sutton, L.; Gandjbakhch, I.; Binet, J.L.; Raphael, M. Posttransplant lymphoproliferative disorders not associated with Epstein-Barr virus: A distinct entity? *J. Clin. Oncol.* **1998**, *16*, 2052–2059. [CrossRef] [PubMed]
97. Jang, S.; Kwon, E.J.; Lee, J.J. Rheumatoid arthritis: Pathogenic roles of diverse immune cells. *Int. J. Mol. Sci.* **2022**, *23*, 905. [CrossRef] [PubMed]
98. McInnes, I.B.; Schett, G. The pathogenesis of rheumatoid arthritis. *N. Engl. J. Med.* **2011**, *365*, 2205–2219. [CrossRef] [PubMed]
99. Smitten, A.L.; Simon, T.A.; Hochberg, M.C.; Suissa, S. A meta-analysis of the incidence of malignancy in adult patients with rheumatoid arthritis. *Arthritis Res. Ther.* **2008**, *10*, R45. [CrossRef] [PubMed]
100. Huang, W.K.; Chiou, M.J.; Kuo, C.F.; Lin, Y.C.; Yu, K.H.; See, L.C. No overall increased risk of cancer in patients with rheumatoid arthritis: A nationwide dynamic cohort study in Taiwan. *Rheumatol. Int.* **2014**, *34*, 1379–1386. [CrossRef] [PubMed]

101. Beydon, M.; Pinto, S.; De Rycke, Y.; Fautrel, B.; Mariette, X.; Seror, R.; Tubach, F. Risk of cancer for patients with rheumatoid arthritis versus general population: A national claims database cohort study. *Lancet Reg. Health Eur.* **2023**, *35*, 100768. [CrossRef] [PubMed]
102. Simon, T.A.; Thompson, A.; Gandhi, K.K.; Hochberg, M.C.; Suissa, S. Incidence of malignancy in adult patients with rheumatoid arthritis: A meta-analysis. *Arthritis Res. Ther.* **2015**, *17*, 212. [CrossRef] [PubMed]
103. Sugimoto, N.; Tanaka, E.; Inoue, E.; Abe, M.; Sugano, E.; Sugitani, N.; Saka, K.; Ochiai, M.; Higuchi, Y.; Yamaguchi, R.; et al. Trends in risks of malignancies in Japanese patients with rheumatoid arthritis: Analyses from a 14-year observation of the IORRA cohort. *Mod. Rheumatol.* **2023**, *33*, 715–722. [CrossRef] [PubMed]
104. Yamada, T.; Nakajima, A.; Inoue, E.; Tanaka, E.; Taniguchi, A.; Momohara, S.; Yamanaka, H. Incidence of malignancy in Japanese patients with rheumatoid arthritis. *Rheumatol. Int.* **2011**, *31*, 1487–1492. [CrossRef] [PubMed]
105. Hemminki, K.; Li, X.; Sundquist, K.; Sundquist, J. Cancer risk in hospitalized rheumatoid arthritis patients. *Rheumatology* **2008**, *47*, 698–701. [CrossRef] [PubMed]
106. Ramadan, S.M.; Fouad, T.M.; Summa, V.; Hasan, S.K.h.; Lo-Coco, F. Acute myeloid leukemia developing in patients with autoimmune diseases. *Haematologica* **2012**, *97*, 805–817. [CrossRef] [PubMed]
107. Mercer, L.K.; Green, A.C.; Galloway, J.B.; Davies, R.; Lunt, M.; Dixon, W.G.; Watson, K.D.; British Society for Rheumatology Biologics Register Control Centre Consortium; Symmons, D.P.M.; Hyrich, K.L.; et al. The influence of anti-TNF therapy upon incidence of keratinocyte skin cancer in patients with rheumatoid arthritis: Longitudinal results from the British Society for Rheumatology Biologics Register. *Ann. Rheum. Dis.* **2012**, *71*, 869–874. [CrossRef] [PubMed]
108. Chakravarty, E.F.; Michaud, K.; Wolfe, F. Skin cancer, rheumatoid arthritis, and tumor necrosis factor inhibitors. *J. Rheumatol.* **2005**, *32*, 2130–2135. [PubMed]
109. Mercer, L.K.; Davies, R.; Galloway, J.B.; Low, A.; Lunt, M.; Dixon, W.G.; Watson, K.D.; Symmons, D.P.; Hyrich, K.L.; The British Society for Rheumatology Biologics Register (BSRBR) Control Centre Consortium. Risk of cancer in patients receiving non-biologic disease-modifying therapy for rheumatoid arthritis compared with the UK general population. *Rheumatology* **2013**, *52*, 91–98. [CrossRef] [PubMed]
110. Edmunds, J.J. Anti-Inflammatory and Immunomodulatory Drugs. In *Drug Discovery, Practives, Processes, and Perspectives*; Li, J.J., Corey, E.J., Eds.; John Wiley & Sons Inc.: Hoboken, NJ, USA, 2013; pp. 337–388.
111. Wang, D.; Dubois, R.N. Eicosanoids and cancer. *Nat. Rev. Cancer* **2010**, *10*, 181–193. [CrossRef] [PubMed]
112. Rostom, A.; Dubé, C.; Lewin, G.; Tsertsvadze, A.; Barrowman, N.; Code, C.; Sampson, M.; Moher, D. US Preventive Services Task Force. Nonsteroidal anti-inflammatory drugs and cyclooxygenase-2 inhibitors for primary prevention of colorectal cancer: A systematic review prepared for the U.S. Preventive Services Task Force. *Ann. Intern. Med.* **2007**, *146*, 376–389. [CrossRef] [PubMed]
113. Harris, R.E. Cyclooxygenase-2 (cox-2) blockade in the chemoprevention of cancers of the colon, breast, prostate, and lung. *Inflammopharmacology* **2009**, *17*, 55–67. [CrossRef] [PubMed]
114. Honda, S.; Sakai, R.; Inoue, E.; Majima, M.; Konda, N.; Takada, H.; Kihara, M.; Yajima, N.; Nanki, T.; Yamamoto, K.; et al. Association of methotrexate use and lymphoproliferative disorder in patients with rheumatoid arthritis: Results from a Japanese multi-institutional retrospective study. *Mod. Rheumatol.* **2022**, *32*, 16–23. [CrossRef] [PubMed]
115. Kauppi, M.; Pukkala, E.; Isomäki, H. Low incidence of colorectal cancer in patients with rheumatoid arthritis. *Clin. Exp. Rheumatol.* **1996**, *14*, 551–553. [PubMed]
116. Wessels, J.A.; Huizinga, T.W.; Guchelaar, H.J. Recent insights in the pharmacologicalactions of methotrexate in the treatment of rheumatoid arthritis. *Rheumatology* **2008**, *47*, 249–255. [CrossRef] [PubMed]
117. Feng, W.H.; Cohen, J.I.; Fischer, S.; Li, L.; Sneller, M.; Goldbach-Mansky RvRaab-Traub, N.; Delecluse, H.J.; Kenney, S.C. Reactivation of latent Epstein–Barr virus by methotrexate. A potential contributor to methotrexate-associated lymphomas. *J. Natl. Cancer Inst.* **2004**, *96*, 1691–1702. [CrossRef] [PubMed]
118. Wolfe, F.; Michaud, K. Lymphoma in rheumatoid arthritis: The effect of methotrexate and anti-tumor necrosis factor therapy in 18,572 patients. *Arthritis Rheum.* **2004**, *50*, 1740–1751. [CrossRef] [PubMed]
119. Wolfe, F.; Michaud, K. Biologic treatment of rheumatoid arthritis and the risk of malignancy: Analyses from a large US observational study. *Arthritis Rheum.* **2007**, *56*, 2886–2895. [CrossRef] [PubMed]
120. Mariette, X.; Cazals-Hatem, D.; Warszawki, J.; Liote, F.; Balandraud, N.; Sibilia, J. Investigators of the Club Rhumatismes et Inflammation. Lymphomas in rheumatoid arthritis patients treated with methotrexate: A 3-year prospective study in France. *Blood* **2002**, *99*, 3909–3915. [CrossRef] [PubMed]
121. Franklin, J.; Lunt, M.; Bunn, D.; Symmons, D.; Silman, A. Incidence of lymphoma in a large primary care derived cohort of cases of inflammatory polyarthritis. *Ann. Rheum. Dis.* **2006**, *65*, 617–622. [CrossRef] [PubMed]

122. Hoshida, Y.; Ohshima, S.; Saeki, Y.; Katayama, M.; Miyamura, T.; Hashimoto, A.; Higa, S.; Oshima, H.; Yagita, M.; Hiramatsu, Y.; et al. Multi-center analyses on 518 cases with rheumatoid arthritis developing lymphoproliferative disorders (RA-LPD): The prognostic factors and the influence of anti-rheumatic drugs on LPD development. *Arthritis Rheumatol.* **2019**, *71* (Suppl. S10), 2364, (abstract).
123. Balkwill, F. Tumour necrosis factor and cancer. *Nat. Rev. Cancer* **2009**, *9*, 361–371. [CrossRef] [PubMed]
124. Mercer, L.K.; Lunt, M.; Low, A.L.; Dixon, W.G.; Watson, K.D.; Symmons, D.P.; Hyrich, K.L. BSRBR Control Centre Consortium. Risk of solid cancer in patients exposed to anti-tumour necrosis factor therapy: Results from the British Society for Rheumatology Biologics Register for Rheumatoid Arthritis. *Ann. Rheum. Dis.* **2015**, *74*, 1087–1093. [CrossRef] [PubMed]
125. Mercer, L.K.; Galloway, J.B.; Lunt, M.; Davies, R.; Low, A.L.; Dixon, W.G.; Watson, K.D.; Symmons, D.P.; Hyrich, K.L.; BSRBR Control Centre Consortium. Risk of lymphoma in patients exposed to antitumour necrosis factor therapy: Results from the British Society for Rheumatology Biologics Register for Rheumatoid Arthritis. *Ann Rheum Dis.* **2017**, *76*, 497–503. [CrossRef] [PubMed]
126. Askling, J.; van Vollenhoven, R.F.; Granath, F.; Raaschou, P.; Fored, C.M.; Baecklund, E.; Dackhammar, C.; Feltelius, N.; Cöster, L.; Geborek, P.; et al. Cancer risk in patients with rheumatoid arthritis treated with anti-tumor necrosis factor alpha therapies: Does the risk change with the time since start of treatment? *Arthritis Rheum.* **2009**, *60*, 3180–3189. [CrossRef] [PubMed]
127. Thompson, A.E.; Rieder, S.W.; Pope, J.E. Tumor necrosis factor therapy and the risk of serious infection and malignancy in patients with early rheumatoid arthritis: A meta-analysis of randomized controlled trials. *Arthritis Rheum.* **2011**, *63*, 1479–1485. [CrossRef] [PubMed]
128. Lopez-Olivo, M.A.; Tayar, J.H.; Martinez-Lopez, J.A.; Pollono, E.N.; Cueto, J.P.; Gonzales-Crespo, M.R.; Fulton, S.; Suarez-Almazor, M.E. Risk of malignancies in patients with rheumatoid arthritis treated with biologic therapy: A meta-analysis. *JAMA* **2012**, *308*, 898–908. [CrossRef] [PubMed]
129. Askling, J.; Fored, C.M.; Baecklund, E.; Brandt, L.; Backlin, C.; Ekbom, A.; Sundström, C.; Bertilsson, L.; Cöster, L.; Geborek, P.; et al. Haematopoietic malignancies in rheumatoid arthritis: Lymphoma risk and characteristics after exposure to tumour necrosis factor antagonists. *Ann. Rheum. Dis.* **2005**, *64*, 1414–1420. [CrossRef] [PubMed]
130. Hellgren, K.; Di Giuseppe, D.; Smedby, K.E.; Sundström, C.; Askling, J.; Baecklund, E.; ARTIS study group. Lymphoma risks in patients with rheumatoid arthritis treated with biological drugs-a Swedish cohort study of risks by time, drug and lymphoma subtype. *Rheumatology* **2021**, *60*, 809–819. [CrossRef] [PubMed]
131. Dreyer, L.; Mellemkjær, L.; Andersen, A.R.; Bennett, P.; Poulsen, U.E.; Ellingsen, T.J.; Hansen, T.H.; Jensen, D.V.; Linde, L.; Lindegaard, H.M.; et al. Incidences of overall and site specific cancers in TNFα inhibitor treated patients with rheumatoid arthritis and other arthritides—A follow-up study from the DANBIO Registry. *Ann. Rheum. Dis.* **2013**, *72*, 79–82. [CrossRef] [PubMed]
132. Mariette, X.; Tubach, F.; Bagheri, H.; Bardet, M.; Berthelot, J.M.; Gaudin, P.; Heresbach, D.; Martin, A.; Schaeverbeke, T.; Salmon, D.; et al. Lymphoma in patients treated with anti-TNF: Results of the 3-year prospective French RATIO registry. *Ann. Rheum. Dis.* **2010**, *69*, 400–408. [CrossRef] [PubMed]
133. Mariette, X.; Matucci-Cerinic, M.; Pavelka, K.; Taylor, P.; van Vollenhoven, R.; Heatley, R.; Walsh, C.; Lawson, R.; Reynolds, A.; Emery, P. Malignancies associated with tumour necrosis factor inhibitors in registries and prospective observational studies: A systematic review and meta-analysis. *Ann. Rheum. Dis.* **2011**, *70*, 1895–1904. [CrossRef] [PubMed]
134. Dommasch, E.D.; Abuabara, K.; Shin, D.B.; Nguyen, J.; Troxel, A.B.; Gelfand, J.M. The risk of infection and malignancy with tumor necrosis factor antagonists in adults with psoriatic disease: A systematic review and meta-analysis of randomized controlled trials. *J. Am. Acad. Dermatol.* **2011**, *64*, 1035–1050. [CrossRef] [PubMed]
135. Askling, J.; Baecklund, E.; Granath, F.; Geborek, P.; Fored, M.; Backlin, C.; Bertilsson, L.; Cöster, L.; Jacobsson, L.T.; Lindblad, S.; et al. Anti-tumour necrosis factor therapy in rheumatoid arthritis and risk of malignant lymphomas: Relative risks and time trends in the Swedish Biologics Register. *Ann. Rheum. Dis.* **2009**, *68*, 648–653. [CrossRef] [PubMed]
136. Huss, V.; Bower, H.; Wadström, H.; Frisell, T.; Askling, J. ARTIS group. Short- and longer-term cancer risks with biologic and targeted synthetic disease-modifying antirheumatic drugs as used against rheumatoid arthritis in clinical practice. *Rheumatology* **2022**, *61*, 1810–1818. [CrossRef] [PubMed]
137. Bongartz, T.; Sutton, A.J.; Sweeting, M.J.; Buchan, I.; Matteson, E.L.; Montori, V. Anti-TNF antibody therapy in rheumatoid arthritis and the risk of serious infections and malignancies: Systematic review and meta-analysis of rare harmful effects in randomized controlled trials. *JAMA* **2006**, *295*, 2275–2285. [CrossRef] [PubMed]
138. Solomon, D.H.; Kremer, J.M.; Fisher, M.; Curtis, J.R.; Furer, V.; Harrold, L.R.; Hochberg, M.C.; Reed, G.; Tsao, P.; Greenberg, J.D. Comparative cancer risk associated with methotrexate, other non-biologic and biologic disease-modifying anti-rheumatic drugs. *Semin. Arthritis Rheum.* **2014**, *43*, 489–497. [CrossRef] [PubMed]
139. Geborek, P.; Bladström, A.; Turesson, C.; Gulfe, A.; Petersson, I.F.; Saxne, T.; Olsson, H.; Jacobsson, L.T. Tumour necrosis factor blockers do not increase overall tumour risk in patients with rheumatoid arthritis, but may be associated with an increased risk of lymphomas. *Ann. Rheum. Dis.* **2005**, *64*, 699–703. [CrossRef] [PubMed]

140. Askling, J.; Fahrbach, K.; Nordstrom, B.; Ross, S.; Schmid, C.H.; Symmons, D. Cancer risk with tumor necrosis factor alpha (TNF) inhibitors: Meta-analysis of randomized controlled trials of adalimumab, etanercept, and infliximab using patient level data. *Pharmacoepidemiol. Drug Saf.* **2011**, *20*, 119–130. [CrossRef] [PubMed]
141. Raaschou, P.; Simard, J.F.; Holmqvist, M.; Askling, J. ARTISStudy Group Rheumatoid arthritis anti-tumour necrosis factor therapy risk of malignant melanoma: Nationwide population based prospective cohort study from Sweden. *BMJ* **2013**, *346*, f1939. [CrossRef] [PubMed]
142. McLaughlin, P.; Grillo-López, A.J.; Link, B.K.; Levy, R.; Czuczman, M.S.; Williams, M.E.; Heyman, M.R.; Bence-Bruckler, I.; White, C.A.; Cabanillas, F.; et al. Rituximab chimeric anti-CD20 monoclonal antibody therapy for relapsed indolent lymphoma: Half of patients respond to a four-dose treatment program. *J. Clin. Oncol.* **1998**, *16*, 2825–2833. [CrossRef] [PubMed]
143. Finn, O.J. Cancer immunology. *N. Engl. J. Med.* **2008**, *358*, 2704–2715. [CrossRef] [PubMed]
144. Tao, L.; Clarke, C.A.; Rosenberg, A.S.; Advani, R.H.; Jonas, B.A.; Flowers, C.R.; Keegan, T.H.M. Subsequent primary malignancies after diffuse large B-cell lymphoma in the modern treatment era. *Br. J. Haematol.* **2017**, *178*, 72–80. [CrossRef] [PubMed]
145. Fleury, I.; Chevret, S.; Pfreundschuh, M.; Salles, G.; Coiffier, B.; van Oers, M.H.; Gisselbrecht, C.; Zucca, E.; Herold, M.; Ghielmini, M.; et al. Rituximab and risk of second primary malignancies in patients with non-Hodgkin lymphoma: A systematic review and meta-analysis. *Ann. Oncol.* **2016**, *27*, 390–397. [CrossRef] [PubMed]
146. Montastruc, F.; Renoux, C.; Dell'Aniello, S.; Simon, T.A.; Azoulay, L.; Hudson, M.; Suissa, S. Abatacept initiation in rheumatoid arthritis and the risk of cancer: A population-based comparative cohort study. *Rheumatology* **2019**, *58*, 683–691. [CrossRef] [PubMed]
147. de Germay, S.; Bagheri, H.; Despas, F.; Rousseau, V.; Montastruc, F. Abatacept in rheumatoid arthritis and the risk of cancer: A world observational post-marketing study. *Rheumatology* **2020**, *59*, 2360–2367. [CrossRef] [PubMed]
148. Wadström, H.; Frisell, T.; Askling, J. Anti-Rheumatic Therapy in Sweden (ARTIS) Study Group. Malignant neoplasms in patients with rheumatoid arthritis treated with tumor necrosis factor inhibitors, tocilizumab, abatacept, or rituximab in clinical practice: A nationwide cohort study from Sweden. *JAMA Intern. Med.* **2017**, *177*, 1605–1612. [CrossRef] [PubMed]
149. Kim, S.C.; Pawar, A.; Desai, R.J.; Solomon, D.H.; Gale, S.; Bao, M.; Sarsour, K.; Schneeweiss, S. Risk of malignancy associated with use of tocilizumab versus other biologics in patients with rheumatoid arthritis: A multi-database cohort study. *Semin. Arthritis Rheum.* **2019**, *49*, 222–228. [CrossRef] [PubMed]
150. Ozen, G.; Pedro, S.; Schumacher, R.; Simon, T.A.; Michaud, K. Safety of abatacept compared with other biologic and conventional synthetic disease-modifying antirheumatic drugs in patients with rheumatoid arthritis: Data from an observational study. *Arthritis Res. Ther.* **2019**, *21*, 141. [CrossRef] [PubMed]
151. Tokunaga, K.; Matsui, K.; Oshikawa, H.; Matsui, T.; Tohma, S. Risk of serious infection, malignancy, or death in Japanese rheumatoid arthritis patients treated with a combination of abatacept and tacrolimus: A retrospective cohort study. *Clin. Rheumatol.* **2021**, *40*, 1811–1817. [CrossRef] [PubMed]
152. Simon, T.A.; Smitten, A.L.; Franklin, J.; Askling, J.; Lacaille, D.; Wolfe, F.; Hochberg, M.C.; Qi, K.; Suissa, S. Malignancies in the rheumatoid arthritis abatacept clinical development programme: An epidemiological assessment. *Ann. Rheum. Dis.* **2009**, *68*, 1819–1826. [CrossRef] [PubMed]
153. Wolchok, J.D.; Chiarion-Sileni, V.; Rutkowski, P.; Cowey, C.L.; Schadendorf, D.; Wagstaff, J.; Queirolo, P.; Dummer, R.; Butler, M.O.; Hill, A.G.; et al. Final, 10-year outcomes with Nivolumab plus Ipilimumab in advanced melanoma. *N. Engl. J. Med.* **2025**, *392*, 11–22. [CrossRef] [PubMed]
154. Sato, K.; Tsuchiya, M.; Saldanha, J.; Koishihara, Y.; Ohsugi, Y.; Kishimoto, T.; Bendig, M.M. Reshaping a human antibody to inhibit the interleukin 6-dependent tumor cell growth. *Cancer Res.* **1993**, *53*, 51–56.
155. Soler, M.F.; Abaurrea, A.; Azcoaga, P.; Araujo, A.M.; Caffarel, M.M. New perspectives in cancer immunotherapy: Targeting IL-6 cytokine family. *J. Immunother. Cancer* **2023**, *11*, e007530. [CrossRef] [PubMed]
156. Morel, J.; Wetzman, A.; Wendling, D.; Soubrier, M.; Hoang, S.; Briançon, D.; Roth, O.; Goupille, P.; Gottenberg, J.E.; Mariette, X.; et al. Risk of cancer in patients with rheumatoid arthritis under tocilizumab: Data from the French national registry REGATE. *Jt. Bone Spine* **2025**, *92*, 105900. [CrossRef] [PubMed]
157. Rubbert-Roth, A.; Sebba, A.; Brockwell, L.; Kelman, A.; Porter-Brown, B.; Pulley, J.; Napalkov, P.; van Vollenhoven, R.F. Malignancy rates in patients with rheumatoid arthritis treated with tocilizumab. *RMD Open.* **2016**, *2*, e000213. [CrossRef] [PubMed]
158. Buchert, M.; Burns, C.J.; Ernst, M. Targeting JAK kinase in solid tumors: Emerging opportunities and challenges. *Oncogene* **2016**, *35*, 939–951. [CrossRef] [PubMed]
159. Sonbol, M.B.; Firwana, B.; Zarzour, A.; Morad, M.; Rana, V.; Tiu, R.V. Comprehensive review of JAK inhibitors in myeloproliferative neoplasms. *Ther. Adv. Hematol.* **2013**, *4*, 15–35. [CrossRef] [PubMed]
160. Harrison, C.; Kiladjian, J.J.; Al-Ali, H.K.; Gisslinger, H.; Waltzman, R.; Stalbovskaya, V.; McQuitty, M.; Hunter, D.S.; Levy, R.; Knoops, L.; et al. JAK inhibition with ruxolitinib versus best available therapy for myelofibrosis. *N. Engl. J. Med.* **2012**, *366*, 787–798. [CrossRef] [PubMed]

161. O'Shea, J.J.; Schwartz, D.M.; Villarino, A.V.; Gadina, M.; McInnes, I.B.; Laurence, A. The JAK-STAT pathway: Impact on human disease and therapeutic intervention. *Annu. Rev. Med.* **2015**, *66*, 311–328. [CrossRef] [PubMed]
162. Yoshida, S.; Miyata, M.; Suzuki, E.; Kanno, T.; Sumichika, Y.; Saito, K.; Matsumoto, H.; Temmoku, J.; Fujita, Y.; Matsuoka, N.; et al. Safety of JAK and IL-6 inhibitors in patients with rheumatoid arthritis: A multicenter cohort study. *Front. Immunol.* **2023**, *14*, 1267749. [CrossRef] [PubMed]
163. Huss, V.; Bower, H.; Hellgren, K.; Frisell, T.; Askling, J.; Ahlenius, G.M.; Baecklund, E.; Chatzidionysiou, K.; Feltelius, N.; Forsblad-d'Elia, H.; et al. Cancer risks with JAKi and biological disease-modifying antirheumatic drugs in patients with rheumatoid arthritis or psoriatic arthritis: A national real-world cohort study. *Ann. Rheum. Dis.* **2023**, *82*, 911–919. [CrossRef] [PubMed]
164. Genovese, M.C.; Smolen, J.S.; Takeuchi, T.; Burmester, G.; Brinker, D.; Rooney, T.P.; Zhong, J.; Daojun, M.; Saifan, C.; Cardoso, A.; et al. Safety profile of baricitinib for the treatment of rheumatoid arthritis over a median of 3 years of treatment: An updated integrated safety analysis. *Lancet Rheumatol.* **2020**, *2*, e347–e357. [CrossRef] [PubMed]
165. Mok, C.C.; So, H.; Yim, C.W.; To, C.H.; Lao, W.N.; Wong, S.P.Y.; Ng, H.Y.; Lee, J.M.Y.; Lee, P.M.L.; Ying, S.K.Y.; et al. Safety of the JAK and TNF inhibitors in rheumatoid arthritis: Real world data from the Hong Kong Biologics Registry. *Rheumatology* **2024**, *63*, 358–365. [CrossRef] [PubMed]
166. Cohen, S.B.; van Vollenhoven, R.F.; Winthrop, K.L.; Zerbini, C.A.F.; Tanaka, Y.; Bessette, L.; Zhang, Y.; Khan, N.; Hendrickson, B.; Enejosa, J.V.; et al. Safety profile of upadacitinib in rheumatoid arthritis: Integrated analysis from the SELECT phase III clinical programme. *Ann. Rheum. Dis.* **2021**, *80*, 304–311. [CrossRef] [PubMed]
167. Cohen, S.B.; Tanaka, Y.; Mariette, X.; Curtis, J.R.; Lee, E.B.; Nash, P.; Winthrop, K.L.; Charles-Schoeman, C.; Thirunavukkarasu, K.; DeMasi, R.; et al. Long-term safety of tofacitinib for the treatment of rheumatoid arthritis up to 8.5 years: Integrated analysis of data from the global clinical trials. *Ann. Rheum. Dis.* **2017**, *76*, 1253–1262. [CrossRef] [PubMed]
168. Kremer, J.M.; Bingham, C.O., III; Cappelli, L.C.; Greenberg, J.D.; Madsen, A.M.; Geier, J.; Rivas, J.L.; Onofrei, A.M.; Barr, C.J.; Pappas, D.A.; et al. Postapproval comparative safety study of Tofacitinib and biological disease-modifying antirheumatic drugs: 5-year results from a United States-based rheumatoid arthritis registry. *ACR Open Rheumatol.* **2021**, *3*, 173–184. [CrossRef] [PubMed]
169. Ytterberg, S.R.; Bhatt, D.L.; Mikuls, T.R.; Koch, G.G.; Fleischmann, R.; Rivas, J.L.; Germino, R.; Menon, S.; Sun, Y.; Wang, C.; et al. Cardiovascular and cancer risk with Tofacitinib in rheumatoid arthritis. *N. Engl. J. Med.* **2022**, *386*, 316–326. [CrossRef] [PubMed]
170. Bezzio, C.; Vernero, M.; Ribaldone, D.G.; Alimenti, E.; Manes, G.; Saibeni, S. Cancer Risk in Patients Treated with the JAK Inhibitor Tofacitinib: Systematic Review and Meta-Analysis. *Cancers* **2023**, *15*, 2197. [CrossRef] [PubMed]
171. Khosrow-Khavar, F.; Desai, R.J.; Lee, H.; Lee, S.B.; Kim, S.C. Tofacitinib and risk of malignancy: Results from the safety of Tofacitinib in routine care patients with rheumatoid arthritis (STAR-RA) study. *Arthritis Rheumatol.* **2022**, *74*, 1648–1659. [CrossRef] [PubMed]
172. Russell, M.D.; Stovin, C.; Alveyn, E.; Adeyemi, O.; Chan, C.K.D.; Patel, V.; Adas, M.A.; Atzeni, F.; Ng, K.K.H.; Rutherford, A.I.; et al. JAK inhibitors and the risk of malignancy: A meta-analysis across disease indications. *Ann. Rheum. Dis.* **2023**, *82*, 1059–1067. [CrossRef] [PubMed]
173. Kuwana, M.; Sugiyama, N.; Momohara, S.; Atsumi, T.; Takei, S.; Tamura, N.; Harigai, M.; Fujii, T.; Matsuno, H.; Takeuchi, T.; et al. Six-month safety and effectiveness of tofacitinib in patients with rheumatoid arthritis in Japan: Interim analysis of post-marketing surveillance. *Mod. Rheumatol.* **2024**, *34*, 272–286. [CrossRef] [PubMed]
174. Schaefer, M.; Purschke, A.; Zietemann, V.; Rudi, T.; Meissner, Y.; Richter, A.; Berger, S.; Rockwitz, K.; Krüger, K.; Schneider, K.M.; et al. Comparative risk of incident malignancies in rheumatoid arthritis patients treated with Janus kinase inhibitors or bDMARDs: Observational data from the German RABBIT register. *Ann. Rheum. Dis.* **2025**, *Epub ahead of print*. [CrossRef] [PubMed]
175. Curtis, J.R.; Yamaoka, K.; Chen, Y.H.; Bhatt, D.L.; Gunay, L.M.; Sugiyama, N.; Connell, C.A.; Wang, C.; Wu, J.; Menon, S.; et al. Malignancy risk with tofacitinib versus TNF inhibitors in rheumatoid arthritis: Results from the open-label, randomised controlled ORAL Surveillance trial. *Ann. Rheum. Dis.* **2023**, *82*, 331–343. [CrossRef] [PubMed]
176. Llorca, J.; Lopez-Diaz, M.J.; Gonzalez-Juanatey, C.; Ollier, W.E.; Martin, J.; Gonzalez-Gay, M.A. Persistent chronic inflammation contributes to the development of cancer in patients with rheumatoid arthritis from a defined population of northwestern Spain. *Semin. Arthritis Rheum.* **2007**, *7*, 31–38. [CrossRef] [PubMed]
177. Kamel, O.W.; van de Rijn, M.; Weiss, L.M.; Zoppo, G.J.D.; Hench, P.K.; Robbins, B.A.; Montgomery, P.G.; Warnke, R.A.; Dorfman, R.F. Brief report: Reversible lymphomas associated with Epstein-Barr virus occurring during therapy for rheumatoid arthritis and dermatomyositis. *N. Engl. J. Med.* **1993**, *328*, 1317–1321. [CrossRef] [PubMed]
178. Harigai, M. Lymphoproliferative disorders in patients with rheumatoid arthritis in the era of widespread use of methotrexate: A review of the literature and current perspective. *Mod. Rheumatol.* **2018**, *28*, 1–8. [CrossRef] [PubMed]
179. Hoshida, Y.; Xu, J.X.; Fujita, S.; Nakamichi, I.; Ikeda, J.; Tomita, Y.; Nakatsuka, S.; Tamaru, J.; Iizuka, A.; Takeuchi, T.; et al. Lymphoproliferative disorders in rheumatoid arthritis: Clinicopathological analysis of 76 cases in relation to methotrexate medication. *J. Rheumatol.* **2007**, *34*, 322–331. [PubMed]

180. Salloum, E.; Cooper, D.L.; Howe, G.; Lacy, J.; Tallini, G.; Crouch, J.; Schultz, M.; Murren, J. Spontaneous regression of lymphoproliferative disorders in patients treated with methotrexate for rheumatoid arthritis and other rheumatic diseases. *J. Clin. Oncol.* **1996**, *14*, 1943–1949. [CrossRef] [PubMed]
181. Banko, A.; Miljanovic, D.; Lazarevic, I.; Jeremic, I.; Despotovic, A.; Grk, M.; Cirkovic, A. New Evidence of Significant Association between EBV Presence and Lymphoproliferative Disorders Susceptibility in Patients with Rheumatoid Arthritis: A Systematic Review with Meta-Analysis. *Viruses* **2022**, *14*, 115. [CrossRef] [PubMed]
182. Inui, Y.; Matsuoka, H.; Yakushijin, K.; Okamura, A.; Shimada, T.; Yano, S.; Takeuchi, M.; Ito, M.; Murayama, T.; Yamamoto, K.; et al. Methotrexate-associated lymphoproliferative disorders: Management by watchful waiting and observation of early lymphocyte recovery after methotrexate withdrawal. *Leuk. Lymphoma* **2015**, *56*, 3045–3051. [CrossRef] [PubMed]
183. Tokuhira, M.; Saito, S.; Okuyama, A.; Suzuki, K.; Higashi, M.; Momose, S.; Shimizu, T.; Mori, T.; Anan-Nemoto, T.; Amano, K.; et al. Clinicopathologic investigation of ethotrexate-induced lymphoproliferative disorders, with a focus on regression. *Leuk. Lymphoma* **2018**, *59*, 1143–1152. [CrossRef] [PubMed]
184. Yamada, K.; Oshiro, Y.; Okamura, S.; Fujisaki, T.; Kondo, S.; Nakayama, Y.; Suematsu, E.; Tamura, K.; Takeshita, M. Clinicopathological characteristics and rituximab addition to cytotoxic therapies in patients with rheumatoid arthritis and methotrexate-associated large B lymphoproliferative disorders. *Histopathology* **2015**, *67*, 70–80. [CrossRef] [PubMed]
185. Nakano, K.; Saito, K.; Nawata, A.; Hanami, K.; Kubo, S.; Miyagawa; Fujino, Y.; Nakayamada, S.; Tanaka, Y. Clinical aspects in patients with rheumatoid arthritis complicated with lymphoproliferative disorders without regression after methotrexate withdrawal and treatment for arthritis after regression of lymphoproliferative disorders. *Mod. Rheumatol.* **2021**, *31*, 94–100. [CrossRef] [PubMed]
186. Fujimoto, K.; Hatanaka, K.C.; Hatanaka, Y.; Kasahara, I.; Yamamoto, S.; Tsuji, T.; Nakata, M.; Takakuwa, Y.; Haseyama, Y.; Oyamada, Y.; et al. Association of Epstein-Barr virus with regression after withdrawal of immunosuppressive drugs and subsequent progression of iatrogenic immunodeficiency-associated lymphoproliferative disorders in patients with autoimmune diseases. *Hematol. Oncol.* **2020**, *38*, 799–807. [CrossRef] [PubMed]
187. Katsuyama, T.; Sada, K.E.; Yan, M.; Zeggar, S.; Hiramatsu, S.; Miyawaki, Y.; Ohashi, K.; Morishita, M.; Watanabe, H.; Katsuyama, E.; et al. Prognostic factors of methotrexate-associated lymphoproliferative disorders associated with rheumatoid arthritis and plausible application of biological agents. *Mod. Rheumatol.* **2017**, *27*, 773–777. [CrossRef] [PubMed]
188. Harada, T.; Iwasaki, H.; Muta, T.; Urata, S.; Sakamoto, A.; Kohno, K.; Takase, K.; Miyamura, T.; Sawabe, T.; Asaoku, H.; et al. Outcomes of methotrexate-associated lymphoproliferative disorders in rheumatoid arthritis patients treated with disease-modifying anti-rheumatic drugs. *Br. J. Haematol.* **2021**, *194*, 101–110. [CrossRef] [PubMed]
189. Brown, S.L.; Greeene, M.H.; Gershon, S.K.; Edward, E.T.; Braum, M.M. Tumor necrosis factor antagonist therapy and lymphoma development: Twenty-six cases reported to the Food and Drug Administration. *Arthritis Rheum.* **2002**, *46*, 3151–3158. [CrossRef] [PubMed]
190. Hoshida, Y.; Yamamoto, S.; Wada, N.; Xu, J.X.; Sasaki, T.; Aozasa, K. Infliximab-associated lymphoproliferative disorders. *Int. J. Hematol.* **2005**, *81*, 356–357. [CrossRef] [PubMed]
191. Hoshida, Y.; Tsujii, A.; Ohshima, S.; Saeki, Y.; Yagita, M.; Miyamura, T.; Katayama, M.; Hiramatsu, Y.; Oshima, H.; Murayama, T.; et al. Rheumatoid Arthritis Associated Lymphoproliferative Disorders: Current Features and It's Changing Pattern Due to the Influence of Anti-rheumatic Drugs. *Arthritis Rheumatol.* **2022**, *74* (Suppl. S9), 3953–3957, (abstract).
192. Nocturne, G.; Seror, R.; Mariette, X. Does the risk of lymphoma in patients with RA treated with TNF inhibitors differ according to the histological subtype and the type of TNF inhibitor? *Ann. Rheum. Dis.* **2017**, *76*, e3. [CrossRef] [PubMed]
193. Mercer, L.K.; Regierer, A.C.; Mariette, X.; Dixon, W.G.; Baecklund, E.; Hellgren, K.; Dreyer, L.; Hetland, M.L.; Cordtz, R.; Hyrich, K.; et al. Spectrum of lymphomas across different drug treatment groups in rheumatoid arthritis: A European registries collaborative project. *Ann. Rheum. Dis.* **2017**, *76*, 2025–2030. [CrossRef] [PubMed]
194. Scallon, B.; Cai, A.; Solowski, N.; Rosenberg, A.; Song, X.Y.; Shealy, D.; Wagner, C. Binding and functional comparisons of two types of tumor necrosis factor antagonists. *J. Pharmacol. Exp. Ther.* **2002**, *301*, 418–426. [CrossRef] [PubMed]
195. Furst, D.E. The risk of infections with biologic therapies for rheumatoid arthritis. *Semin. Arthritis Rheum.* **2010**, *39*, 327–346. [CrossRef] [PubMed]
196. Salmon-Ceron, D.; Tubach, F.; Lortholary, O.; Chosidow, O.; Bretagne, S.; Nicolas, N.; Cuillerier, E.; Fautrel, B.; Michelet, C.; Morel, J.; et al. Drug-specific risk of non-tuberculosis opportunistic infections in patients receiving anti-TNF therapy reported to the 3-year prospective French RATIO registry. *Ann. Rheum. Dis.* **2011**, *70*, 616–623. [CrossRef] [PubMed]
197. Sandborn, W.J.; Hanauer, S.B.; Kart, S.; Safdi, M.; Wolf, D.G.; Baerg, R.D.; Tremaine, W.J.; Johnson, T.; Diehl, N.N.; Zinsmeister, A.R. Etanercept for active Crohn's disease: A randomized, double-blind, placebo-controlled trial. *Gastroenterology* **2001**, *121*, 1088–1094. [CrossRef] [PubMed]
198. Guignard, S.; Grossec, L.; Salliot, C.; Ruyssen-Witrand, A.; Luc, M.; Duclos, M.; Dougados, M. Efficacy of tumor necrosis factor blockers in reducing uveitis flares in patients with spondylathropathy: A retrospective study. *Ann. Rheum. Dis.* **2006**, *65*, 1631–1634. [CrossRef] [PubMed]

199. Saliu, O.Y.; Sofer, C.; Stein, D.S.; Schwander, S.K.; Wallis, R.S. Tumor-necrosis-factor blockers: Differential effects on mycobacterial immunity. *J. Infect. Dis.* **2006**, *194*, 486–492. [CrossRef] [PubMed]
200. Mariette, X.; Chen, C.; Biswas, P.; Kwok, K.; Boy, M.G. Lymphoma in the Tofacitinib rheumatoid arthritis clinical development program. *Arthritis Care Res.* **2018**, *70*, 685–694. [CrossRef] [PubMed]
201. Porpaczy, E.; Tripolt, S.; Hoelbl-Kovacic, A.; Gisslinger, B.; Bago-Horvath, Z.; Casanova-Hevia, E.; Clappier, E.; Decker, T.; Fajmann, S.; Fux, D.A.; et al. Aggressive B-cell lymphomas in patients with myelofibrosis receiving JAK1/2 inhibitor therapy. *Blood* **2018**, *132*, 694–706. [CrossRef] [PubMed]
202. Alspaugh, M.A.; Henle, G.; Lennette, E.T.; Henle, W. Elevated levels of antibodies to Epstein-Barr virus antigens in sera and synovial fluids of patients with rheumatoid arthritis. *J. Clin. Investig.* **1981**, *67*, 1134–1140. [CrossRef] [PubMed]
203. Balandraud, N.; Guis, S.; Meynard, J.B.; Auger, I.; Roudier, J.; Roudier, C. Long-term treatment with methotrexate or tumor necrosis factor alpha inhibitors does not increase Epstein-Barr virus load in patients with rheumatoid arthritis. *Arthritis Rheum.* **2007**, *57*, 762–767. [CrossRef] [PubMed]
204. Mercer, L.K.; Galloway, J.B.; Lunt, M.; Davies, R.; Low, A.A.; Dixon, W.G.; Watson, K.D.; Symmons, D.P.; Hyrich, K.L. Response to: 'Does the risk of lymphoma in patients with RA treated with TNF inhibitors differ according to the histological subtype and the type of TNF inhibitor?' by Nocturne et al. *Ann. Rheum. Dis.* **2017**, *76*, e4. [CrossRef] [PubMed]

Journal of
Clinical Medicine

MDPI

Review

Pathogenic Role of Cytokines in Rheumatoid Arthritis

Sho Fujimoto and Hiroaki Niiro *

Department of Medical Education, Faculty of Medical Sciences, Kyushu University, Fukuoka 812-8582, Japan; fujimoto.sho.366@m.kyushu-u.ac.jp
* Correspondence: niiro.hiroaki.811@m.kyushu-u.ac.jp; Tel.: +81-92-642-6678

Abstract: Rheumatoid arthritis (RA) is a systemic autoimmune disease characterized by a multistep pathogenesis, from the preclinical phase of autoantibody emergence to the clinical onset of synovitis and joint destruction. Cytokines play central roles throughout this progression by orchestrating immune cell activation, tissue inflammation, and bone erosion. In the preclinical phase, several cytokines, including IL-12, IL-6, IL-21 and TGF-β, promote Tfh and Tph cell differentiation, helping autoreactive B cells to produce ACPA. During the clinical phase, TNF-α, IL-6, and IL-1β drive synovitis by activating macrophages and fibroblast-like synoviocytes, while also promoting RANKL (Receptor Activator of Nuclear factor κB Ligand) expression and osteoclast differentiation. This review highlights the pathogenic role of cytokines in RA and discusses their relevance as biomarkers and therapeutic targets. A better understanding of cytokine networks may offer new opportunities for early intervention and disease prevention in RA.

Keywords: rheumatoid arthritis; cytokines; autoimmunity; synovitis; joint destruction

1. Introduction

Rheumatoid arthritis (RA) is an autoimmune disease characterized by chronic synovial inflammation and progressive bone destruction and resulting in severe joint deformity and functional impairment. The underlying pathogenesis involves an aberrant immune response in which the immune system, originally intended to protect the host from external threats, mistakenly targets self-tissues. The pathogenesis of RA is orchestrated by a complex network of immune cells and soluble mediators, among which cytokines play a central role. The significance of cytokines in RA is evident from the high efficacy of cytokine-targeted therapies such as tumor necrosis factor (TNF)-α inhibitors and interleukin (IL)-6 inhibitors. In this review, we sought to divide the pathogenesis of autoantibody-positive RA into a pre-arthritis (preclinical) phase and an arthritis (clinical) phase, and discuss the roles of cytokines in terms of the 'initiation of autoimmunity', 'development and persistence of synovitis', and 'progression of joint destruction'. In particular, we focus on cytokines that play central roles in RA pathogenesis across these stages, including IL-6 and TNF-α as major drivers of inflammation and joint damage, IL-1β and IL-17 as amplifiers of synovitis, IL-21 as a key mediator of T follicular helper cell (Tfh)/T peripheral helper cells (Tph)–B cell interactions, B cell-activating factor (BAFF) and A proliferation-inducing ligand (APRIL) as regulators of B cell survival and autoantibody production, and type I interferon (IFN) as a critical factor in the preclinical phase. To enhance the comprehensiveness of this narrative review, we conducted a literature search using PubMed. The keywords used included "rheumatoid arthritis," "cytokines," "autoimmunity," "synovitis," and "bone destruction." We included both original and review articles published in English, mainly between January 2000 and June 2025. Articles were selected based on their relevance to the immunopathogenesis of RA, particularly those describing cytokine function, immune cell interactions, and tissue damage. Case reports and non-peer-reviewed sources were excluded.

2. Pre-Arthritis (Preclinical) Phase of RA

The pre-arthritis phase of RA refers to the stage before the onset of clinical symptoms, during which autoimmunity has already begun, characterized by the appearance of autoantibodies such as anti-cyclic citrullinated peptide antibody (ACPA) and rheumatoid factor (RF) [1]. In this RA risk phase, genetic and environmental factors interact to drive disease progression (Figure 1). Genetic factors include susceptibility genes such as HLA-DR (Human Leukocyte Antigen-DR) shared-epitope (SE) alleles and the peptidyl arginine deiminase 4 (PADI4) gene, which encodes peptidyl arginine deiminase, involved in citrullination [2,3]. Environmental factors such as smoking, periodontitis and gut dysbiosis activate PADI4 in neutrophils, leading to the abundant production of citrullinated self-proteins [4–6]. These self-proteins are presented as citrullinated peptides by dendritic cell HLA-DR SE molecules, inducing the activation of naïve CD4^{+} T cells, thereby initiating autoimmunity [7]. Concurrently, the activation of naïve B cells reactive to these autoantigens is also induced [8]. In autoimmune diseases like RA, a breakdown of B cell tolerance results in an increased presence of autoreactive naïve B cells compared to healthy individuals [9].

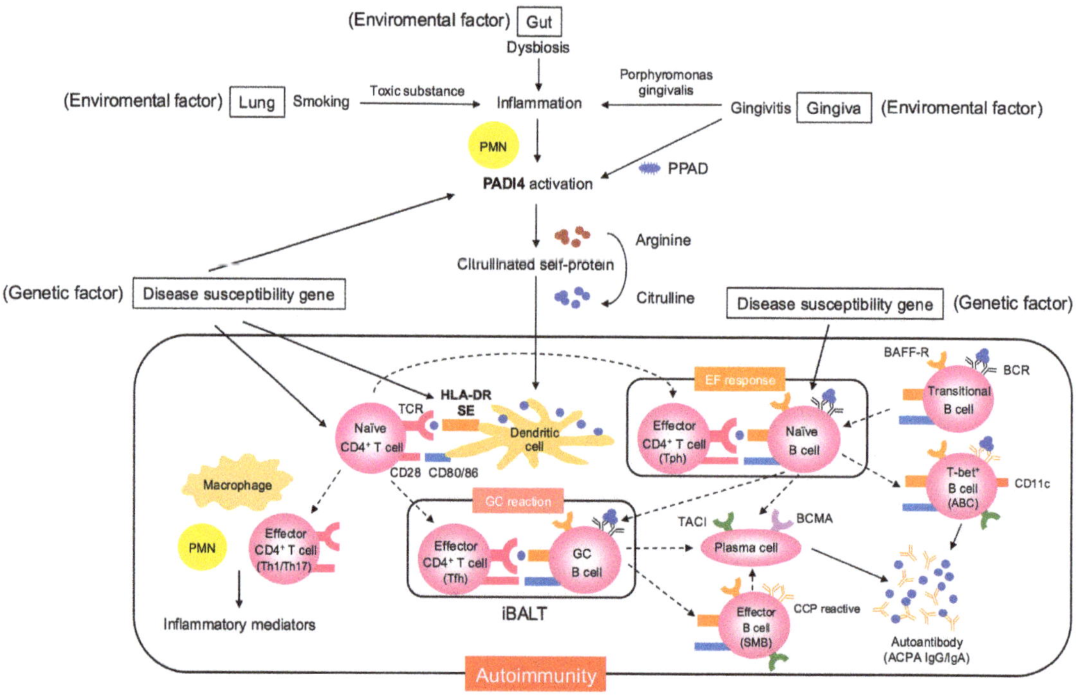

Figure 1. Pathologic mechanisms linking environmental and genetic factors to autoimmunity in the preclinical phase of RA. This figure details the interplay between genetic susceptibility (e.g., disease risk genes including PADI4) and environmental insults such as smoking, gingivitis caused by Porphyromonas gingivalis, and gut dysbiosis. It describes how these factors drive post-translational

modification of self-proteins, notably citrullination catalyzed by PPAD and PADI4, creating neoantigens that breach immune tolerance. The process involves tissue sites such as the lung, gingiva, and gut, and depicts the initial activation of innate immune cells (e.g., neutrophils and dendritic cells), subsequent T and B cell activation through antigen presentation (via HLA-DR molecules and costimulatory signals such as CD28/CD80/86), and the fostering of local and systemic autoimmune responses and inflammation. ABC, age-associated B cell; ACPA, anti-citrullinated protein antibody; BAFF-R, B-cell-activating factor-receptor; BCMA, B-cell maturation antigen; EF, extrafollicular; GC, germinal center; iBALT, inducible bronchus-associated lymphoid tissue; PADI, peptidyl arginine deaminase; PPAD, porphyromonas gingivalis peptidylarginine deiminase; PMN polymorphonuclear neutrophil; TACI, transmembrane activator and CAML interactor; Tfh, T follicular helper; Tph, T peripheral helper.

Cytokines are critical for the functional maturation (differentiation into effectors) of both T and B cells. The activation of naïve $CD4^+$ T cells requires antigen recognition via T cell receptor (TCR) (signal 1) and co-stimulation via CD28 (signal 2); however, differentiation into effector $CD4^+$ T cells with specific cytokine-producing profiles requires additional cytokine stimulation (signal 3) (Figure 2). In local tissues, such as the lungs, differentiation into Th1 or Th17 subsets and the subsequent production of inflammatory mediators is observed, but a key feature in this stage is the production of autoantibody ACPA. This process critically involves Tfh and Tph subsets, which exhibit a strong B cell-helper capacity (Figure 2). Multiple cytokines are involved in Tfh differentiation, and in humans, as in Th1 cells, IL-12 plays an essential role; indeed, Tfh differentiation is impaired in individuals with IL-12 receptor β1 chain (IL12RB1) deficiency [10]. In addition to IL-12, cytokines such as transforming growth factor (TGF)-β are also important for human Tfh differentiation. Moreover, the marked reduction in circulating Tfh (cTfh) cells in patients with Signal Transducer and Activator of Transcription 3 (STAT3) deficiency suggests that the cytokines acting via the STAT3 pathway—such as IL-6 and IL-21—are also crucial [11]. Among the cytokines produced by Tfh cells, IL-21 is of central importance. B cells require cytokine stimulation to exert effector functions (Figure 3). IL-21 activates STAT3 in B cells and induces the transcription factor B lymphocyte-induced maturation protein 1 (BLIMP-1), which is critical for plasma cell differentiation [12].

As previously mentioned, RA patients harbor abundant autoreactive naïve B cells. These cells are influenced not only by T cell-derived IL-21 but also by other cytokines that disrupt their self-tolerance. Innate immune cells such as neutrophils, macrophages, and dendritic cells produce key B cell-modulating cytokines, including BAFF, APRIL, and IL-10 (Figure 3). BAFF promotes the differentiation, survival, and maturation of B cells [13]. Since naïve B cells express the BAFF receptor (BAFF-R), excessive BAFF availability may support the persistence of autoreactive B cells [14]. APRIL is critical for the long-term survival of plasma cells, which express its receptors the transmembrane activator and CAML interactor (TACI) and B-cell maturation antigens (BCMAs) [15,16]. Unlike BAFF and APRIL, IL-10 can also be produced by B cells themselves. It promotes plasma cell differentiation via STAT3 activation [17]. Interestingly, although APRIL facilitates the differentiation and survival of pathogenic (autoreactive) B cells, it has also been reported to promote IL-10-producing regulatory B cells (Bregs). Under APRIL stimulation, IgA^+ Bregs are induced, which suppress T cell and macrophage-mediated inflammation through IL-10 and programmed death-ligand 1 (PD-L1) expression [18,19]. This duality of APRIL—supporting both pathogenic and regulatory B cell subsets—has important implications for therapeutic targeting and adverse event prediction in RA [20].

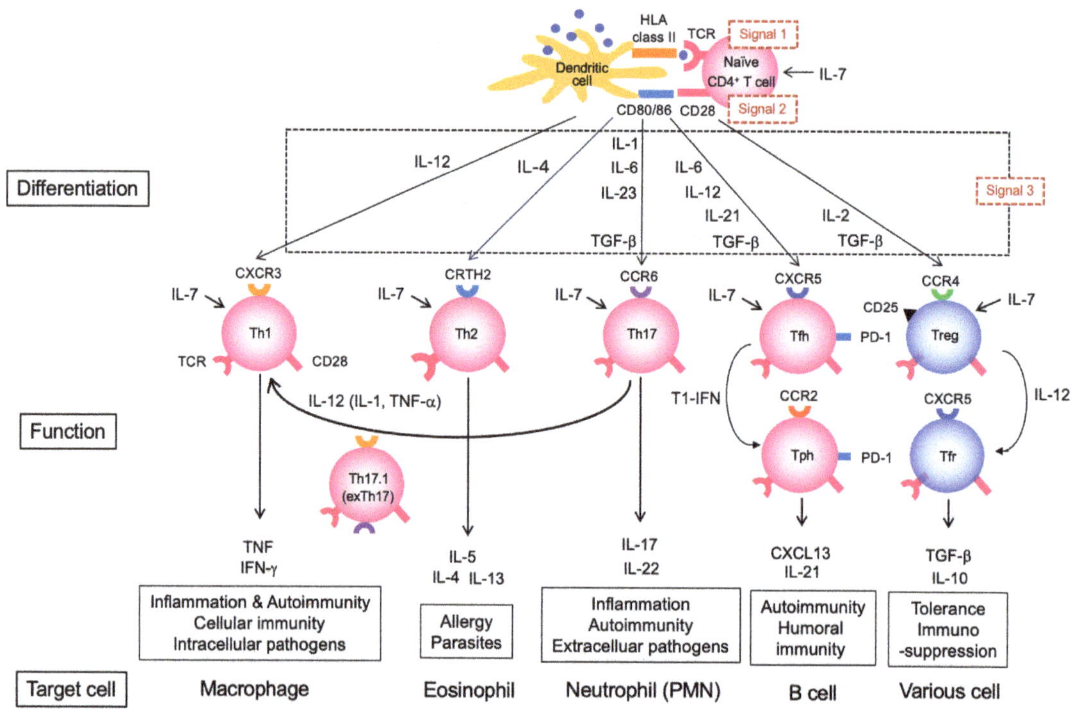

Figure 2. Differentiation and functions of CD4⁺ T cell subsets and their roles in autoimmunity. This figure outlines the differentiation pathways of naïve CD4⁺ T cells into effector subsets (Th1, Th17.1, Th2, Th17, Tfh, Tph, Treg, Tfr), driven by different cytokines and environmental cues. The specific functions and characteristic markers of each subset are diagrammed, including their involvement in cellular and humoral immunity, inflammation, immunosuppression, and tolerance. TCR, T cell receptor; Tfh, T follicular helper; Tfr, T follicular regulatory cell: Tph, T peripheral helper; Treg, regulatory T cell.

Tph cells were originally identified in RA joints as IL-21-producing PD-1^{hi} $CD4^{+}$ T cells distinct from Tfh cells [21]. Notably, while Tfh cells express CXCR5, Tph cells express CCR2, indicating that Tfh cells are involved in B cell-help within lymphoid tissues, whereas Tph cells function in inflamed tissues such as synovial tissues in RA [22] (Figure 2). Interestingly, Tph cells themselves also produce CXCL13, a ligand for CXCR5, suggesting that they may recruit Tfh cells to inflammatory sites. Recent studies suggest that type I IFN can induce a shift from Tfh to Tph cells, a phenomenon that could potentially occur in inflammatory environments [23]. Tfh cells are involved in the germinal center (GC) reaction and promote somatic hypermutation (SHM) and class-switch recombination in GC B cells, mainly via IL-4 and IL-21 [24]. On the other hand, Tph cells induce the differentiation of naïve B cells into a distinct $CD11c^{+}$ T-bet^{+} subset known as age-associated B cells (ABC) [25]. These T-bet^{+} B cells are frequently autoreactive [26], strongly implicating them in autoimmunity. In addition to IL-21, IFN-γ is crucial for their differentiation, as T-bet^{+} B cells are reduced when IFN-γ signaling is impaired [27]. IFN-γ signaling is also essential for the expression of CXCR3 on T-bet^{+} B cells, promoting their recruitment to inflammatory sites [28]. Interestingly, IFN-γ and IL-4 act antagonistically in driving T-bet^{+} B cell development, suggesting that the cytokine milieu may influence the choice between GC and extrafollicular pathways [29].

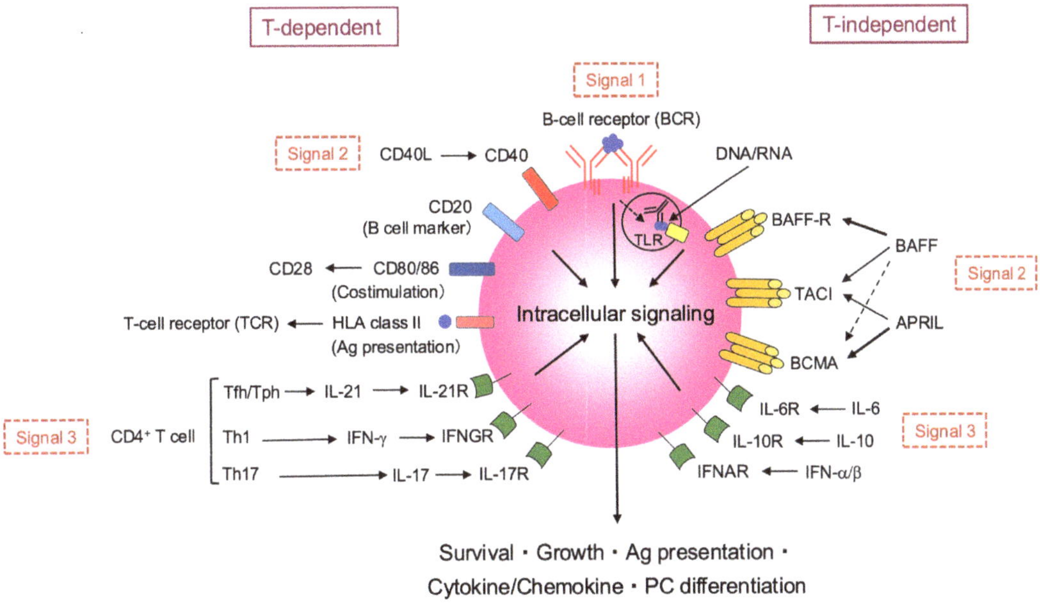

Figure 3. B cell activation, differentiation, and effector functions in autoimmune responses. This figure provides an overview of B cell activation via T-dependent and T-independent pathways. T-dependent activation requires three signals: antigen binding to the B-cell receptor (BCR) (Signal 1), co-stimulation via CD40-CD40L and CD28-CD80/86 interactions with CD4$^+$ T cells (Signal 2), and cytokine signaling (Signal 3) from Tfh/Tph, Th1, or Th17 cells. T-independent activation also involves antigen/TLR binding (Signal 1) and additional signals (Signal 2) from BAFF/APRIL binding to BAFF-R, TACI, and BCMA, along with cytokine signaling (Signal 3) from IL-6, IL-10, and IFN-α/β. All these pathways converge on intracellular signaling to promote B cell survival, growth, and antigen presentation, cytokine/chemokine production, and plasma cell differentiation. BAFF, B-cell-activating factor; BCMA, B-cell maturation antigen; IFN, interferon; TACI, transmembrane activator and CAML interactor; PC, plasma cell.

What, then, is the contribution of Tfh and Tph cells to pathogenesis during the preclinical phase? In RA lung lesions, structures resembling secondary lymphoid organs called inducible bronchus-associated lymphoid tissue (iBALT) are observed [30], suggesting that GC reactions mediated by Tfh cells may be occurring (Figure 1), though direct evidence is currently limited. ACPA is known to undergo variable domain glycosylation (VDG), which progressively increases even before the onset of arthritis and is already fully established by the time of clinical manifestation. Since this glycosylation is introduced through SHM [31], it again suggests the importance of GC reactions driven by Tfh cells during the preclinical phase. On the other hand, although much remains unclear regarding Tph cells, an increase in Tph cells has been observed in the peripheral blood of ACPA-positive individuals in the preclinical phase, suggesting their potential involvement in RA development [32,33]. Although this pertains to the clinical phase, Tph cells have also been reported in the sputum and lung tissues of RA patients [34]. Additionally, since elevated type I IFN are present in ACPA-positive individuals prior to RA onset [35], Tph differentiation may also occur during this phase. The presence of Tph cells implies possible co-localization with T-bet$^+$ B cells. An analysis of bronchoalveolar lavage (BAL) fluid from ACPA-positive individuals in the preclinical phase revealed the presence of double-negative (IgD$^-$ CD27$^-$) B cells, possibly including T-bet$^+$ B cells, in lung tissues, suggesting their involvement in autoantibody production [36]. These findings collectively support the notion that autoantibody production reflecting underlying autoimmunity begins during the preclinical phase.

Omics analyses in the preclinical phase of RA have provided evidence for the critical role of type I IFN. Notably, transcriptomic studies have demonstrated that ACPA-positive individuals and those with arthralgia prior to RA onset exhibit an type I IFN signature—defined as the upregulation of type I IFN-responsive genes—which is significantly associated with increased risk of progression to RA [37,38]. Individuals with high type I IFN signature expression had approximately twice the risk of developing RA, independent of the presence of autoantibodies such as ACPA and RF. This type I IFN signature also correlates with autoantibody titers and is implicated in immunological alterations such as immune cell activation and B cell proliferation. In addition, serum proteomic analyses conducted around the time of RA onset have revealed changes in molecular networks associated with IFN-α responses and lipid metabolism pathways [39]. Furthermore, proteomic analyses of sera from ACPA-positive individuals have shown that cytokines such as IL-1, IL-2, and IFN-γ correlate with ACPA variable-domain glycosylation (VDG), and cases that progressed to inflammatory arthritis exhibited strong activation of the JAK-STAT pathway [40].

To date, no studies have shown that the inhibition of specific cytokines during the preclinical phase can prevent the onset of RA. For instance, the administration of TNF-α inhibitors during the preclinical stage does not suppress disease development, likely because TNF-α plays a more prominent role during the arthritis (clinical) phase, as discussed later. In contrast, IL-6, which promotes the differentiation of Tfh and Tph cells as described above, may hold promise as a preventive target. Results from some studies suggest that IL-6 inhibitors and JAK inhibitors may have the potential to suppress disease progression in high-risk individuals—such as those who are autoantibody-positive or exhibit subclinical inflammation [41]. Notably, JAK inhibitors are of particular interest as a potential therapeutic strategy in the preclinical phase due to their capacity to regulate the activity of type I IFN, as described above. However, there is currently no evidence supporting its use for disease prevention, and further research is needed [42].

3. Arthritis (Clinical) Phase of RA

3.1. Autoimmunity

Even during the clinical phase of RA, T cells and B cells continue to mediate autoimmune responses within the joint. The RA synovium harbors diverse T cell subsets—particularly Tph cells—as well as B cells, which undergo clonal expansion, recognize self-antigens, produce cytokines, and promote plasma cell differentiation [4]. Comprehensive analyses comparing immune cell profiles between synovial tissue and peripheral blood in patients with early, treatment-naïve RA have shown that Tph cell-associated signatures serve as important biomarkers for treatment response and prognosis [43]. Circulating Tfh (cTfh) and Tph cells in RA patients exhibit distinct metabolic profiles: cTfh cells show heightened glucose metabolism, particularly glycolysis, and are more potent in B cell activation and antibody production, whereas Tph cells demonstrate elevated mitochondrial reactive oxygen species (mtROS) and express high levels of cytotoxicity-related molecules such as BLIMP-1 and T-bet, as well as markers of cellular senescence [44]. Moreover, synovial Tph cells show stronger recent TCR activation signatures and more pronounced clonal expansion compared to Tfh cells [45]. Interestingly, recent studies have identified two functionally and spatially distinct Tph subsets in RA: stem-like Tph (S-Tph) and effector Tph (E-Tph). S-Tph cells possess self-renewal and B cell-helping capacity within tertiary lymphoid structures (TLS), while E-Tph cells contribute to inflammation and tissue damage. Differentiation from S-Tph to E-Tph occurs within RA tissues [46]. Human Tph cells also produce a primate-specific secreted factor, insulin-like growth factor-like family member 2 (IGFL2), which correlates with RA disease activity [47]. IGFL2 functions as a cytokine that cooperates with TGF-β stimulation to promote CXCL13 production and induces the expression of numerous inflammatory and IFN-related genes (e.g., CXCL9/10/11) in monocytes and macrophages (Figure 4).

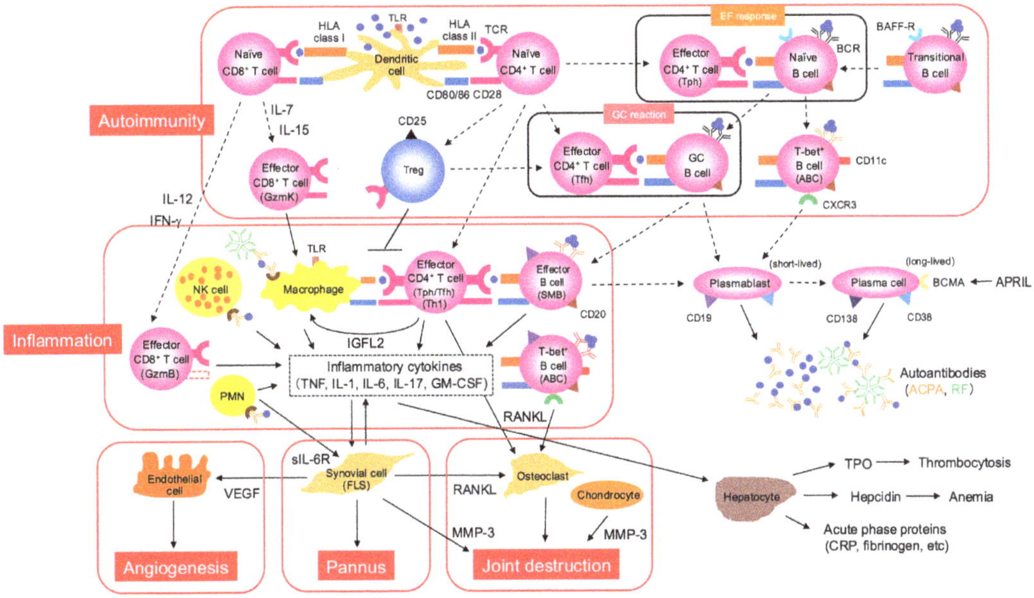

Figure 4. Pathogenesis of clinical phase of RA is characterized by autoimmunity, synovitis, and joint destruction. This figure delineates the intricate cellular and molecular events in autoimmunity, inflammation, pannus formation, and joint destruction. In the context of autoimmunity, dendritic cells activate naïve CD8⁺ T cells and naïve CD4⁺ T cells via HLA class I and HLA class II, respectively. These activated T cells can differentiate into effector CD8⁺ T cells (GzmK) and effector CD4⁺ T cells (Tfh). The EF response involves the interaction between effector CD4⁺ T cells (Tph) and naïve B cells, thereby generating T-bet⁺ B cells. The GC reaction involves effector CD4⁺ T cells (Tfh) and GC B cells. Ultimately, plasmablasts (short-lived) and plasma cells (long-lived), characterized by CD19, CD138, CD38, BCMA, and APRIL, produce autoantibodies such as ACPA and RF. Inflammation is driven by macrophages and NK cells, activated via TLR, leading to the stimulation of effector CD4⁺ T cells (Tph/Tfh/Th1) and effector B cells (SMB). PMNs and effector CD8+ T cells (GzmB) also contribute to the release of inflammatory cytokines like TNF, IL-1, IL-6, and IL-8. T-bet⁺ B cells are also implicated in the inflammatory process. These inflammatory processes contribute directly to pannus formation and subsequent joint destruction. Synovial cells (FLS), osteoclasts, and chondrocytes, through pathways involving RANKL and MMP-3, drive the development of pannus and eventual joint degradation. Additionally, inflammatory cytokines influence hepatocytes, leading to the production of acute phase proteins (CRP, fibrinogen, etc.) and hepcidin, which is associated with anemia. ABC, age-associated B cell; ACPA, anti-citrullinated protein antibody; APRIL, a proliferation-inducing ligand; BAFF, B-cell-activating factor; BCR, B cell receptor; BCMA, B-cell maturation antigen; FLS, fibroblast-like synoviocyte; Gzm, granzyme; IGFL2, insulin-like growth factor-like family member 2; MMP, matrix metalloproteinase; PMN, polymorphonuclear neutrophil; RANKL receptor activator of nuclear factor kappa B ligand; RF, rheumatoid factor; TPO, thrombopoietin; VEGF, vascular endothelial growth factor.

In patients with early RA who are DMARD-naïve, ABCs highly express chemokine receptors such as CXCR3 and adhesion molecules involved in homing to inflamed tissues, and represent a dominant B cell subset in synovial fluid [48]. Single-cell RNA sequencing analysis of ABCs in peripheral blood of RA patients revealed that the proportion of ABCs correlates with disease activity and serum TNF-α levels, and identified spleen tyrosine kinase (Syk) as a key regulator of the myeloid-like phenotype of ABCs [49]. The aberrant expansion of ABCs is implicated in RA pathogenesis and represents a potential therapeutic target [50].

As described earlier, IL-6 plays a critical role in the differentiation of both Tfh and Tph cells; in addition, IL-6 directly acts on B cells, promoting plasma cell differentiation via STAT3 activation (Figures 3 and 4). In this phase, members of the TNF cytokine family, BAFF and APRIL, are also upregulated in RA serum and synovial tissue (Figure 4) [14]. However, ACPA titers show only weak correlation with RA disease activity and treatment response, and generally remain stable over time. This may be partly explained by the fact that ACPA-producing B cells have already acquired immunological memory—as evidenced by VDG—before the onset of arthritis [51]. Moreover, as ACPA-producing cells, $CXCR3^+$ switched memory B cells (SMB), plasmablasts, and long-lived plasma cells residing in the bone marrow have been implicated, rather than the aforementioned $T\text{-bet}^+$ B cells (Figure 4) [52,53]. In contrast, rheumatoid factor (RF), which is typically an IgM autoantibody targeting the Fc region of IgG, appears to be produced through mechanisms that involve innate immune signaling, unlike ACPA [54].

3.2. Development and Maintenance of Synovitis

In addition to autoimmunity, the clinical phase is marked by synovial inflammation. At this stage, not only T and B cells, but also innate immune cells such as macrophages and fibroblast-like synoviocytes (FLS), play key roles. Synovial macrophages play a central role in promoting chronic synovitis and joint destruction by producing pro-inflammatory cytokines—particularly TNF-α, IL-1β, and IL-6 (Figure 4). Synovial macrophages are classified into M1 (pro-inflammatory) and M2 (anti-inflammatory) phenotypes; in RA, there is a predominance of M1 macrophages, which are characterized by the elevated production of TNF-α and IL-1β [55]. Among the cytokines, IFN-γ, secreted by Th1 cells, potently drives M1 polarization, while granulocyte–macrophage colony-stimulating factor (GM-CSF), which is highly expressed in the synovium, is also critical for maintaining the M1 phenotype in monocyte-derived macrophages. TNF-α and IL-1β secreted by M1 macrophages further amplify the inflammatory loop [56–58].

FLS, when stimulated by cytokines such as TNF-α, IL-1β, IL-6, and TGF-β, increase the expression of adhesion molecules (e.g., ICAM-1) and enhance crosstalk with immune cells—particularly $CD4^+$ T cells and macrophages—leading to elevated production of inflammatory cytokines and chemokines [59]. Under TNF-α stimulation, FLS particularly promote direct cellular interactions with T cells and enhance their activation and differentiation. Moreover, FLS contribute to bone destruction through the production of receptor activator of nuclear factor κB ligand (RANKL), and a subset of $ITGA5^+$ FLS expressing TGF-β, periostin (POSTN), and CCL5 has been implicated in promoting Tph differentiation and forming inflammatory niches [60]. Interactions between FLS and macrophages further increase the production of inflammatory cytokines and matrix metalloproteinases (MMP2 and MMP9), exacerbating chronic inflammation and tissue damage. Recent single-cell and spatial transcriptomic analyses have revealed the functional heterogeneity of FLS subsets, highlighting their emerging importance as therapeutic targets in RA [61].

In addition to Th1 cells, Th17 cells produce IL-17A and other cytokines that stimulate FLS and macrophages, thereby amplifying inflammation. Under inflammatory conditions (e.g., in the presence of IL-12, IL-1 or TNF-α), Th17 cells may transdifferentiate into Th17.1 (or exTh17) cells, which co-produce IFN-γ (Figure 2). These Th17.1 cells are increased in RA synovial fluid and have been reported to be more pro-inflammatory and treatment-resistant than classical Th17 cells [62].

In early RA, synovial T cells exhibit a Th1-skewed profile, with high production of inflammatory cytokines such as IFN-γ, while IL-4 and Th2 cells are relatively scarce. Nonetheless, IL-4 production is detectable in the synovium of early RA and may contribute to both anti-inflammatory effects and enhanced antibody production through B cell activation. IL-4 promotes B cell differentiation and antibody production—particularly IgE and autoantibodies—and may be involved in the autoimmune processes of RA. It also modulates inflammatory cytokine secretion from synovial fibroblasts and neutrophils [63]. In chronic or advanced RA, however, a Th1/Th17-dominant milieu prevails, and synovial T cells become resistant to Th2 polarization, thereby limiting IL-4's anti-inflammatory function. Nevertheless, IL-4 can still suppress neutrophil infiltration into the joints and enhance FcγR2b expression, contributing to inflammation control [64,65]. As previously noted, Tph cells play a central role in RA synovium, but Tfh cells are also present. Tfh cells can be subdivided into Tfh1, Tfh2, and Tfh17 subsets based on their cytokine profiles. During the clinical phase, Tfh2 cells—which produce IL-21 and IL-4—are considered more functionally relevant than Tfh1 cells, which produce IL-21 and IFN-γ. Tfh2 cells strongly contribute to B cell activation and autoantibody production [66]. Moreover, in peripheral blood of RA patients, increases in Tfh2 and Tfh17 (producing IL-21 and IL-17) subsets have been observed, whereas Tfh1 cells appear to have lower B cell-helper activity.

In contrast to pathogenic subsets, regulatory CD4$^+$ T cell subsets also exist (Figure 2). T regulatory (Treg) cells are induced by IL-2 and TGF-β and secrete immunosuppressive cytokines such as IL-10 and TGF-β. Tregs maintain immune homeostasis by suppressing effector T cell responses. In co-culture experiments with human conventional CD4$^+$ T cells (Tconv), Tregs have been shown to strongly suppress both the proliferation and cytokine production of Tconv cells. This suppression is primarily contact-dependent, as the effect is abolished when Tregs and Tconv cells are separated by a transwell, indicating that direct cell–cell interactions, in addition to soluble factors, are essential [67]. Moreover, the suppressive capacity of Tregs varies by subset. Memory-type Tregs (CD45RA$^-$ FoxP3^{hi}) potently inhibit early Tconv activation—such as activation marker expression and cytokine secretion—whereas their ability to suppress proliferation is comparable to that of naive Tregs [68]. Tregs that express follicular-homing molecules such as CXCR5, migrate into follicles, and acquire suppressive functions are referred to as T follicular regulatory (Tfr) cells. Recent human studies have shown that low-dose IL-12 induces Tfr differentiation programs in activated Tregs by activating STAT4 and upregulating Tfr-associated genes (Figure 2) [69]. In untreated early RA patients, Treg cells are significantly reduced, showing negative correlations with disease activity and autoantibody titers [70]. Additionally, peripheral Tfr cells are decreased in active RA compared to remission [71]. These findings suggest reductions in both Treg and Tfr populations during the clinical phase of RA (Figure 4). In humans, impaired Treg function and numerical deficiency contribute to the breakdown of peripheral B cell tolerance checkpoints, leading to the accumulation of autoreactive B cells and subsequent autoantibody production [72]. Interestingly, TNF inhibitors restore Treg populations in RA [73], and IL-6 inhibitors have been shown to restore both Treg and Tfr cells [74,75]. Meanwhile, T-bet$^+$ B cells, which express CXCR3, are abundant in the joint and contribute to the inflammatory milieu by producing TNF-α and IL-6 [76] (Figure 4).

IL-8 produced by macrophages promotes the migration and activation of neutrophils, playing a critical role in sustaining chronic inflammation in RA [77]. Recent single-cell analyses have demonstrated the expansion of IL1B$^+$ pro-inflammatory macrophages in the RA synovium [78]. FLS also contribute to IL-1β production. In addition to these cytokines, TNF-α and IL-6 are especially important in the inflamed joint microenvironment. TNF-α acts on various synovial cell types, with FLS being particularly important targets. TNF-α stimulates FLS to produce inflammatory cytokines and chemokines, promotes their proliferation and migration, enhances resistance to apoptosis, and collectively drives chronic synovitis [79].

IL-6, on the other hand, plays a central role in amplifying inflammation and inducing tissue damage in the joint. IL-6 signaling proceeds via two primary pathways: classic signaling and trans-signaling. In classic signaling, IL-6 acts on cells that express membrane-bound IL-6 receptor (mIL-6R), such as neutrophils, macrophages, and hepatocytes. In trans-signaling, IL-6 forms a complex with soluble IL-6R (sIL-6R), allowing it to act on nearly all cells that express the signal transducer gp130. This pathway leads to broader and sustained inflammation and is considered more relevant to RA pathogenesis [80]. In RA, concentrations of IL-6 and sIL-6R are elevated in the joint, enabling IL-6 to transmit inflammatory signals to cells such as FLS and chondrocytes that lack mIL-6R. Current IL-6 inhibitors target IL-6R and therefore block both classic and trans-signaling. Neutrophils are considered a major source of sIL-6R in the joint, generated via shedding of mIL-6R (Figure 4).

What, then, are the primary sources of IL-6 in the joint? Recent single-cell studies have identified THY1 (CD90)$^+$ sublining FLS as the main producers of IL-6 [78]. These findings underscore the central role of FLS in driving inflammation in the clinical phase of RA. Beyond local effects, IL-6 also contributes to systemic inflammation by inducing the hepatic production of hepcidin and thrombopoietin (TPO), leading to anemia of chronic disease and thrombocytosis. IL-6 further stimulates the acute-phase response, promoting the synthesis of C-reactive protein (CRP), fibrinogen, and other proteins (Figure 4).

Omics technologies, including transcriptomics and single-cell RNA sequencing, have been widely employed to elucidate RA pathogenesis. These analyses have revealed that multiple cytokines—such as TNF-α, IL-6, IL-17, IL-1β, and GM-CSF—play central roles in inflammation and tissue destruction in RA. The cytokine profiling of blood from RA patients has also demonstrated correlations between disease activity and levels of cytokines such as IL-17A and TNF-α [4,81]. Furthermore, plasma proteomics comparing RA patients and healthy controls has uncovered abnormalities in molecular networks centered around immune regulation, intracellular signaling, hematopoiesis, and cytokine modulation, including STAT1, TNF, and CD40. In addition, altered levels of osteocalcin (involved in bone metabolism), apolipoprotein A-I, and metallothionein-2 (an antioxidant protein) were also observed [82]. Proteomic analyses of neutrophils in RA synovial tissue have revealed a highly activated state, characterized by the massive release of myeloperoxidase (MPO) and ROS, which are major contributors to local protein carbamylation. Since carbamylated proteins can become targets of autoantibodies, they may contribute to the progression of RA [83].

Although the focus thus far has been on CD4$^+$ T cells, CD8$^+$ T cells also play important roles in RA pathogenesis (Figure 4). Recent single-cell studies have revealed expansions of cytotoxic CD8$^+$ T cells, particularly granzyme B (GzmB)$^+$ cells, in the peripheral blood and synovial tissue of ACPA-positive RA patients. These cells are activated by citrullinated antigens and contribute to synovitis and tissue destruction [84]. GzmB degrades components of the synovial extracellular matrix—such as tenascin-C—thereby generating pro-inflammatory fragments [85]. In contrast, a distinct subset of GzmK$^+$ CD8$^+$ T cells have recently gained attention. These cells are abundant in the sublining regions of RA synovium and exhibit limited cytotoxicity, but maintain chronic inflammation by producing inflammatory cytokines such as IFN-γ, activating complementary cells, and interacting with stromal cells [86]. The differentiation of these two CD8$^+$ T cell subsets is also distinct

(Figure 4): GzmK⁺ cells predominantly display central memory (CM) or effector memory (EM) phenotypes and respond strongly to cytokines such as IL-7 and IL-15. Under TCR stimulation, they downregulate GzmK and upregulate GzmB [87]. In contrast, $GzmB^{+}$ cells represent more terminally differentiated effector phenotypes and are primarily induced via TCR stimulation, with IL-12 and IFN-γ acting as key cytokines [88]. We have also identified a subset of $CD8^{+}$ T cells with B cell-helper capacity. These cells produce cytokines such as IFN-γ and IL-21 and share functional characteristics with Tph cells. They are abundant in the joints of autoantibody-positive RA patients [89]. Intriguingly, age-associated $CD4^{+}$ T cells (ThA) were recently reported to possess a dual functionality, exhibiting both cytotoxic properties like $CD8^{+}$ T cells and B cell-helper functions, supporting autoantibody production [90].

In addition to $CD8^{+}$ T cells, NK cells also play important roles within RA joints. $CD16^{+}$ NK cells are increased in RA synovial tissue and are activated through immune complexes to produce IFN-γ. This NK-derived IFN-γ promotes the expansion of $CD90^{+}$ FLS, which express high levels of HLA-DR and inflammatory cytokines such as IL-6. These activated FLS enhance $CD4^{+}$ T cell activation via antigen presentation and contribute to the maintenance of chronic inflammation and autoimmunity in RA [91].

Angiogenesis in RA synovium is promoted by various factors, including vascular endothelial growth factor (VEGF), TNF-α, IL-6, and IL-17. Among these, VEGF is considered the principal pro-angiogenic factor in RA [92]. FLS constitutively express VEGF, and their expression is further enhanced by hypoxia and pro-inflammatory cytokines [93]. TNF and IL-6 inhibitors, such as infliximab and tocilizumab, suppress VEGF production and are positively correlated with reductions in synovitis severity, as assessed by ultrasound [92].

3.3. Progression of Joint Destruction

During the clinical phase of RA, joint destruction progresses and ultimately leads to irreversible deformity and functional impairment. TNF-α and IL-1β induce FLS and chondrocytes to express MMP-3, which contributes to cartilage matrix degradation [94]. Furthermore, IL-6–mediated trans-signaling promotes RANKL expression by FLS, thereby inducing osteoclast differentiation and bone resorption [4].

IFN-γ, in addition to modulating FLS function, enhances their motility and invasiveness, contributing to the destructive remodeling of joint tissues. This process is mediated via the JAK2–FAK signaling pathway and is suppressed by JAK inhibitors [95]. Osteoclasts are central to bone erosion. TNF-α, IL-6, IL-1β, and IL-17 upregulate RANKL expression in FLS, promoting osteoclastogenesis and activation. IL-1β enhances the bone-resorbing activity of osteoclasts and also contributes to RANKL-independent activation [96]. Moreover, TNF-α, in the presence of M-CSF, can induce osteoclast differentiation from murine macrophages independently of RANKL [97]; however, in human monocytes, synergistic actions with other cytokines—particularly IL-6 and TGF-β—are considered essential [98,99]. Since FLS do not express mIL-6R, trans-signaling is again critical for IL-6-induced RANKL expression in these cells [100]. Transcription factors such as Ets2 and SOX5 are also activated under IL-6 trans-signaling and contribute to RANKL upregulation [101].

Although FLS are the primary source of RANKL in RA, we showed that double-negative B cells—including T-bet⁺ subsets—and switched memory B cells also express RANKL [102]. In untreated RA patients, the frequency of T-bet⁺ B cells correlates with bone erosions, joint space narrowing, and modified total sharp score (mTSS) [103]. In addition, T cells can also serve as a source of RANKL in RA (Figure 4). $CD4^{+}$ T cells from RA patients have been shown to express RANKL upon stimulation with inflammatory cytokines such as IL-21 and IL-23, thereby contributing to bone destruction [104]. However, recent molecular analyses have demonstrated that the majority of RANKL-producing cells in RA synovium are FLS [105]. Interestingly, the inhibition of RANKL alone effectively suppresses bone erosion but does not sufficiently control synovitis, suggesting that the mechanisms of joint inflammation and bone destruction are at least partially distinct [106].

4. Conclusions

RA represents a paradigm of chronic inflammation in which cytokine networks orchestrate the continuum from autoimmunity to synovitis and joint destruction. Our synthesis of current evidence highlights that although TNF-α and IL-6 remain the most dominant and therapeutically validated cytokines, a broader spectrum—including IL-1β, IL-17, BAFF/APRIL, type I IFN, and novel mediators identified by single-cell and proteomic technologies—collectively shape disease progression. This complexity underscores why blockade of a single cytokine may fail in a subset of patients and points to the need for strategies that can modulate multiple signaling pathways simultaneously, as exemplified by JAK inhibitors.

From the authors' perspective, one of the most pressing frontiers is the preclinical phase. Cytokine perturbations clearly precede the onset of arthritis, yet reliable biomarkers that predict transition to overt disease remain elusive, and preventive interventions have not been firmly established. Deeper exploration of this "window of opportunity," through longitudinal profiling and molecular stratification, may ultimately allow us to intercept disease before irreversible tissue injury occurs. At the same time, heterogeneity within the synovium—such as FLS subsets driving fibrosis, or pathogenic Tph/T-bet$^+$ B cell interactions sustaining chronicity—reminds us that RA is not a uniform condition. Future therapies will likely need to account for such endotype-specific differences.

In conclusion, while cytokine-targeted therapies have already transformed RA management, the continued integration of omics technologies, spatial immunology, and clinical observation holds the promise of a more precise and preventive approach. We envision a future in which cytokine signatures not only guide treatment selection but also enable early intervention strategies, redefining the trajectory of RA from inevitable progression to a potentially preventable disease.

Author Contributions: Conceptualization: H.N. Writing—original draft preparation: S.F. and H.N. Writing—review and editing: S.F. and H.N. Supervision: H.N. All authors have read and agreed to the published version of the manuscript.

Funding: This work was supported by JSPS KAKENHI: grant number 24K11597 for H.N.

Acknowledgments: We are indebted to the lab members for their helpful discussions on this review.

Conflicts of Interest: H.N. has received research grants from Chugai and Asahi-Kasei, as well as receiving speaking fees from Chugai, Asahi-Kasei, Bristol-Myers Squibb, Eli Lilly, Glaxo Smith Kline, Mitsubishi-Tanabe, AstraZeneca.

References

1. Nielen, M.M.J.; van Schaardenburg, D.; Reesink, H.W.; van de Stadt, R.J.; van der Horst-Bruinsma, I.E.; de Koning, M.H.M.T.; Habibuw, M.R.; Vandenbroucke, J.P.; Dijkmans, B.A.C. Specific Autoantibodies Precede the Symptoms of Rheumatoid Arthritis: A Study of Serial Measurements in Blood Donors. *Arthritis Rheum.* **2004**, *50*, 380–386. [CrossRef] [PubMed]
2. Raychaudhuri, S.; Sandor, C.; Stahl, E.A.; Freudenberg, J.; Lee, H.-S.; Jia, X.; Alfredsson, L.; Padyukov, L.; Klareskog, L.; Worthington, J.; et al. Five Amino Acids in Three HLA Proteins Explain Most of the Association between MHC and Seropositive Rheumatoid Arthritis. *Nat. Genet.* **2012**, *44*, 291–296. [CrossRef] [PubMed]
3. Snir, O.; Gomez-Cabrero, D.; Montes, A.; Perez-Pampin, E.; Gómez-Reino, J.J.; Seddighzadeh, M.; Klich, K.U.; Israelsson, L.; Ding, B.; Catrina, A.I.; et al. Non-HLA Genes PTPN22, CDK6 and PADI4 Are Associated with Specific Autoantibodies in HLA-Defined Subgroups of Rheumatoid Arthritis. *Arthritis Res. Ther.* **2014**, *16*, 414. [CrossRef] [PubMed]

4. Gravallese, E.M.; Firestein, G.S. Rheumatoid Arthritis—Common Origins, Divergent Mechanisms. *N. Engl. J. Med.* **2023**, *388*, 529–542. [CrossRef] [PubMed]
5. Möller, B.; Kollert, F.; Sculean, A.; Villiger, P.M. Infectious Triggers in Periodontitis and the Gut in Rheumatoid Arthritis (RA): A Complex Story About Association and Causality. *Front. Immunol.* **2020**, *11*, 1108. [CrossRef]
6. Lu, J.; Wang, Y.; Wu, J.; Duan, Y.; Zhang, H.; Du, H. Linking Microbial Communities to Rheumatoid Arthritis: Focus on Gut, Oral Microbiome and Their Extracellular Vesicles. *Front. Immunol.* **2025**, *16*, 1503474. [CrossRef]
7. James, E.A.; Rieck, M.; Pieper, J.; Gebe, J.A.; Yue, B.B.; Tatum, M.; Peda, M.; Sandin, C.; Klareskog, L.; Malmström, V.; et al. Citrulline-Specific Th1 Cells Are Increased in Rheumatoid Arthritis and Their Frequency Is Influenced by Disease Duration and Therapy. *Arthritis Rheumatol.* **2014**, *66*, 1712–1722. [CrossRef] [PubMed]
8. Scherer, H.U.; Huizinga, T.W.J.; Krönke, G.; Schett, G.; Toes, R.E.M. The B Cell Response to Citrullinated Antigens in the Development of Rheumatoid Arthritis. *Nat. Rev. Rheumatol.* **2018**, *14*, 157–169. [CrossRef]
9. Samuels, J.; Ng, Y.-S.; Coupillaud, C.; Paget, D.; Meffre, E. Impaired Early B Cell Tolerance in Patients with Rheumatoid Arthritis. *J. Exp. Med.* **2005**, *201*, 1659–1667. [CrossRef]
10. Schmitt, N.; Ueno, H. Regulation of Human Helper T Cell Subset Differentiation by Cytokines. *Curr. Opin. Immunol.* **2015**, *34*, 130–136. [CrossRef]
11. Ma, C.S.; Wong, N.; Rao, G.; Avery, D.T.; Torpy, J.; Hambridge, T.; Bustamante, J.; Okada, S.; Stoddard, J.L.; Deenick, E.K.; et al. Monogenic Mutations Differentially Affect the Quantity and Quality of T Follicular Helper Cells in Patients with Human Primary Immunodeficiencies. *J. Allergy Clin. Immunol.* **2015**, *136*, 993–1006.e1. [CrossRef]
12. Avery, D.T.; Deenick, E.K.; Ma, C.S.; Suryani, S.; Simpson, N.; Chew, G.Y.; Chan, T.D.; Palendira, U.; Bustamante, J.; Boisson-Dupuis, S.; et al. B Cell-Intrinsic Signaling through IL-21 Receptor and STAT3 Is Required for Establishing Long-Lived Antibody Responses in Humans. *J. Exp. Med.* **2010**, *207*, 155–171. [CrossRef]
13. Eslami, M.; Schneider, P. Function, Occurrence and Inhibition of Different Forms of BAFF. *Curr. Opin. Immunol.* **2021**, *71*, 75–80. [CrossRef]
14. Shabgah, A.G.; Shariati-Sarabi, Z.; Tavakkol-Afshari, J.; Mohammadi, M. The Role of BAFF and APRIL in Rheumatoid Arthritis. *J. Cell. Physiol.* **2019**, *234*, 17050–17063. [CrossRef]
15. Lee, L.; Draper, B.; Chaplin, N.; Philip, B.; Chin, M.; Galas-Filipowicz, D.; Onuoha, S.; Thomas, S.; Baldan, V.; Bughda, R.; et al. An APRIL-Based Chimeric Antigen Receptor for Dual Targeting of BCMA and TACI in Multiple Myeloma. *Blood* **2018**, *131*, 746–758. [CrossRef] [PubMed]
16. Stephenson, S.; Care, M.A.; Doody, G.M.; Tooze, R.M. APRIL Drives a Coordinated but Diverse Response as a Foundation for Plasma Cell Longevity. *J. Immunol. Baltim.* **2022**, *209*, 926–937. [CrossRef] [PubMed]
17. Rodríguez-Bayona, B.; Ramos-Amaya, A.; López-Blanco, R.; Campos-Caro, A.; Brieva, J.A. STAT-3 Activation by Differential Cytokines Is Critical for Human in Vivo-Generated Plasma Cell Survival and Ig Secretion. *J. Immunol. Baltim.* **2013**, *191*, 4996–5004. [CrossRef] [PubMed]
18. Hua, C.; Audo, R.; Yeremenko, N.; Baeten, D.; Hahne, M.; Combe, B.; Morel, J.; Daïen, C. A Proliferation Inducing Ligand (APRIL) Promotes IL-10 Production and Regulatory Functions of Human B Cells. *J. Autoimmun.* **2016**, *73*, 64–72. [CrossRef]
19. Fehres, C.M.; van Uden, N.O.; Yeremenko, N.G.; Fernandez, L.; Franco Salinas, G.; van Duivenvoorde, L.M.; Huard, B.; Morel, J.; Spits, H.; Hahne, M.; et al. APRIL Induces a Novel Subset of IgA+ Regulatory B Cells That Suppress Inflammation via Expression of IL-10 and PD-L1. *Front. Immunol.* **2019**, *10*, 1368. [CrossRef]
20. Poznyak, A.V.; Gerasimova, E.V.; Orekhov, N.A.; Karimova, A.E.; Vergun, M.A.; Lapshina, K.O.; Sukhorukov, V.N.; Orekhov, A.N. Exploring the Role of APRIL in Autoimmunity: Implications for Therapeutic Targeting in Systemic Lupus Erythematosus, Rheumatoid Arthritis, and Sjögren's Syndrome. *Front. Immunol.* **2025**, *16*, 1523392. [CrossRef]
21. Rao, D.A.; Gurish, M.F.; Marshall, J.L.; Slowikowski, K.; Fonseka, C.Y.; Liu, Y.; Donlin, L.T.; Henderson, L.A.; Wei, K.; Mizoguchi, F.; et al. Pathologically Expanded Peripheral T Helper Cell Subset Drives B Cells in Rheumatoid Arthritis. *Nature* **2017**, *542*, 110–114. [CrossRef] [PubMed]
22. Yoshitomi, H.; Ueno, H. Shared and Distinct Roles of T Peripheral Helper and T Follicular Helper Cells in Human Diseases. *Cell. Mol. Immunol.* **2021**, *18*, 523–527. [CrossRef] [PubMed]
23. Tanemura, S.; Tsujimoto, H.; Seki, N.; Kojima, S.; Miyoshi, F.; Sugahara, K.; Yoshimoto, K.; Suzuki, K.; Kaneko, Y.; Chiba, K.; et al. Role of Interferons (IFNs) in the Differentiation of T Peripheral Helper (Tph) Cells. *Int. Immunol.* **2022**, *34*, 519–532. [CrossRef]
24. Gonzalez, D.G.; Cote, C.M.; Patel, J.R.; Smith, C.B.; Zhang, Y.; Nickerson, K.M.; Zhang, T.; Kerfoot, S.M.; Haberman, A.M. Nonredundant Roles of IL-21 and IL-4 in the Phased Initiation of Germinal Center B Cells and Subsequent Self-Renewal Transitions. *J. Immunol. Baltim.* **2018**, *201*, 3569–3579. [CrossRef]
25. Huang, Y.; Ba, X.; Han, L.; Wang, H.; Lin, W.; Chen, Z.; Tu, S. T Peripheral Helper Cells in Autoimmune Diseases: What Do We Know? *Front. Immunol.* **2023**, *14*, 1145573. [CrossRef]

26. Maul, R.W.; Catalina, M.D.; Kumar, V.; Bachali, P.; Grammer, A.C.; Wang, S.; Yang, W.; Hasni, S.; Ettinger, R.; Lipsky, P.E.; et al. Transcriptome and IgH Repertoire Analyses Show That CD11chi B Cells Are a Distinct Population with Similarity to B Cells Arising in Autoimmunity and Infection. *Front. Immunol.* **2021**, *12*, 649458. [CrossRef]
27. Chodisetti, S.B.; Fike, A.J.; Domeier, P.P.; Singh, H.; Choi, N.M.; Corradetti, C.; Kawasawa, Y.I.; Cooper, T.K.; Caricchio, R.; Rahman, Z.S.M. Type II but Not Type I IFN Signaling Is Indispensable for TLR7-Promoted Development of Autoreactive B Cells and Systemic Autoimmunity. *J. Immunol. Baltim.* **2020**, *204*, 796–809. [CrossRef]
28. Nakayama, T.; Yoshimura, M.; Higashioka, K.; Miyawaki, K.; Ota, Y.; Ayano, M.; Kimoto, Y.; Mitoma, H.; Ono, N.; Arinobu, Y.; et al. Type 1 Helper T Cells Generate CXCL9/10-Producing T-Bet+ Effector B Cells Potentially Involved in the Pathogenesis of Rheumatoid Arthritis. *Cell. Immunol.* **2021**, *360*, 104263. [CrossRef]
29. Naradikian, M.S.; Myles, A.; Beiting, D.P.; Roberts, K.J.; Dawson, L.; Herati, R.S.; Bengsch, B.; Linderman, S.L.; Stelekati, E.; Spolski, R.; et al. Cutting Edge: IL-4, IL-21, and IFN-γ Interact To Govern T-Bet and CD11c Expression in TLR-Activated B Cells. *J. Immunol. Baltim.* **2016**, *197*, 1023–1028. [CrossRef]
30. Rangel-Moreno, J.; Hartson, L.; Navarro, C.; Gaxiola, M.; Selman, M.; Randall, T.D. Inducible Bronchus-Associated Lymphoid Tissue (iBALT) in Patients with Pulmonary Complications of Rheumatoid Arthritis. *J. Clin. Investig.* **2006**, *116*, 3183–3194. [CrossRef] [PubMed]
31. Scherer, H.U.; van der Woude, D.; Toes, R.E.M. From Risk to Chronicity: Evolution of Autoreactive B Cell and Antibody Responses in Rheumatoid Arthritis. *Nat. Rev. Rheumatol.* **2022**, *18*, 371–383. [CrossRef]
32. Takada, H.; Demoruelle, M.K.; Deane, K.D.; Nakamura, S.; Katsumata, Y.; Ikari, K.; Buckner, J.H.; Robinson, W.H.; Seifert, J.A.; Feser, M.L.; et al. Expansion of HLA-DR Positive Peripheral Helper T and Naive B Cells in Anticitrullinated Protein Antibody-Positive Individuals At Risk for Rheumatoid Arthritis. *Arthritis Rheumatol.* **2024**, *76*, 1023–1035. [CrossRef] [PubMed]
33. Inamo, J.; Keegan, J.; Griffith, A.; Ghosh, T.; Horisberger, A.; Howard, K.; Pulford, J.F.; Murzin, E.; Hancock, B.; Dominguez, S.T.; et al. Deep Immunophenotyping Reveals Circulating Activated Lymphocytes in Individuals at Risk for Rheumatoid Arthritis. *J. Clin. Investig.* **2025**, *135*, e185217. [CrossRef] [PubMed]
34. Yokoi, E.; Wakahara, K.; Nakamura, S.; Fukutani, E.; Asai, S.; Takahashi, N.; Kojima, T.; Iwano, S.; Shimada, S.; Chen-Yoshikawa, T.F.; et al. Increased Sputum Peripheral Helper T Cells Are Associated with the Severity of Rheumatoid Arthritis but Not with the Severity of Airway Disease. *Front. Immunol.* **2025**, *16*, 1526881. [CrossRef] [PubMed]
35. Ridgley, L.A.; Anderson, A.E.; Pratt, A.G. What Are the Dominant Cytokines in Early Rheumatoid Arthritis? *Curr. Opin. Rheumatol.* **2018**, *30*, 207–214. [CrossRef]
36. Joshua, V.; Loberg Haarhaus, M.; Hensvold, A.; Wähämaa, H.; Gerstner, C.; Hansson, M.; Israelsson, L.; Stålesen, R.; Sköld, M.; Grunewald, J.; et al. Rheumatoid Arthritis-Specific Autoimmunity in the Lung Before and at the Onset of Disease. *Arthritis Rheumatol.* **2023**, *75*, 1910–1922. [CrossRef]
37. Castañeda-Delgado, J.E.; Bastián-Hernandez, Y.; Macias-Segura, N.; Santiago-Algarra, D.; Castillo-Ortiz, J.D.; Alemán-Navarro, A.L.; Martínez-Tejada, P.; Enciso-Moreno, L.; Garcia-De Lira, Y.; Olguín-Calderón, D.; et al. Type I Interferon Gene Response Is Increased in Early and Established Rheumatoid Arthritis and Correlates with Autoantibody Production. *Front. Immunol.* **2017**, *8*, 285. [CrossRef]
38. Lübbers, J.; Brink, M.; van de Stadt, L.A.; Vosslamber, S.; Wesseling, J.G.; van Schaardenburg, D.; Rantapää-Dahlqvist, S.; Verweij, C.L. The Type I IFN Signature as a Biomarker of Preclinical Rheumatoid Arthritis. *Ann. Rheum. Dis.* **2013**, *72*, 776–780. [CrossRef]
39. Brink, M.; Lundquist, A.; Alexeyenko, A.; Lejon, K.; Rantapää-Dahlqvist, S. Protein Profiling and Network Enrichment Analysis in Individuals before and after the Onset of Rheumatoid Arthritis. *Arthritis Res. Ther.* **2019**, *21*, 288. [CrossRef]
40. O'Neil, L.J.; Meng, X.; Mcfadyen, C.; Fritzler, M.J.; El-Gabalawy, H.S. Serum Proteomic Networks Associate with Pre-Clinical Rheumatoid Arthritis Autoantibodies and Longitudinal Outcomes. *Front. Immunol.* **2022**, *13*, 958145. [CrossRef]
41. Isaacs, J.D.; Iqbal, K. Potential Pharmacologic Targets for the Prevention of Rheumatoid Arthritis. *Clin. Ther.* **2019**, *41*, 1312–1322. [CrossRef]
42. Deane, K.D.; Holers, V.M.; Emery, P.; Mankia, K.; El-Gabalawy, H.; Sparks, J.A.; Costenbader, K.H.; Schett, G.; van der Helm-van Mil, A.; van Schaardenburg, D.; et al. Therapeutic Interception in Individuals at Risk of Rheumatoid Arthritis to Prevent Clinically Impactful Disease. *Ann. Rheum. Dis.* **2025**, *84*, 14–28. [CrossRef] [PubMed]
43. Rivellese, F.; Pontarini, E.; Fossati-Jimack, L.; Moura, R.A.; Romão, V.C.; Fonseca, J.E.; Nerviani, A.; Çubuk, C.; Goldmann, K.; Giorli, G.; et al. Comparative Analysis of Circulating and Synovial Immune Cells in Early Untreated Rheumatoid Arthritis and Their Relationship with Molecular Pathology and Disease Outcomes. *Arthritis Rheumatol.* **2025**. [CrossRef] [PubMed]
44. Bai, Z.; Yang, S.; Ren, J.; Zhang, C.; Chen, X.; Huang, H.; Wang, G.; Tang, Y.; Qi, J.; Li, X. Exploring the Differential Functions of Circulating Follicular Helper T and Peripheral Helper T Cells in Rheumatoid Arthritis Based on Metabolism Patterns. *Front. Immunol.* **2025**, *16*, 1608675. [CrossRef]
45. Sowerby, J.M.; Rao, D.A. T Cell-B Cell Interactions in Human Autoimmune Diseases. *Curr. Opin. Immunol.* **2025**, *93*, 102539. [CrossRef]

46. Masuo, Y.; Murakami, A.; Akamine, R.; Iri, O.; Uno, S.; Murata, K.; Nishitani, K.; Ito, H.; Watanabe, R.; Fujii, T.; et al. Stem-like and Effector Peripheral Helper T Cells Comprise Distinct Subsets in Rheumatoid Arthritis. *Sci. Immunol.* **2025**, *10*, eadt3955. [CrossRef]
47. Murakami, A.; Akamine, R.; Tanaka, S.; Murata, K.; Nishitani, K.; Ito, H.; Watanabe, R.; Fujii, T.; Iwasaki, T.; Masuo, Y.; et al. Human CD4+ T Cells Regulate Peripheral Immune Responses in Rheumatoid Arthritis via Insulin-like Growth Factor-like Family Member 2. *Sci. Immunol.* **2025**, *10*, eadr3838. [CrossRef] [PubMed]
48. Vidal-Pedrola, G.; Naamane, N.; Cameron, J.A.; Pratt, A.G.; Mellor, A.L.; Isaacs, J.D.; Scheel-Toellner, D.; Anderson, A.E. Characterization of Age-Associated B Cells in Early Drug-Naïve Rheumatoid Arthritis Patients. *Immunology* **2023**, *168*, 640–653. [CrossRef]
49. Kim, J.G.; Kim, M.; Hong, B.-K.; Choe, Y.-H.; Kim, J.-R.; Lee, N.; You, S.; Lee, S.-I.; Kim, W.-U. Circulatory Age-Associated B Cells: Their Distinct Transcriptomic Characteristics and Clinical Significance in Drug-Naïve Patients with Rheumatoid Arthritis. *Clin. Immunol.* **2025**, *271*, 110425. [CrossRef]
50. Li, Z.-Y.; Cai, M.-L.; Qin, Y.; Chen, Z. Age/Autoimmunity-Associated B Cells in Inflammatory Arthritis: An Emerging Therapeutic Target. *Front. Immunol.* **2023**, *14*, 1103307. [CrossRef]
51. Pelzek, A.J.; Grönwall, C.; Rosenthal, P.; Greenberg, J.D.; McGeachy, M.; Moreland, L.; Rigby, W.F.C.; Silverman, G.J. Persistence of Disease-Associated Anti-Citrullinated Protein Antibody-Expressing Memory B Cells in Rheumatoid Arthritis in Clinical Remission. *Arthritis Rheumatol.* **2017**, *69*, 1176–1186. [CrossRef]
52. Reijm, S.; Kwekkeboom, J.C.; Blomberg, N.J.; Suurmond, J.; van der Woude, D.; Toes, R.E.; Scherer, H.U. Autoreactive B Cells in Rheumatoid Arthritis Include Mainly Activated CXCR3+ Memory B Cells and Plasmablasts. *JCI Insight* **2023**, *8*, e172006. [CrossRef] [PubMed]
53. Hensvold, A.; Horuluoglu, B.; Sahlström, P.; Thyagarajan, R.; Diaz Boada, J.S.; Hansson, M.; Mathsson-Alm, L.; Gerstner, C.; Sippl, N.; Israelsson, L.; et al. The Human Bone Marrow Plasma Cell Compartment in Rheumatoid Arthritis—Clonal Relationships and Anti-Citrulline Autoantibody Producing Cells. *J. Autoimmun.* **2023**, *136*, 103022. [CrossRef] [PubMed]
54. Lu, D.R.; McDavid, A.N.; Kongpachith, S.; Lingampalli, N.; Glanville, J.; Ju, C.-H.; Gottardo, R.; Robinson, W.H. T Cell-Dependent Affinity Maturation and Innate Immune Pathways Differentially Drive Autoreactive B Cell Responses in Rheumatoid Arthritis. *Arthritis Rheumatol.* **2018**, *70*, 1732–1744. [CrossRef]
55. Kurowska-Stolarska, M.; Alivernini, S. Synovial Tissue Macrophages in Joint Homeostasis, Rheumatoid Arthritis and Disease Remission. *Nat. Rev. Rheumatol.* **2022**, *18*, 384–397. [CrossRef] [PubMed]
56. Cutolo, M.; Campitiello, R.; Gotelli, E.; Soldano, S. The Role of M1/M2 Macrophage Polarization in Rheumatoid Arthritis Synovitis. *Front. Immunol.* **2022**, *13*, 867260. [CrossRef]
57. Kennedy, A.; Fearon, U.; Veale, D.J.; Godson, C. Macrophages in Synovial Inflammation. *Front. Immunol.* **2011**, *2*, 52. [CrossRef]
58. Chen, J.; Zhan, M.; Zhao, Y.; Xu, H.; Feng, F.; Bai, Z.; Zhang, K.; Fu, L.; Wang, F.; Cheng, Y.; et al. GM-CSF Potentiates Macrophages to Retain an Inflammatory Feature from Their Circulating Monocyte Precursors in Rheumatoid Arthritis. *J. Transl. Med.* **2025**, *23*, 883. [CrossRef]
59. Kugler, M.; Dellinger, M.; Kartnig, F.; Müller, L.; Preglej, T.; Heinz, L.X.; Simader, E.; Göschl, L.; Puchner, S.E.; Weiss, S.; et al. Cytokine-Directed Cellular Cross-Talk Imprints Synovial Pathotypes in Rheumatoid Arthritis. *Ann. Rheum. Dis.* **2023**, *82*, 1142–1152. [CrossRef]
60. Zheng, L.; Gu, M.; Li, X.; Hu, X.; Chen, C.; Kang, Y.; Pan, B.; Chen, W.; Xian, G.; Wu, X.; et al. ITGA5+ Synovial Fibroblasts Orchestrate Proinflammatory Niche Formation by Remodelling the Local Immune Microenvironment in Rheumatoid Arthritis. *Ann. Rheum. Dis.* **2025**, *84*, 232–252. [CrossRef]
61. Nygaard, G.; Firestein, G.S. Restoring Synovial Homeostasis in Rheumatoid Arthritis by Targeting Fibroblast-like Synoviocytes. *Nat. Rev. Rheumatol.* **2020**, *16*, 316–333. [CrossRef]
62. van Hamburg, J.P.; Tas, S.W. Molecular Mechanisms Underpinning T Helper 17 Cell Heterogeneity and Functions in Rheumatoid Arthritis. *J. Autoimmun.* **2018**, *87*, 69–81. [CrossRef] [PubMed]
63. Aldridge, J.; Ekwall, A.-K.H.; Mark, L.; Bergström, B.; Andersson, K.; Gjertsson, I.; Lundell, A.-C.; Rudin, A. T Helper Cells in Synovial Fluid of Patients with Rheumatoid Arthritis Primarily Have a Th1 and a CXCR3+Th2 Phenotype. *Arthritis Res. Ther.* **2020**, *22*, 245. [CrossRef]
64. Panda, S.K.; Wigerblad, G.; Jiang, L.; Jiménez-Andrade, Y.; Iyer, V.S.; Shen, Y.; Boddul, S.V.; Guerreiro-Cacais, A.O.; Raposo, B.; Kasza, Z.; et al. IL-4 Controls Activated Neutrophil FcγR2b Expression and Migration into Inflamed Joints. *Proc. Natl. Acad. Sci. USA* **2020**, *117*, 3103–3113. [CrossRef] [PubMed]
65. Isomäki, P.; Luukkainen, R.; Lassila, O.; Toivanen, P.; Punnonen, J. Synovial Fluid T Cells from Patients with Rheumatoid Arthritis Are Refractory to the T Helper Type 2 Differentiation-Inducing Effects of Interleukin-4. *Immunology* **1999**, *96*, 358–364. [CrossRef]
66. Arroyo-Villa, I.; Bautista-Caro, M.-B.; Balsa, A.; Aguado-Acín, P.; Bonilla-Hernán, M.-G.; Plasencia, C.; Villalba, A.; Nuño, L.; Puig-Kröger, A.; Martín-Mola, E.; et al. Constitutively Altered Frequencies of Circulating Follicullar Helper T Cell Counterparts and Their Subsets in Rheumatoid Arthritis. *Arthritis Res. Ther.* **2014**, *16*, 500. [CrossRef] [PubMed]

67. Ho, T.H.; Pfeffer, K.; Weiss, G.J.; Ruiz, Y.; Lake, D.F. Identification of a CD4+ T Cell Line with Treg-like Activity. *Hum. Immunol.* **2022**, *83*, 281–294. [CrossRef]
68. Lei, H.; Kuchenbecker, L.; Streitz, M.; Sawitzki, B.; Vogt, K.; Landwehr-Kenzel, S.; Millward, J.; Juelke, K.; Babel, N.; Neumann, A.; et al. Human CD45RA(-) FoxP3(Hi) Memory-Type Regulatory T Cells Show Distinct TCR Repertoires with Conventional T Cells and Play an Important Role in Controlling Early Immune Activation. *Am. J. Transplant.* **2015**, *15*, 2625–2635. [CrossRef]
69. Castaño, D.; Wang, S.; Atencio-Garcia, S.; Shields, E.J.; Rico, M.C.; Sharpe, H.; Bustamante, J.; Feng, A.; Le Coz, C.; Romberg, N.; et al. IL-12 Drives the Differentiation of Human T Follicular Regulatory Cells. *Sci. Immunol.* **2024**, *9*, eadf2047. [CrossRef]
70. Avdeeva, A.; Rubtsov, Y.; Dyikanov, D.; Popkova, T.; Nasonov, E. Regulatory T Cells in Patients with Early Untreated Rheumatoid Arthritis: Phenotypic Changes in the Course of Methotrexate Treatment. *Biochimie* **2020**, *174*, 9–17. [CrossRef]
71. Liu, C.; Wang, D.; Lu, S.; Xu, Q.; Zhao, L.; Zhao, J.; Song, Y.; Wang, H. Increased Circulating Follicular Treg Cells Are Associated with Lower Levels of Autoantibodies in Patients with Rheumatoid Arthritis in Stable Remission. *Arthritis Rheumatol.* **2018**, *70*, 711–721. [CrossRef]
72. Meffre, E.; O'Connor, K.C. Impaired B-Cell Tolerance Checkpoints Promote the Development of Autoimmune Diseases and Pathogenic Autoantibodies. *Immunol. Rev.* **2019**, *292*, 90–101. [CrossRef]
73. Ehrenstein, M.R.; Evans, J.G.; Singh, A.; Moore, S.; Warnes, G.; Isenberg, D.A.; Mauri, C. Compromised Function of Regulatory T Cells in Rheumatoid Arthritis and Reversal by Anti-TNFα Therapy. *J. Exp. Med.* **2004**, *200*, 277–285. [CrossRef] [PubMed]
74. Thiolat, A.; Semerano, L.; Pers, Y.M.; Biton, J.; Lemeiter, D.; Portales, P.; Quentin, J.; Jorgensen, C.; Decker, P.; Boissier, M.-C.; et al. Interleukin-6 Receptor Blockade Enhances CD39+ Regulatory T Cell Development in Rheumatoid Arthritis and in Experimental Arthritis. *Arthritis Rheumatol.* **2014**, *66*, 273–283. [CrossRef]
75. Niu, Q.; Huang, Z.-C.; Wu, X.-J.; Jin, Y.-X.; An, Y.-F.; Li, Y.-M.; Xu, H.; Yang, B.; Wang, L.-L. Enhanced IL-6/Phosphorylated STAT3 Signaling Is Related to the Imbalance of Circulating T Follicular Helper/T Follicular Regulatory Cells in Patients with Rheumatoid Arthritis. *Arthritis Res. Ther.* **2018**, *20*, 200. [CrossRef] [PubMed]
76. Qin, Y.; Cai, M.-L.; Jin, H.-Z.; Huang, W.; Zhu, C.; Bozec, A.; Huang, J.; Chen, Z. Age-Associated B Cells Contribute to the Pathogenesis of Rheumatoid Arthritis by Inducing Activation of Fibroblast-like Synoviocytes via TNF-α-Mediated ERK1/2 and JAK-STAT1 Pathways. *Ann. Rheum. Dis.* **2022**, *81*, 1504–1514. [CrossRef] [PubMed]
77. Koch, A.E.; Kunkel, S.L.; Burrows, J.C.; Evanoff, H.L.; Haines, G.K.; Pope, R.M.; Strieter, R.M. Synovial Tissue Macrophage as a Source of the Chemotactic Cytokine IL-8. *J. Immunol. Baltim.* **1991**, *147*, 2187–2195. [CrossRef]
78. Zhang, F.; Wei, K.; Slowikowski, K.; Fonseka, C.Y.; Rao, D.A.; Kelly, S.; Goodman, S.M.; Tabechian, D.; Hughes, L.B.; Salomon-Escoto, K.; et al. Defining Inflammatory Cell States in Rheumatoid Arthritis Joint Synovial Tissues by Integrating Single-Cell Transcriptomics and Mass Cytometry. *Nat. Immunol.* **2019**, *20*, 928–942. [CrossRef]
79. Suto, T.; Tosevska, A.; Dalwigk, K.; Kugler, M.; Dellinger, M.; Stanic, I.; Platzer, A.; Niederreiter, B.; Sevelda, F.; Bonelli, M.; et al. TNFR2 Is Critical for TNF-Induced Rheumatoid Arthritis Fibroblast-like Synoviocyte Inflammation. *Rheumatology* **2022**, *61*, 4535–4546. [CrossRef]
80. Rose-John, S.; Jenkins, B.J.; Garbers, C.; Moll, J.M.; Scheller, J. Targeting IL-6 Trans-Signalling: Past, Present and Future Prospects. *Nat. Rev. Immunol.* **2023**, *23*, 666–681. [CrossRef] [PubMed]
81. Dissanayake, K.; Jayasinghe, C.; Wanigasekara, P.; Sominanda, A. Potential Applicability of Cytokines as Biomarkers of Disease Activity in Rheumatoid Arthritis: Enzyme-Linked Immunosorbent Spot Assay-Based Evaluation of TNF-α, IL-1β, IL-10 and IL-17A. *PLoS ONE* **2021**, *16*, e0246111. [CrossRef]
82. Masood, A.; Benabdelkamel, H.; Alfadda, A.A.; Alarfaj, A.S.; Fallata, A.; Joy, S.S.; Al Mogren, M.; Rahman, A.M.A.; Siaj, M. Proteomic Profiling Reveals Novel Molecular Insights into Dysregulated Proteins in Established Cases of Rheumatoid Arthritis. *Proteomes* **2025**, *13*, 32. [CrossRef]
83. Chen, X.; Du, R.; Wang, P.; Qiu, W.; Chen, L.; Wan, J.; Qiu, H.; Xiong, L.; Nandakumar, K.S.; Holmdahl, R.; et al. Proteomic Analysis of Infiltrating Neutrophils from Rheumatoid Arthritis Synovial Fluid and Their Contribution to Protein Carbamylation. *Front. Immunol.* **2025**, *16*, 1563426. [CrossRef]
84. Moon, J.-S.; Younis, S.; Ramadoss, N.S.; Iyer, R.; Sheth, K.; Sharpe, O.; Rao, N.L.; Becart, S.; Carman, J.A.; James, E.A.; et al. Cytotoxic CD8+ T Cells Target Citrullinated Antigens in Rheumatoid Arthritis. *Nat. Commun.* **2023**, *14*, 319. [CrossRef]
85. Aubert, A.; Liu, A.; Kao, M.; Goeres, J.; Richardson, K.C.; Nierves, L.; Jung, K.; Nabai, L.; Zhao, H.; Orend, G.; et al. Granzyme B Cleaves Tenascin-C to Release Its C-Terminal Domain in Rheumatoid Arthritis. *JCI Insight* **2024**, *9*, e181935. [CrossRef]
86. Guo, C.-L.; Wang, C.-S.; Wang, X.-H.; Yu, D.; Liu, Z. GZMK+CD8+ T Cells: Multifaceted Roles beyond Cytotoxicity. *Trends Immunol.* **2025**, *46*, 562–572. [CrossRef]
87. Duquette, D.; Harmon, C.; Zaborowski, A.; Michelet, X.; O'Farrelly, C.; Winter, D.; Koay, H.-F.; Lynch, L. Human Granzyme K Is a Feature of Innate T Cells in Blood, Tissues, and Tumors, Responding to Cytokines Rather than TCR Stimulation. *J. Immunol. Baltim.* **2023**, *211*, 633–647. [CrossRef] [PubMed]
88. Pham, N.-L.; Badovinac, V.; Harty, J. Differential Role of "Signal 3" Inflammatory Cytokines in Regulating CD8 T Cell Expansion and Differentiation in Vivo. *Front. Immunol.* **2011**, *2*, 4. [CrossRef]

89. Higashioka, K.; Yoshimura, M.; Sakuragi, T.; Ayano, M.; Kimoto, Y.; Mitoma, H.; Ono, N.; Arinobu, Y.; Kikukawa, M.; Yamada, H.; et al. Human PD-1hiCD8+ T Cells Are a Cellular Source of IL-21 in Rheumatoid Arthritis. *Front. Immunol.* **2021**, *12*, 654623. [CrossRef] [PubMed]
90. Goto, M.; Takahashi, H.; Yoshida, R.; Itamiya, T.; Nakano, M.; Nagafuchi, Y.; Harada, H.; Shimizu, T.; Maeda, M.; Kubota, A.; et al. Age-Associated CD4+ T Cells with B Cell-Promoting Functions Are Regulated by ZEB2 in Autoimmunity. *Sci. Immunol.* **2024**, *9*, eadk1643. [CrossRef] [PubMed]
91. Zhao, S.; Grieshaber-Bouyer, R.; Rao, D.A.; Kolb, P.; Chen, H.; Andreeva, I.; Tretter, T.; Lorenz, H.-M.; Watzl, C.; Wabnitz, G.; et al. Effect of JAK Inhibition on the Induction of Proinflammatory HLA-DR+CD90+ Rheumatoid Arthritis Synovial Fibroblasts by Interferon-γ. *Arthritis Rheumatol.* **2022**, *74*, 441–452. [CrossRef]
92. Kim, J.-W.; Kong, J.-S.; Lee, S.; Yoo, S.-A.; Koh, J.H.; Jin, J.; Kim, W.-U. Angiogenic Cytokines Can Reflect the Synovitis Severity and Treatment Response to Biologics in Rheumatoid Arthritis. *Exp. Mol. Med.* **2020**, *52*, 843–853. [CrossRef]
93. Jackson, J.R.; Minton, J.A.; Ho, M.L.; Wei, N.; Winkler, J.D. Expression of Vascular Endothelial Growth Factor in Synovial Fibroblasts Is Induced by Hypoxia and Interleukin 1beta. *J. Rheumatol.* **1997**, *24*, 1253–1259.
94. Goldring, S.R. Pathogenesis of Bone and Cartilage Destruction in Rheumatoid Arthritis. *Rheumatology* **2003**, *42*, ii11–ii16. [CrossRef] [PubMed]
95. Karonitsch, T.; Beckmann, D.; Dalwigk, K.; Niederreiter, B.; Studenic, P.; Byrne, R.A.; Holinka, J.; Sevelda, F.; Korb-Pap, A.; Steiner, G.; et al. Targeted Inhibition of Janus Kinases Abates Interfon Gamma-Induced Invasive Behaviour of Fibroblast-like Synoviocytes. *Rheumatology* **2018**, *57*, 572–577. [CrossRef]
96. O' Gradaigh, D.; Ireland, D.; Bord, S.; Compston, J.E. Joint Erosion in Rheumatoid Arthritis: Interactions between Tumour Necrosis Factor Alpha, Interleukin 1, and Receptor Activator of Nuclear Factor kappaB Ligand (RANKL) Regulate Osteoclasts. *Ann. Rheum. Dis.* **2004**, *63*, 354–359. [CrossRef]
97. Kobayashi, K.; Takahashi, N.; Jimi, E.; Udagawa, N.; Takami, M.; Kotake, S.; Nakagawa, N.; Kinosaki, M.; Yamaguchi, K.; Shima, N.; et al. Tumor Necrosis Factor Alpha Stimulates Osteoclast Differentiation by a Mechanism Independent of the ODF/RANKL-RANK Interaction. *J. Exp. Med.* **2000**, *191*, 275–286. [CrossRef] [PubMed]
98. Xia, Y.; Inoue, K.; Du, Y.; Baker, S.J.; Reddy, E.P.; Greenblatt, M.B.; Zhao, B. TGFβ Reprograms TNF Stimulation of Macrophages towards a Non-Canonical Pathway Driving Inflammatory Osteoclastogenesis. *Nat. Commun.* **2022**, *13*, 3920. [CrossRef]
99. Yokota, K.; Sato, K.; Miyazaki, T.; Aizaki, Y.; Tanaka, S.; Sekikawa, M.; Kozu, N.; Kadono, Y.; Oda, H.; Mimura, T. Characterization and Function of Tumor Necrosis Factor and Interleukin-6-Induced Osteoclasts in Rheumatoid Arthritis. *Arthritis Rheumatol.* **2021**, *73*, 1145–1154. [CrossRef] [PubMed]
100. Hashizume, M.; Hayakawa, N.; Mihara, M. IL-6 Trans-Signalling Directly Induces RANKL on Fibroblast-like Synovial Cells and Is Involved in RANKL Induction by TNF-Alpha and IL-17. *Rheumatology* **2008**, *47*, 1635–1640. [CrossRef]
101. Singh, A.K.; Haque, M.; Madarampalli, B.; Shi, Y.; Wildman, B.J.; Basit, A.; Khuder, S.A.; Prasad, B.; Hassan, Q.; Ouseph, M.M.; et al. Ets-2 Propagates IL-6 Trans-Signaling Mediated Osteoclast-Like Changes in Human Rheumatoid Arthritis Synovial Fibroblast. *Front. Immunol.* **2021**, *12*, 746503. [CrossRef]
102. Ota, Y.; Niiro, H.; Ota, S.-I.; Ueki, N.; Tsuzuki, H.; Nakayama, T.; Mishima, K.; Higashioka, K.; Jabbarzadeh-Tabrizi, S.; Mitoma, H.; et al. Generation Mechanism of RANKL(+) Effector Memory B Cells: Relevance to the Pathogenesis of Rheumatoid Arthritis. *Arthritis Res. Ther.* **2016**, *18*, 67. [CrossRef]
103. McGrath, S.; Grimstad, K.; Thorarinsdottir, K.; Forslind, K.; Glinatsi, D.; Leu Agelii, M.; Aranburu, A.; Sundell, T.; Jonsson, C.A.; Camponeschi, A.; et al. Correlation of Professional Antigen-Presenting Tbet+CD11c+ B Cells with Bone Destruction in Untreated Rheumatoid Arthritis. *Arthritis Rheumatol.* **2024**, *76*, 1263–1277. [CrossRef]
104. Bhattacharya, G.; Sengupta, S.; Jha, R.; Shaw, S.K.; Jogdand, G.M.; Barik, P.K.; Padhan, P.; Parida, J.R.; Devadas, S. IL-21/23 Axis Modulates Inflammatory Cytokines and RANKL Expression in RA CD4+ T Cells via p-Akt1 Signaling. *Front. Immunol.* **2023**, *14*, 1235514. [CrossRef] [PubMed]
105. Matsuda, K.; Shiba, N.; Hiraoka, K. New Insights into the Role of Synovial Fibroblasts Leading to Joint Destruction in Rheumatoid Arthritis. *Int. J. Mol. Sci.* **2023**, *24*, 5173. [CrossRef]
106. Takeuchi, T.; Tanaka, Y.; Soen, S.; Yamanaka, H.; Yoneda, T.; Tanaka, S.; Nitta, T.; Okubo, N.; Genant, H.K.; van der Heijde, D. Effects of the Anti-RANKL Antibody Denosumab on Joint Structural Damage in Patients with Rheumatoid Arthritis Treated with Conventional Synthetic Disease-Modifying Antirheumatic Drugs (DESIRABLE Study): A Randomised, Double-Blind, Placebo-Controlled Phase 3 Trial. *Ann. Rheum. Dis.* **2019**, *78*, 899–907. [CrossRef] [PubMed]

Journal of
Clinical Medicine

MDPI

Review

The Interplay Between Rheumatoid Arthritis and Chronic Kidney Disease: From Mechanisms to Treatment

Kunihiro Ichinose [1,2]

[1] Department of Rheumatology, Faculty of Medicine, Shimane University, 89-1 Enya-cho, Izumo 693-8501, Japan; kichinose@med.shimane-u.ac.jp; Tel.: +81-853-20-2196; Fax: +81-853-20-2194

[2] Integrated Kidney Research and Advance, Faculty of Medicine, Shimane University, 89-1 Enya-cho, Izumo 693-8501, Japan

Abstract

Chronic kidney disease (CKD) is a frequent and clinically significant comorbidity in patients with rheumatoid arthritis (RA), with a reported prevalence ranging from 20% to 50% depending on the cohort and definition applied. The high burden of CKD in RA reflects the complex interplay between traditional risk factors (aging, hypertension, diabetes, and dyslipidemia) and RA-specific factors such as persistent systemic inflammation, immune complex deposition, and long-term exposure to nephrotoxic agents, including older DMARDs (gold, D-penicillamine) and calcineurin inhibitors. Histopathologically, RA-associated kidney involvement encompasses a broad spectrum of conditions, including mesangial proliferative glomerulonephritis, membranous nephropathy, AA amyloidosis, and drug-induced interstitial nephritis. Recent advances in RA therapy, particularly the widespread use of biologic DMARDs, have markedly reduced the incidence of AA amyloidosis and may exert indirect renoprotective effects through stringent inflammation control. However, targeted synthetic DMARDs such as Janus kinase (JAK) inhibitors require careful dose adjustment in CKD and heightened infection vigilance. CKD in RA is a strong predictor of cardiovascular events, serious infections, and all-cause mortality. Importantly, recent data indicate that even low-grade albuminuria below the traditional microalbuminuria threshold is associated with excess mortality in RA. Early detection through routine monitoring of eGFR and urinary albumin-to-creatinine ratio (uACR), combined with individualized pharmacologic adjustment and close collaboration with nephrologists, is essential for optimizing long-term outcomes. This review provides an updated synthesis of the epidemiology, pathophysiological mechanisms, therapeutic strategies, and prognostic implications of CKD in RA, with a particular focus on both Japanese and international evidence.

Keywords: rheumatoid arthritis; chronic kidney disease; renal impairment; inflammation; biologics; TNF inhibitor; IL-6 inhibitor; JAK inhibitor; nephroprotection

1. Introduction

Rheumatoid arthritis (RA) is a chronic autoimmune inflammatory disease that primarily affects the synovial joints; however, its systemic nature often leads to extra-articular manifestations, including renal involvement. Chronic kidney disease (CKD) has emerged as a clinically relevant comorbidity in patients with RA, contributing to increased morbidity, mortality, and therapeutic complexity. The prevalence of CKD among patients with RA is significantly higher than that in the general population, with estimates ranging from 20% to 50%, depending on the study design and definitions employed [1–3].

Several mechanisms have been proposed to explain this increased susceptibility, including traditional risk factors such as aging, hypertension, diabetes, and dyslipidemia, as well as RA-specific factors such as persistent systemic inflammation, long-term use of nephrotoxic agents such as nonsteroidal anti-inflammatory drugs (NSAIDs), and adverse effects of disease-modifying anti-rheumatic drugs (DMARDs) [1,4,5]. The histopathological findings in RA-associated nephropathy are diverse, ranging from mesangial proliferative glomerulonephritis and membranous nephropathy to AA amyloidosis and drug-induced tubulointerstitial nephritis [6–9].

Advances in RA management, particularly the widespread use of biological and targeted synthetic DMARDs, have improved disease control and may help mitigate renal complications in patients with RA. Interleukin-6 (IL-6) inhibitors have shown promise in preserving renal function, particularly in patients with AA amyloidosis [10–12]. Nevertheless, the presence of CKD complicates therapeutic decision-making and requires careful dose adjustment and interdisciplinary collaboration.

This review aimed to provide a comprehensive overview of the epidemiology, pathophysiology, clinical management strategies, and prognostic implications of CKD in patients with RA by synthesizing evidence from clinical studies and basic research across diverse populations.

2. Methods (Literature Search Strategy)

This narrative review was conducted based on a comprehensive literature search of PubMed and Embase databases. The search included articles published up to March 2025. The following key terms and their combinations were used: "rheumatoid arthritis", "chronic kidney disease", "renal impairment", "albuminuria", "biologic DMARDs", "IL-6 inhibitor", "TNF inhibitor", "JAK inhibitor", "SGLT2 inhibitor", and "glomerulonephritis".

Only English-language articles were included. Both observational and interventional studies, as well as relevant systematic reviews and meta-analyses, were considered. Case reports were included only when they provided mechanistic insights or addressed rare renal manifestations. Editorials and non-peer-reviewed articles were excluded. Reference lists of key publications were also manually screened to identify additional relevant studies.

3. Epidemiological Background

Chronic kidney disease (CKD) is increasingly recognized as a frequent and clinically significant comorbidity in patients with RA. Epidemiological studies have reported a wide range of CKD prevalence in RA, with rates varying from 20% to 50%, depending on the population and diagnostic criteria used [3]. For example, the French COMEDRA cohort reported that 8.8% of patients with RA had an estimated glomerular filtration rate (eGFR) below 60 mL/min/1.73 m^2 and 9% had proteinuria [1]. In a Japanese retrospective cohort study of 1077 patients with RA, the baseline prevalence of CKD, defined as an eGFR <60 or proteinuria $\geq$1+, was 24.5%, and the cumulative incidence over 10 years was 60% [2].

The growing burden of CKD in patients with RA is partly attributable to the aging RA population and improved survival resulting from early diagnosis and better disease control. Indeed, the average age of patients with RA has been rising globally, and comorbid conditions such as hypertension and diabetes, which are key risk factors for CKD, are more prevalent in older adults. Long-term follow-up studies have shown that patients with RA are more likely to progress to CKD than age- and sex-matched non-RA controls. For instance, in a 20-year cohort study, approximately 25% of patients with RA developed an eGFR < 60, compared to 20% in non-RA individuals [13].

Several risk factors for the development and progression of CKD in patients with RA have been identified. A multicenter Japanese study demonstrated that advanced age

https://doi.org/10.3390/jcm15010108

(≥65 years; odds ratio [OR], 5.19), hypertension (OR, 3.05), diabetes mellitus (OR, 1.52), dyslipidemia (OR, 1.53), and higher cumulative glucocorticoid exposure (OR, 1.45) were independently associated with a reduced eGFR [4].

In addition, the frequent use of nonsteroidal anti-inflammatory drugs (NSAIDs) increases the risk of new-onset CKD by approximately 1.4-fold and may increase all-cause mortality [1]. Genetic susceptibility may further influence the risk of developing CKD. For example, the HLA-DRB1*DR6 allele is associated with a higher CKD prevalence in Japanese patients with RA [14].

A substantial proportion of patients with RA exhibit low-grade albuminuria, and values below the traditional microalbuminuria range may provide prognostic information for these patients. In the National Health and Nutritional Examination Surveys (NHANES) from 1999 to 2018, the uACR–mortality curve in RA showed an L-shaped threshold near ~6 mg/g, suggesting that "normal-high" albuminuria warrants attention [15]. Independent cohorts have also been associated with microalbuminuria (uACR 30–300 mg/g) and higher mortality [16]. These data support the incorporation of albuminuria, not just eGFR, into risk appraisal.

From a measurement standpoint, Kidney Disease: Improving Global Outcomes (KDIGO) 2024 recommends staging CKD according to eGFR categories (G1–G5) and albuminuria categories (A1–A3), emphasizing periodic screening in at-risk populations in which annual eGFR/uACR is reasonable, and more frequent testing is justified in patients with active disease, nephrotoxic analgesic use, or existing CKD [17–19]. Finally, the therapeutic era matters: the decline of AA amyloidosis with modern anti-cytokine strategies likely alters the renal epidemiology of RA; however, drug-related nephrotoxicity (e.g., chronic NSAID exposure) remains a modifiable contributor to the CKD burden [17,20].

In Japanese data, concomitant CKD independently increased the risk of hospitalized infections among patients with RA, and infections (including sepsis) were the leading reasons for Intensive Care Unit (ICU) admission in a Japanese ICU cohort of patients with RA, underscoring infection vulnerability when renal impairment coexists [21,22].

Together, these findings suggest that both traditional and RA-specific factors interact to increase the risk of CKD in patients with RA. In particular, older patients with RA have a higher prevalence of renal impairment than younger patients. However, recent evidence suggests that maintaining a low disease activity may attenuate the rate of eGFR decline. A large prospective study showed that patients with RA with sustained low disease activity had slower renal function loss than those with high disease activity, highlighting the importance of inflammation control in preserving renal outcomes [23]. Over the past two decades, improved survival in patients with RA due to earlier diagnosis and the adoption of treat-to-target strategies has paradoxically increased the clinical burden of age-related comorbidities, including CKD. In Japan, the average age of patients with RA has increased considerably, further amplifying the impact of age-associated renal risks.

4. Pathophysiology

Renal involvement in RA occurs through both inflammatory and drug-induced mechanisms. Systemic inflammation in RA leads to elevated circulating cytokines, such as tumor necrosis factor-alpha (TNF-α) and IL-6, which contribute to glomerular injury, vascular dysfunction, and interstitial fibrosis. IL-6 levels are markedly elevated in advanced CKD and play a key role in promoting proteinuria, glomerular permeability, and renal fibrosis [24]. Cytokine-induced disruption of the glomerular basement membrane (GBM) can cause podocyte injury and loss of charge selectivity, resulting in proteinuria [25–27]. Beyond serving as a marker of glomerular injury, proteinuria itself actively contributes to the progression of kidney damage. Excessive filtration of albumin leads to its uptake by proximal

 https://doi.org/10.3390/jcm15010108

tubular epithelial cells via endocytic pathways, triggering cellular stress responses and the release of pro-inflammatory and pro-fibrotic mediators. Extracellular vesicles (EVs), including exosomes as a major subclass, have emerged as important mediators of intercellular communication in the kidney. Experimental and translational studies have demonstrated that albumin overload induces the release of these EVs from tubular epithelial cells. These vesicles carry cytokines, chemokines, and microRNAs that propagate local inflammation, activate interstitial fibroblasts, and promote tubulointerstitial fibrosis. Thus, albuminuria represents not only a consequence of glomerular injury but also a direct driver of tubular inflammation and chronic kidney disease progression [26,27].

In RA, chronic systemic inflammation contributes directly to glomerular and tubulointerstitial injuries. Activated T lymphocytes and macrophages infiltrate the glomeruli and release cytokines, such as IL-6, TNF-α, and interferon-γ. These mediators enhance the permeability of the glomerular basement membrane (GBM), leading to protein leakage and mesangial activation. Immune complexes containing rheumatoid factor or anti-citrullinated protein antibodies may deposit along the subepithelial or mesangial regions, triggering complement activation and subsequent podocyte injury.

Furthermore, podocytes can internalize IgG via the neonatal Fc receptor (FcRn), amplifying local inflammation and proteinuria. Collectively, these immunological events promote mesangial proliferation, endothelial activation, and progressive glomerular damage, as illustrated in Figure 1.

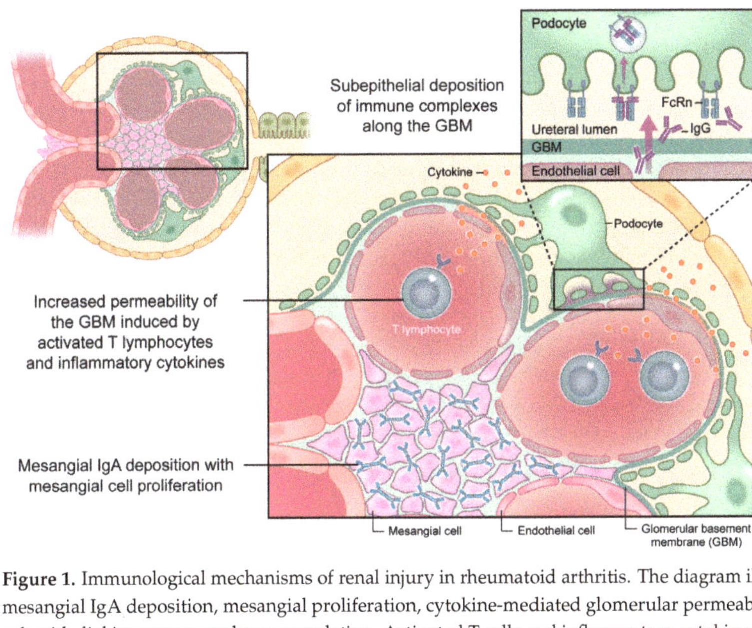

Figure 1. Immunological mechanisms of renal injury in rheumatoid arthritis. The diagram illustrates mesangial IgA deposition, mesangial proliferation, cytokine-mediated glomerular permeability, and subepithelial immune complex accumulation. Activated T cells and inflammatory cytokines damage the glomerular basement membrane (GBM) and podocytes, while FcRn-mediated IgG trafficking perpetuates proteinuria. Abbreviations: GBM, glomerular basement membrane; FcRn, neonatal Fc receptor; IgG, immunoglobulin G; IgA, immunoglobulin A.

4.1. Immune-Complex-Mediated Renal Injury in Rheumatoid Arthritis

Renal involvement in rheumatoid arthritis (RA) has traditionally been attributed to immune-complex-mediated mechanisms. Circulating immune complexes containing rheumatoid factor and other autoantibodies may deposit within glomerular structures, leading to complement activation and inflammatory cell infiltration. Histopathological

https://doi.org/10.3390/jcm15010108

studies have demonstrated that membranous nephropathy and mesangial proliferative glomerulonephritis represent typical renal manifestations associated with these immune-mediated processes in RA [7,9]. Although the overall incidence of such classical immune-complex-mediated glomerular lesions has declined in the biologic era, these entities remain relevant, particularly in patients with long-standing or inadequately controlled disease [2, 4].

4.2. *AA Amyloidosis in the Biologic Era*

AA amyloidosis has historically been a major cause of chronic kidney disease (CKD) and progression to end-stage renal disease in patients with poorly controlled RA. Persistent systemic inflammation results in sustained elevation of serum amyloid A, which promotes amyloid deposition within renal tissue and leads to progressive proteinuria and renal dysfunction [28]. The introduction and widespread use of biologic DMARDs, especially IL-6 inhibitors, have dramatically reduced the incidence and progression of AA amyloidosis in RA, as demonstrated in both Japanese and international cohorts [9–11]. Nevertheless, AA amyloidosis remains clinically relevant in selected patient populations, including those with delayed diagnosis, limited access to biologic therapy, or refractory inflammatory disease [12].

4.3. *Drug-Induced Renal Injury and Nephrotoxicity*

Drug-related nephrotoxicity continues to play an important role in the development and progression of CKD in patients with RA. Nonsteroidal anti-inflammatory drugs are well recognized to cause hemodynamic renal injury through inhibition of prostaglandin synthesis, leading to reduced renal perfusion and acute or chronic kidney dysfunction [29]. In addition, older disease-modifying anti-rheumatic drugs, such as gold salts and D-penicillamine, have been associated with immune-mediated interstitial nephritis and proteinuric renal disease [30]. Calcineurin inhibitors, including tacrolimus, may induce dose-dependent nephrotoxicity through sustained vasoconstriction, endothelial dysfunction, and promotion of renal fibrosis, particularly with long-term exposure [31]. These observations underscore the importance of careful drug selection and regular renal monitoring in patients with RA, especially those with pre-existing CKD.

4.4. *Emerging Molecular Pathways Linking RA-Associated Inflammation and Renal Injury*

Beyond classical immune-complex-mediated mechanisms, recent experimental studies have highlighted several molecular pathways that may bridge systemic inflammation and renal parenchymal injury in RA. Oxidative stress and activation of the renin–angiotensin system contribute to endothelial dysfunction, podocyte injury, and progressive glomerulosclerosis [32]. Inflammatory signaling through the IL-17–ERK/AKT pathway has been implicated in amplifying mesangial cell proliferation and tubular epithelial damage [33,34]. In addition, activation of the Wnt1/β-catenin pathway promotes fibroblast activation and renal interstitial fibrosis, thereby accelerating CKD progression [35].

At present, most supporting evidence for these pathways derives from experimental and preclinical studies, and their direct relevance to human RA-associated CKD requires validation through future translational and clinical investigations.

4.5. *Summary of Mechanistic Pathways*

Taken together, RA-associated renal injury reflects a complex interplay between immune-complex deposition, chronic inflammation, drug-related nephrotoxicity, and emerging molecular pathways that promote endothelial dysfunction and renal fibrosis. These mechanisms are summarized schematically in Figure 2 and provide a biological rationale for early inflammation control and integrated renoprotective strategies.

https://doi.org/10.3390/jcm15010108

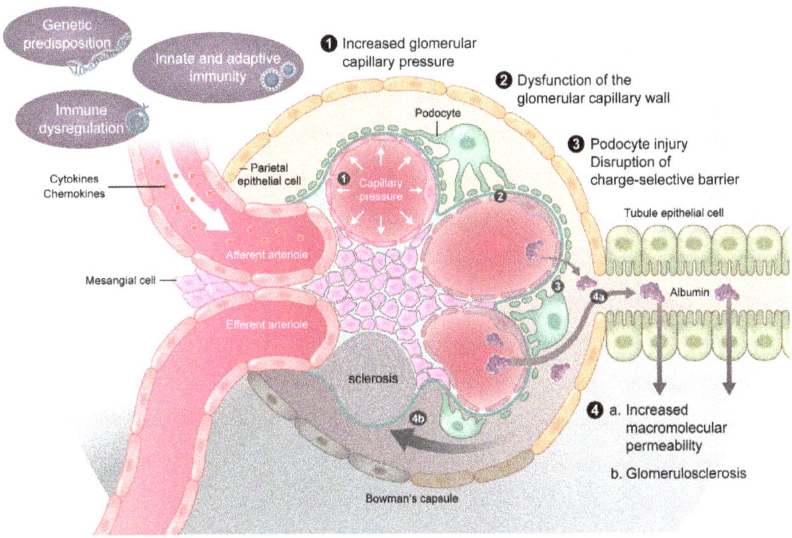

Figure 2. Conceptual framework illustrating the pathophysiological links between rheumatoid arthritis (RA) and chronic kidney disease (CKD). This figure summarizes the major mechanisms contributing to renal injury in RA, encompassing immune-mediated pathways (such as chronic systemic inflammation and autoantibody- or immune-complex-mediated glomerular injury) as well as non-immunologic mechanisms, including endothelial dysfunction, hemodynamic stress, and cardiometabolic factors. The framework highlights the bidirectional interaction between RA disease activity and CKD progression, integrating inflammatory and hemodynamic processes within a unified conceptual model. In addition, proteinuria is depicted as an active pathogenic mediator, whereby excessive albumin uptake by tubular epithelial cells induces the release of extracellular vesicles, including exosomes, which amplify local inflammation and fibrotic responses within the tubulointerstitium.

5. Treatment and Management

Managing RA in patients with coexisting CKD requires a dual approach: effective control of systemic inflammation to prevent further renal injury, and tailored adjustment of pharmacologic regimens to preserve kidney function and avoid drug-induced nephrotoxicity. Tight disease control has been shown to slow the decline in renal function in RA, supporting the treat-to-target strategy, even in patients with impaired kidney function [23].

5.1. Adjustment of Anti-Rheumatic Medications

Methotrexate (MTX), a cornerstone drug used in RA management, is primarily excreted renally. In patients with CKD, especially those with eGFR < 30 mL/min/1.73 m^2, MTX accumulation can lead to serious toxicity, such as bone marrow suppression, necessitating dose reduction or discontinuation [36,37]. Leflunomide, which is hepatically metabolized, should be used with caution in patients with CKD, although its active metabolite can accumulate in advanced renal dysfunction [38]. Sulfasalazine and hydroxychloroquine have relatively favorable renal safety profiles and may be continued in mild to moderate CKD, although adjustments may be required in end-stage renal disease or dialysis [37,39–41].

Calcineurin inhibitors, such as tacrolimus, although used in some refractory RA cases, should generally be avoided in patients with progressive CKD because of their dose-dependent nephrotoxicity [37,42]. If renal impairment develops during treatment,

 https://doi.org/10.3390/jcm15010108

alternative treatment agents should be considered. Glucocorticoids require careful tapering because prolonged use can exacerbate hypertension and diabetes, indirectly worsening renal outcomes [2]. The risk of infection with glucocorticoid therapy has also increased in patients with CKD.

5.2. Pain Management and NSAID Use

Nonsteroidal anti-inflammatory drugs (NSAIDs) are commonly used for pain control in RA; however, they pose a significant risk to patients with CKD. NSAIDs impair glomerular perfusion by inhibiting prostaglandin synthesis, potentially leading to acute kidney injury (AKI), particularly in the context of volume depletion or coadministration with renin–angiotensin system inhibitors. Chronic NSAID use can cause interstitial nephritis and accelerate the progression of CKD. Therefore, NSAIDs should be minimized or avoided when possible, and if used, they should be prescribed at the lowest effective dose for the shortest duration, with close monitoring of renal function, urine output, and blood pressure [17]. Acetaminophen and weak opioids may be considered as alternative analgesics, with dose adjustments based on renal clearance.

5.3. Renal Protective Strategies (Clinical Implementation)

A risk-based CKD care plan aligned with KDIGO 2024 guidelines should be incorporated into routine RA management. First, we recommend at least annual eGFR and uACR screening (more frequent screening is required in patients with active disease, pre-existing CKD, or nephrotoxin exposure) and stage by G1–G5 and A1–A3 to guide risk-based care [18,19]. Because low-range albuminuria already has prognostic value in RA, "high-normal" uACR should be considered, even when eGFR is preserved [15]. Blood pressure should be controlled according to the guideline targets using angiotensin-converting enzyme (ACE) inhibitors/angiotensin receptor blockers (ARBs) for albuminuric CKD unless contraindicated [18,19]. Analgesia should be NSAID-sparing. If NSAIDs are unavoidable, the lowest effective dose should be used for the shortest duration with renal monitoring [17].

Renal dosing, avoidance criteria, and recommended monitoring parameters (e.g., complete blood count and serum creatinine for methotrexate) for non-JAK anti-rheumatic agents are summarized in Table 1 (see Table 2 for Janus kinase (JAK) inhibitors).

Table 1. Anti-rheumatic drugs in CKD (non-JAK): dosing/avoidance and renal considerations. Notes: Renal dosing needs and class-specific caveats are summarized; for JAK inhibitors, see Table 2. Abbreviations: AA amyloidosis, amyloid A amyloidosis; CBC, complete blood count; CKD, chronic kidney disease; eGFR, estimated glomerular filtration rate; NSAIDs, nonsteroidal anti-inflammatory drugs; TNF, tumor necrosis factor.

Drug	Renal Adjustment	Use in Advanced CKD (eGFR < 30)	Monitoring Parameters	Key Comments
Methotrexate	Reduce dose or extend interval at eGFR 30–59	Avoid	CBC; serum creatinine	Accumulation risk; myelosuppression
Leflunomide	No adjustment usually required	Use with caution	Liver enzymes; CBC; renal function	Active metabolite long half-life; limited CKD data
Sulfasalazine	No adjustment in mild–moderate CKD	Use with caution	CBC; renal function	Rare interstitial nephritis

https://doi.org/10.3390/jcm15010108

Table 1. *Cont.*

Drug	Renal Adjustment	Use in Advanced CKD (eGFR < 30)	Monitoring Parameters	Key Comments
Hydroxychloroquine	No adjustment usually required	Use with caution	Renal function; ophthalmologic exam	Partial renal clearance; retinal toxicity
Glucocorticoids (low–moderate dose)	No adjustment required	Can be used	Blood pressure; glucose; infection	Long-term metabolic and CV risk
NSAIDs	Avoid or minimize use	Avoid	Serum creatinine; electrolytes	AKI risk; CKD progression
Tacrolimus	Dose adjustment required	Avoid	Serum creatinine; trough level	Dose-dependent nephrotoxicity
TNF inhibitors	No adjustment required	Can be used	Renal function	No intrinsic nephrotoxicity
IL-6 inhibitors	No adjustment required	Can be used	Renal function; CRP	Beneficial for AA amyloidosis
Abatacept	No adjustment required	Can be used	Renal function	Favorable renal safety profile

Table 2. JAK inhibitors: suggested dosing based on renal function in RA. Notes: Dose adjustment recommendations are based on eGFR and refer to adult patients with RA. In patients with advanced CKD, particularly eGFR < 30 mL/min/1.73 m^2, the use of JAK inhibitors should be approached with caution or avoided, depending on the specific agent, due to limited clinical data and altered pharmacokinetics. Baricitinib requires the most stringent renal dose adjustment because of predominant renal elimination, whereas upadacitinib and tofacitinib rely mainly on hepatic metabolism with less renal clearance. Peficitinib is primarily metabolized hepatically and may be used without dose adjustment in mild to moderate CKD; however, evidence in advanced CKD remains limited. Abbreviations: AKI, acute kidney injury; CKD, chronic kidney disease; eGFR, estimated glomerular filtration rate; JAK, Janus kinase; NSAID, nonsteroidal anti-inflammatory drug; RAAS, renin–angiotensin–aldosterone system.

JAK Inhibitor	Renal Elimination	Dose Adjustment in CKD	Use in Advanced CKD (eGFR < 30)	Renal Safety Considerations
Baricitinib	High (~70–75%)	Reduce dose at eGFR 30–59	Not recommended	AKI risk with dehydration, NSAIDs, RAAS blockade
Tofacitinib	Moderate (~30%)	Reduce dose at eGFR < 60	Not recommended	Stable eGFR in trials; monitor during illness
Upadacitinib	Low (<20%)	No adjustment in mild–moderate CKD	Avoid (limited data)	Least renal dependence; infection-related AKI risk
Filgotinib	Moderate (active metabolite)	Reduce dose at eGFR < 60	Not recommended	Limited CKD data; avoid advanced CKD
Peficitinib	Minimal (<15%)	No adjustment in mild–moderate CKD	Use with caution/avoid	Primarily hepatic metabolism; minimal renal exposure

When indicated, sodium-glucose cotransporter 2 (SGLT2) inhibitors can be considered for albuminuric CKD with adequate eGFR, regardless of diabetes status, to slow CKD progression and reduce cardio–renal events, following product-specific eGFR thresholds, and monitor for volume depletion and mycotic infections [18,43,44]. Glucagon-like peptide-1 (GLP-1) receptor agonists are appropriate for patients with type 2 diabetes/obesity and

 https://doi.org/10.3390/jcm15010108

high cardiovascular risk, and may provide kidney benefits (e.g., slower albuminuria progression); they should be considered alongside SGLT2 inhibitors when appropriate [45,46]. Comprehensive multimorbidity management, including lipids, glycemia, weight, smoking cessation, and vaccination (e.g., zoster), is essential to mitigate infection and cardiovascular risk in patients with CKD and those undergoing immunomodulatory therapy [18,19]. Early rheumatology–nephrology co-management is recommended when patients reach CKD stage G3b–G5 and/or exhibit persistent albuminuria of category A2 or higher, as these thresholds identify individuals at substantially increased risk of progression and complications [18,19].

A pragmatic treatment pathway integrating risk staging, DMARD selection, and cotherapy is outlined in Figure 3.

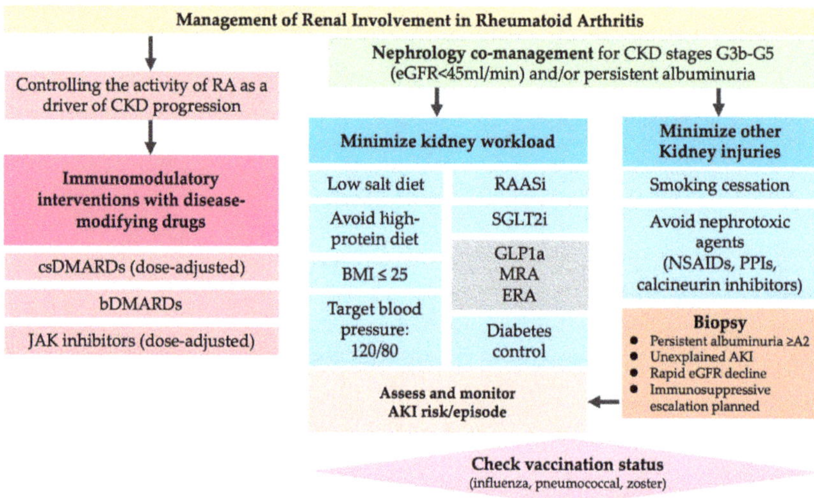

Figure 3. Management pathway for chronic kidney disease in patients with rheumatoid arthritis. This figure illustrates a stepwise management strategy for CKD in patients with RA, integrating immunologic disease control with renoprotective interventions. Initial risk stratification is based on estimated glomerular filtration rate and albuminuria category. Rheumatology–nephrology co-management is recommended for patients with CKD stage G3b–G5 and/or persistent albuminuria of category A2 or higher albuminuria (uACR $\geq$ 30 mg/g). Acute kidney injury risk factors, including NSAID exposure, dehydration, infection, and combined renin–angiotensin system blockade, should be actively assessed. Diagnostic kidney biopsy should be considered in cases of persistent albuminuria, unexplained AKI, or progressive renal dysfunction. Vaccination against influenza, pneumococcus, and herpes zoster is recommended prior to initiation of biologic or JAK inhibitor therapy whenever feasible. RA, rheumatoid arthritis; CKD, chronic kidney disease; csDMARDs, conventional synthetic disease-modifying anti-rheumatic drugs; bDMARDs, biologic DMARDs; JAK, Janus kinase; RAASi, renin–angiotensin–aldosterone system inhibitors; SGLT2i, sodium-glucose cotransporter 2 inhibitors; GLP-1a, glucagon-like peptide-1 receptor agonists; MRA, mineralocorticoid receptor antagonists; ERA, endothelin receptor antagonists; NSAIDs, nonsteroidal anti-inflammatory drugs; PPIs, proton pump inhibitors.

5.4. Acute Kidney Injury, Kidney Biopsy, and Vaccination Strategies

Acute kidney injury represents an important but often underrecognized complication in patients with RA, particularly in the context of dehydration, infection, NSAID exposure, or combined renin–angiotensin system blockade [1,17]. Episodes of AKI may accelerate long-term CKD progression and adversely affect overall prognosis.

 https://doi.org/10.3390/jcm15010108

Regarding diagnostic evaluation, kidney biopsy should be actively considered in patients with RA who present with persistent albuminuria of category A2 or higher (uACR $\geq$ 30 mg/g), especially when the etiology is unclear, proteinuria is progressive, or immunosuppressive therapy is being escalated. Biopsy is also indicated in cases of unexplained AKI, rapidly progressive renal dysfunction, or suspected glomerulonephritis [18,19].

Because both immunosuppression and CKD heighten infection risk, vaccination plays a pivotal role in clinical management. Seasonal influenza, pneumococcal, and recombinant zoster vaccines should be administered according to international recommendations, ideally prior to initiation of biologic or JAK inhibitor therapy [47–50].

5.5. RA Treatment in Dialysis or Transplant Settings

Patients with RA undergoing dialysis require active disease management. As MTX and tacrolimus are contraindicated in end-stage kidney disease (ESKD), treatment regimens typically center on glucocorticoids and biologic agents. In patients with advanced CKD or those on dialysis, biologics do not require renal dose adjustment and demonstrate high treatment retention; vigilance for infection remains essential [51,52]. Balancing immunosuppressive therapy with disease control is challenging for kidney transplant recipients with RA. Escalating glucocorticoid doses should be avoided, if possible, and biologic DMARDs should be introduced to maintain disease remission while minimizing additional immunosuppression. Individualized treatment planning through rheumatology-nephrology collaboration is essential for optimizing both graft survival and RA control [37].

5.6. SGLT2 Inhibitors and GLP-1 Receptor Agonists: Mechanisms and Expected Benefits (Rationale & Evidence)

SGLT2 inhibitors reduce proximal tubular sodium–glucose reabsorption and restore tubuloglomerular feedback, thereby lowering intraglomerular pressure, reducing albuminuria by approximately 30%, and attenuating renal inflammation and fibrosis, which extend to diabetic and non-diabetic CKD [43]. GLP-1 receptor agonists improve weight, blood pressure, lipid levels, and inflammatory adipokine signaling, providing atherosclerotic cardiovascular risk reduction with kidney signals, including slower albuminuria progression [45,46].

Randomized trials have demonstrated disease-modifying kidney effects of SGLT2 inhibitors: DAPA-CKD and EMPA-KIDNEY reduced the composite endpoints of sustained eGFR decline, ESKD, or renal death, including non-diabetic CKD [43]. Large cardiovascular outcome trials of GLP-1 receptor agonists (e.g., LEADER and SUSTAIN-6) have shown reduced major adverse cardiovascular events (MACE) and albuminuria progression, with accumulating evidence of kidney protection [45,46].

Direct RA-CKD randomized trials with renal endpoints are lacking; however, given that the high cardiometabolic burden in RA and the prognostic impact of albuminuria, translating CKD guideline strategies to RA, is reasonable, although disease-specific trials are awaited [18,19,44,46]. Safety requires attention to volume depletion and mycotic infections with SGLT2 inhibitors and gastrointestinal/gallbladder adverse events with GLP-1 receptor agonists; choices should be individualized according to comorbidities and concurrent DMARDs [44,46]. Notably, biologic exposure is associated with a lower incidence of CKD than non-biologic regimens, suggesting that inflammation control and SGLT2i/GLP-1 RA co-therapies may be complementary in reducing residual cardiorenal risk [10,18,19,43–46].

6. Biologic and Targeted Therapies: Renal Implications of TNF Inhibitors, IL-6 Inhibitors, and JAK Inhibitors

The advent of biological disease-modifying anti-rheumatic drugs (bDMARDs) and targeted synthetic DMARDs (tsDMARDs) has revolutionized the treatment of rheumatoid

https://doi.org/10.3390/jcm15010108

arthritis (RA), offering improved joint outcomes and systemic benefits, including potential renoprotection in patients with RA. As chronic inflammation is a key driver of renal impairment in RA, suppression of pro-inflammatory cytokines may confer indirect but meaningful renal protection.

6.1. TNF-α Inhibitors

TNF inhibitors such as infliximab and etanercept have long been used in RA treatment. Their introduction significantly reduces systemic inflammation and acute-phase reactants, thereby contributing to a dramatic decline in the incidence of secondary AA amyloidosis [28]. A large retrospective cohort study using U.S. Veterans Affairs data showed that the use of biological agents, including TNF inhibitors, was associated with a lower incidence of CKD and a slower decline in the estimated glomerular filtration rate (eGFR) compared to non-biological therapies. Specifically, the annual rate of eGFR decline improved from -1.0 mL/min/1.73 m^2/year to -0.4 mL/min/1.73 m^2/year following the initiation of biologic treatment [10].

Contemporary comparative data from a multicenter Japanese cohort similarly suggested a renal benefit signal with TNF blockade: TNF inhibitors were linked to a lower CKD incidence than CTLA4-Ig (abatacept) (HR 0.67, 95% CI 0.46–0.97) [53].

Although TNF inhibitors are generally well tolerated in patients with CKD, rare cases of immune-mediated nephropathies, such as lupus-like nephritis and membranous nephropathy, have been reported, likely due to shifts in immune regulation. Causal inference is limited, but clinicians should monitor for new-onset proteinuria/hematuria during therapy [8,54,55].

6.2. IL-6 Inhibitors

IL-6 plays a central role in inflammation, SAA production, and subsequent amyloid deposition in AA amyloidosis. Tocilizumab, an anti-IL-6 receptor monoclonal antibody, has demonstrated excellent efficacy in controlling systemic inflammation and reducing SAA levels, making it particularly valuable in patients with RA and AA amyloidosis. In a single-center analysis from Heidelberg, patients with renal amyloidosis treated with tocilizumab had significantly better 5-year renal survival rates (71%) than those treated with TNF inhibitors (28%) [12]. These findings suggest superior renal preservation with IL-6 inhibition in the selected populations. Beyond amyloidosis, overall, biologic exposure is associated with a lower incidence of CKD and slower eGFR decline than non-biologic regimens in real-world data [10].

Tocilizumab is also advantageous in patients with CKD, where methotrexate coadministration is contraindicated, as it is highly effective as monotherapy [51,52]. Moreover, treatment persistence rates are higher with IL-6 inhibitors in patients with impaired renal function [52].

6.3. JAK Inhibitors

Janus kinase (JAK) inhibitors, such as tofacitinib, baricitinib, peficitinib, upadacitinib, and filgotinib, block the intracellular signaling of pro-inflammatory cytokines, including IL-6, and exert potent anti-inflammatory effects when administered orally. Their clinical utility has expanded substantially over the past decade; however, use in patients with chronic kidney disease (CKD) requires careful consideration because of differences in renal elimination, potential susceptibility to acute kidney injury (AKI), and an increased risk of infection [24].

https://doi.org/10.3390/jcm15010108

6.3.1. Pharmacokinetics and Renal Elimination

Pharmacokinetic profiles differ substantially among currently available JAK inhibitors. Baricitinib is predominantly eliminated through the kidneys, with approximately 70–75% of the administered dose excreted unchanged in the urine, necessitating strict dose reduction in patients with impaired renal function. In contrast, tofacitinib and upadacitinib are metabolized primarily by hepatic pathways, with renal clearance accounting for a smaller proportion of drug elimination, thereby allowing greater dosing flexibility in patients with mild to moderate CKD.

Despite these differences, dose adjustment is generally recommended for all JAK inhibitors when estimated glomerular filtration rate (eGFR) falls below 60 mL/min/1.73 m^2, and most agents are contraindicated or not recommended in advanced CKD (eGFR < 30 mL/min/1.73 m^2), depending on the specific compound and regulatory guidance.

6.3.2. Renal Safety and Risk of Acute Kidney Injury

Evidence from large randomized controlled trials and post-marketing surveillance suggests that JAK inhibitors are not intrinsically nephrotoxic, and sustained declines in eGFR are uncommon under stable clinical conditions [53]. However, AKI may occur indirectly, particularly in vulnerable clinical settings. Episodes of infection, fever-related volume depletion, concomitant use of nonsteroidal anti-inflammatory drugs, or combined renin–angiotensin system blockade may predispose patients receiving JAK inhibitors to transient renal dysfunction.

Accordingly, baseline assessment and periodic monitoring of serum creatinine and eGFR are essential, especially during treatment initiation, dose escalation, and intercurrent illness.

6.3.3. Infection Risk and Herpes Zoster in Patients with CKD

One of the most clinically relevant safety concerns associated with JAK inhibitors is the increased risk of herpes zoster, which consistently exceeds that observed with biologic DMARDs [50]. This risk is further amplified in patients with CKD, who exhibit baseline immune dysregulation and impaired antiviral immunity. Advanced age, renal impairment, and JAK inhibitor therapy act synergistically to increase the likelihood of severe or disseminated zoster infection.

For this reason, recombinant zoster vaccination should be strongly recommended prior to initiation of JAK inhibitor therapy, particularly in patients with CKD, in accordance with international vaccination guidelines [50].

6.3.4. Comparative Renal Safety Among JAK Inhibitors

Agent-specific pharmacokinetic differences have important clinical implications for renal safety. Baricitinib requires the most stringent renal dose adjustment because of its high dependence on renal elimination, whereas upadacitinib demonstrates the least reliance on renal clearance among currently approved agents. These distinctions should be explicitly considered when selecting therapy for patients with CKD.

At present, no randomized controlled trials have directly compared renal outcomes among different JAK inhibitors in CKD-stratified RA populations. Available data are derived largely from post hoc analyses and observational studies, underscoring the need for cautious interpretation.

6.3.5. Integration with CKD-Specific Management

In patients with RA and CKD, JAK inhibitors should generally be positioned after optimization of conventional synthetic and biologic DMARD therapy. Treatment selection

https://doi.org/10.3390/jcm15010108

should incorporate individualized dose adjustment based on eGFR, careful avoidance of concurrent nephrotoxic exposures, and close collaboration with nephrologists in patients with CKD stage G3b or higher. The dose-adjustment principles summarized in Table 2 provide a practical framework for daily clinical practice.

6.3.6. Evidence Gaps and Future Perspectives

Despite the widespread use of JAK inhibitors, robust evidence regarding their long-term renal safety or potential renoprotective effects remains limited. Most pivotal trials excluded patients with advanced CKD and did not incorporate renal endpoints, such as albuminuria progression or AKI incidence, as primary outcomes. Future prospective RA trials incorporating CKD-specific endpoints and stratified analyses by renal function are urgently needed to inform optimal use of JAK inhibitors in this high-risk population.

The renal dose adjustments for JAK inhibitors are summarized in Table 2.

7. Prognosis and Outcomes

7.1. eGFR Trajectories and Predictors

Higher RA disease activity is consistently associated with faster eGFR decline, underscoring the renoprotective value of tight inflammatory control [23]. Traditional determinants, such as age, hypertension, diabetes, and established CVD, remain salient, but inflammatory biomarkers (e.g., CRP) and albuminuria provide incremental prognostic information in RA [5,15]. Longitudinal data indicate that a meaningful minority of patients with RA transition from preserved function to CKD over time; for example, eGFR < 60 accrued to ~15% at 10 years and ~25% at 20 years in a classic cohort [13].

7.2. Progression to End Stage Kidney Disease (ESKD)

RA increases the risk of kidney failure at the population level. In a nationwide Korean cohort of >930,000 individuals, the incidence of ESKD was 0.81 vs. 0.37 per 1000 person-years in patients with RA versus non-RA, yielding an adjusted HR of 2.10 (95% CI 1.90–2.31) over 7.6 years; thus, the absolute annual risk was low (~0.08%), but the relative risk was roughly doubled [56]. The excess appears more pronounced in younger patients with RA and those with fewer baseline comorbidities, implying that inflammatory mechanisms rather than competing risks dominate in some subgroups [56]. Secondary AA amyloidosis historically accounts for a share of kidney failure in RA; with biologic therapies, its incidence and renal progression have declined, but vigilance remains warranted in persistently inflamed diseases [20].

7.3. Cardiovascular Events and Mortality in RA with CKD

There is a vascular risk of CKD compounds in RA. In a Taiwanese nationwide RA cohort, the presence of CKD was associated with incident ischemic heart disease HR 1.57 (95% CI 1.38–1.79) and stroke HR 1.24 (1.06–1.43) versus RA without CKD [57]. In a Japanese RA cohort, CKD was a predictor of all-cause mortality (HR 1.64 [1.05–2.57]), which increased to HR 4.76 (2.24–9.51) in very high-risk CKD [2]. These data emphasize the need for integrated cardio–renal risk reduction (blood pressure, lipids, glycemia, and smoking cessation) along with inflammation control [4].

7.4. Albuminuria as an Early Prognostic Signal

In patients with RA, albuminuria poses a risk even at low levels. In the NHANES 1999–2018, the uACR–mortality relationship displayed an L-shaped threshold near 6 mg/g; above this level, mortality rose steadily [15]. Additional cohorts have reported approximately 1.5-fold higher mortality with microalbuminuria (30–300 mg/g) [16]. Clinically,

 https://doi.org/10.3390/jcm15010108

routine uACR testing complements eGFR, improves stratification, and can trigger early renoprotective measures.

7.5. Clinical Take-Home Themes

Several themes emerged from these data. First, higher RA disease activity is consistently associated with a steeper decline in kidney function, underscoring the importance of inflammation control as a renoprotective strategy [23]. Second, albuminuria carries prognostic weight even at low ranges. RA cohorts show an L-shaped association between uACR and mortality, with a threshold of approximately 6 mg/g, and microalbuminuria (30–300 mg/g) confers additional risk [15]. Third, although the absolute annual incidence of ESKD among patients with RA is low (~0.08% in contemporary nationwide data), the relative risk is approximately double compared to that in individuals without RA [56]. Fourth, the coexistence of CKD and RA amplifies downstream events, with higher rates of cardiovascular complications and all-cause mortality than in RA without CKD [2,57]. Finally, therapeutic decision-making should adopt KDIGO-aligned, cardio–renal-conscious care—routine eGFR and uACR monitoring, ACEi/ARB for albuminuric disease, and NSAID-sparing analgesia—while integrating co-therapies such as SGLT2 inhibitors or GLP-1 receptor agonists when indicated [18,19,44,46].

8. Future Directions and Unmet Needs

Despite growing recognition of the close bidirectional relationship between rheumatoid arthritis (RA) and chronic kidney disease (CKD), several critical knowledge gaps remain. To date, most randomized controlled trials of disease-modifying anti-rheumatic drugs (DMARDs) have systematically excluded patients with advanced CKD, and renal outcomes have rarely been incorporated as primary or key secondary endpoints. Consequently, evidence guiding treatment decisions in this high-risk population is largely extrapolated from non-CKD cohorts. Future RA trials should therefore prospectively integrate CKD-specific outcomes, including longitudinal changes in estimated glomerular filtration rate (eGFR) slope, albuminuria trajectories, and the incidence of acute kidney injury (AKI), in line with contemporary nephrology trial frameworks.

Second, CKD-stratified trial designs are urgently needed to clarify the comparative renal safety and potential renoprotective effects of biologic and targeted synthetic DMARDs across different stages of kidney dysfunction. Observational studies suggest heterogeneity in renal risk profiles among tumor necrosis factor inhibitors, IL-6 inhibitors, and Janus kinase inhibitors, but robust head-to-head comparisons with renal endpoints are lacking. Stratification by CKD stage would allow more precise and individualized treatment selection in vulnerable populations with RA.

Third, emerging multi-omics technologies, including single-cell transcriptomics, spatial transcriptomics, and proteomics, provide unprecedented opportunities to dissect the cellular and molecular crosstalk between synovial inflammation and renal parenchymal injury. Recent applications of spatially resolved transcriptomic approaches in kidney disease have revealed distinct inflammatory and fibrotic niches that cannot be captured by bulk analyses. Integration of these advanced technologies with well-phenotyped RA cohorts may enable the identification of novel biomarkers and therapeutic targets specific to RA-associated CKD, thereby facilitating translational advances from bench to bedside.

Finally, interventional strategies explicitly targeting cardio–reno–metabolic risk warrant focused investigation in RA-specific CKD populations. Large cardiovascular and renal outcome trials have demonstrated that sodium–glucose cotransporter 2 inhibitors and glucagon-like peptide-1 receptor agonists confer substantial renoprotective and cardioprotective benefits in patients with CKD and diabetes or cardiovascular disease. However,

https://doi.org/10.3390/jcm15010108

patients with systemic inflammatory diseases such as RA have been underrepresented in these studies. Prospective trials evaluating these agents in RA-associated CKD may establish a new paradigm of integrated immunologic and renoprotective management.

9. Conclusions

Chronic kidney disease (CKD) is a frequent and clinically meaningful comorbidity in patients with rheumatoid arthritis, driven by the combined effects of traditional cardio–renal risk factors, persistent systemic inflammation, immune-mediated renal injury, and cumulative drug exposure. Even low-grade albuminuria below conventional microalbuminuria thresholds carries prognostic significance in RA, underscoring the importance of early detection.

Modern RA therapies have substantially reduced the burden of AA amyloidosis and may indirectly confer renal protection through tight inflammatory control. However, dose adjustment and vigilant safety monitoring remain mandatory for several DMARD classes, particularly JAK inhibitors and calcineurin inhibitors.

Routine surveillance of eGFR and uACR, risk-adapted pharmacologic adjustment, timely nephrology co-management, and individualized decisions regarding kidney biopsy are central to optimizing long-term outcomes.

Future RA research must move beyond joint-centered endpoints to incorporate renal and cardio–renal endpoints, thereby establishing truly integrated care strategies for this high-risk population.

Funding: This work was supported by the Japan Agency for Medical Research and Development (AMED) under the FY2025 Medical Research Support Program.

Data Availability Statement: No new data were created or analyzed in this study.

Acknowledgments: We thank those who provided assistance with figure preparation.

Conflicts of Interest: The author declares no conflicts of interest.

References

1. Couderc, M.; Tatar, Z.; Pereira, B.; Tiple, A.; Gilson, M.; Fautrel, B.; Pouplin, S.; Dernis, E.; Gossec, L.; Gaujoux-Viala, C.; et al. Prevalence of Renal Impairment in Patients With Rheumatoid Arthritis: Results From a Cross-Sectional Multicenter Study. *Arthritis Care Res.* **2016**, *68*, 638–644. [CrossRef] [PubMed]
2. Tokoroyama, T.; Ando, M.; Setoguchi, K.; Tsuchiya, K.; Nitta, K. Prevalence, incidence and prognosis of chronic kidney disease classified according to current guidelines: A large retrospective cohort study of rheumatoid arthritis patients. *Nephrol. Dial. Transplant.* **2017**, *32*, 2035–2042. [CrossRef]
3. Oweis, A.O.; Alawneh, K.M.; Alshelleh, S.A.; Alnaimat, F.; Alawneh, D.; Zahran, D.J. Renal dysfunction among rheumatoid arthritis patients: A retrospective cohort study. *Ann. Med. Surg.* **2020**, *60*, 280–284. [CrossRef] [PubMed]
4. Mori, S.; Yoshitama, T.; Hirakata, N.; Ueki, Y. Prevalence of and factors associated with renal dysfunction in rheumatoid arthritis patients: A cross-sectional study in community hospitals. *Clin. Rheumatol.* **2017**, *36*, 2673–2682. [CrossRef] [PubMed]
5. Kochi, M.; Kohagura, K.; Shiohira, Y.; Iseki, K.; Ohya, Y. Inflammation as a Risk of Developing Chronic Kidney Disease in Rheumatoid Arthritis. *PLoS ONE* **2016**, *11*, e0160225. [CrossRef]
6. Nakano, M.; Ueno, M.; Nishi, S.; Shimada, H.; Hasegawa, H.; Watanabe, T.; Kuroda, T.; Sato, T.; Maruyama, Y.; Arakawa, M. Analysis of renal pathology and drug history in 158 Japanese patients with rheumatoid arthritis. *Clin. Nephrol.* **1998**, *50*, 154–160.
7. Makino, H.; Yoshinaga, Y.; Yamasaki, Y.; Morita, Y.; Hashimoto, H.; Yamamura, M. Renal involvement in rheumatoid arthritis: Analysis of renal biopsy specimens from 100 patients. *Mod. Rheumatol.* **2002**, *12*, 148–154. [CrossRef]
8. Piccolo, T.; Lisi, P.; Valicenti, E.; Pannarale, G.; Coratelli, P. Clinical and histological features of lupus nephritis induced by anti-TNFalpha therapy. *NDT Plus* **2008**, *1*, 221–224. [CrossRef]
9. Sawamura, M.; Sawa, N.; Yamanouchi, M.; Ikuma, D.; Sekine, A.; Mizuno, H.; Kawada, M.; Hiramatsu, R.; Hayami, N.; Hasegawa, E.; et al. Use of biologic agents and methotrexate improves renal manifestation and outcome in patients with rheumatoid arthritis: A retrospective analysis. *Clin. Exp. Nephrol.* **2022**, *26*, 341–349. [CrossRef]

https://doi.org/10.3390/jcm15010108

10. Sumida, K.; Molnar, M.Z.; Potukuchi, P.K.; Hassan, F.; Thomas, F.; Yamagata, K.; Kalantar-Zadeh, K.; Kovesdy, C.P. Treatment of rheumatoid arthritis with biologic agents lowers the risk of incident chronic kidney disease. *Kidney Int.* **2018**, *93*, 1207–1216. [CrossRef]
11. Hanaoka, H.; Kikuchi, J.; Hiramoto, K.; Saito, S.; Kondo, Y.; Kaneko, Y. Decreased chronic kidney disease in rheumatoid arthritis in the era of biologic disease-modifying anti-rheumatic drugs. *Clin. Kidney J.* **2022**, *15*, 1373–1378. [CrossRef]
12. Kvacskay, P.; Hegenbart, U.; Lorenz, H.M.; Schonland, S.O.; Blank, N. bDMARD can prevent the progression of AA amyloidosis to end-stage renal disease. *Ann. Rheum. Dis.* **2024**, *83*, 1200–1207. [CrossRef]
13. Hickson, L.J.; Crowson, C.S.; Gabriel, S.E.; McCarthy, J.T.; Matteson, E.L. Development of reduced kidney function in rheumatoid arthritis. *Am. J. Kidney Dis.* **2014**, *63*, 206–213. [CrossRef] [PubMed]
14. Higuchi, T.; Oka, S.; Furukawa, H.; Shimada, K.; Hashimoto, A.; Komiya, A.; Matsui, T.; Fukui, N.; Tohma, S. Associations of HLA Polymorphisms with Chronic Kidney Disease in Japanese Rheumatoid Arthritis Patients. *Genes* **2023**, *14*, 1470. [CrossRef] [PubMed]
15. Tang, M.; Du, L.; Peng, J. Urinary albumin-to-creatinine ratio for predicting risk of all-cause mortality and specific-cause mortality in patients with rheumatoid arthritis: Evidence from NHANES 1999–2018. *Clin. Rheumatol.* **2025**, *44*, 623–633. [CrossRef]
16. Bin, Z.; Shen, R.; Wu, R.; Fan, Y.; Zhang, X.; Gao, C.; Li, X.; Wang, C. Association of urinary albumin excretion with all-cause and cardiovascular mortality among patients with rheumatoid arthritis: A national prospective study. *Front. Immunol.* **2024**, *15*, 1412636. [CrossRef]
17. Baker, M.; Perazella, M.A. NSAIDs in CKD: Are They Safe? *Am. J. Kidney Dis.* **2020**, *76*, 546–557. [CrossRef]
18. Kidney Disease: Improving Global Outcomes, C.K.D.W.G. KDIGO 2024 Clinical Practice Guideline for the Evaluation and Management of Chronic Kidney Disease. *Kidney Int.* **2024**, *105*, S117–S314. [CrossRef] [PubMed]
19. Levin, A.; Ahmed, S.B.; Carrero, J.J.; Foster, B.; Francis, A.; Hall, R.K.; Herrington, W.G.; Hill, G.; Inker, L.A.; Kazancioglu, R.; et al. Executive summary of the KDIGO 2024 Clinical Practice Guideline for the Evaluation and Management of Chronic Kidney Disease: Known knowns and known unknowns. *Kidney Int.* **2024**, *105*, 684–701. [CrossRef]
20. Lane, T.; Gillmore, J.D.; Wechalekar, A.D.; Hawkins, P.N.; Lachmann, H.J. Therapeutic blockade of interleukin-6 by tocilizumab in the management of AA amyloidosis and chronic inflammatory disorders: A case series and review of the literature. *Clin. Exp. Rheumatol.* **2015**, *33*, S46–S53.
21. Higuchi, T.; Tanaka, E.; Inoue, E.; Abe, M.; Saka, K.; Sugano, E.; Sugitani, N.; Higuchi, Y.; Ochiai, M.; Yamaguchi, R.; et al. Impact of concomitant chronic kidney disease on hospitalised infections and remission in patients with rheumatoid arthritis: Results from the IORRA cohort. *Mod. Rheumatol.* **2022**, *32*, 875–884. [CrossRef]
22. Fujiwara, T.; Tokuda, K.; Momii, K.; Shiomoto, K.; Tsushima, H.; Akasaki, Y.; Ikemura, S.; Fukushi, J.I.; Maki, J.; Kaku, N.; et al. Prognostic factors for the short-term mortality of patients with rheumatoid arthritis admitted to intensive care units. *BMC Rheumatol.* **2020**, *4*, 64. [CrossRef]
23. Fukui, S.; Winkelmayer, W.C.; Tedeschi, S.K.; Marrugo, J.; Guan, H.; Harrold, L.; Litman, H.J.; Shinozaki, T.; Solomon, D.H. Disease activity of rheumatoid arthritis and kidney function decline: A large prospective registry study. *Ann. Rheum. Dis.* **2025**, *84*, 201–209. [CrossRef] [PubMed]
24. Hanaoka, H.; Aoki, T.; Kosaka, T.; Yoshinaga, S.; Shibata, A.; Sakai, R.; Kurasawa, T.; Amano, K. Chronic kidney disease and inflammatory cytokines in rheumatoid arthritis: A potential pathogenic link. *Immunol. Med.* **2025**, *48*, 161–170. [CrossRef] [PubMed]
25. Suarez-Fueyo, A.; Bradley, S.J.; Klatzmann, D.; Tsokos, G.C. T cells and autoimmune kidney disease. *Nat. Rev. Nephrol.* **2017**, *13*, 329–343. [CrossRef]
26. Purohit, S.; Piani, F.; Ordonez, F.A.; de Lucas-Collantes, C.; Bauer, C.; Cara-Fuentes, G. Molecular Mechanisms of Proteinuria in Minimal Change Disease. *Front. Med.* **2021**, *8*, 761600. [CrossRef]
27. Romero-Gonzalez, G.; Rodriguez-Chitiva, N.; Canameras, C.; Paul-Martinez, J.; Urrutia-Jou, M.; Troya, M.; Soler-Majoral, J.; Graterol Torres, F.; Sanchez-Baya, M.; Calabia, J.; et al. Albuminuria, Forgotten No More: Underlining the Emerging Role in CardioRenal Crosstalk. *J. Clin. Med.* **2024**, *13*, 777. [CrossRef] [PubMed]
28. Obici, L.; Merlini, G. AA amyloidosis: Basic knowledge, unmet needs and future treatments. *Swiss Med. Wkly.* **2012**, *142*, w13580. [CrossRef]
29. Lim, J.S.; Han, S.; Kim, J.S.; Kim, S.; Oh, B. Effects of NSAIDs on Early CKD Development: A 10-Year Population-Based Study Using the Korean Senior Cohort. *Drugs Aging* **2025**, *42*, 953–961. [CrossRef]
30. Schiff, M.H.; Whelton, A. Renal toxicity associated with disease-modifying antirheumatic drugs used for the treatment of rheumatoid arthritis. *Semin. Arthritis Rheum.* **2000**, *30*, 196–208. [CrossRef]
31. Randhawa, P.S.; Starzl, T.E.; Demetris, A.J. Tacrolimus (FK506)-Associated Renal Pathology. *Adv. Anat. Pathol.* **1997**, *4*, 265–276. [CrossRef]
32. Zha, D.; Gao, P.; Wu, X. Role of Metabolic Abnormalities During the Progression of Chronic Kidney Disease and Preventive Strategies. *Int. J. Med. Sci.* **2025**, *22*, 3543–3555. [CrossRef]

 https://doi.org/10.3390/jcm15010108

33. Pan, D.; Xia, J.; Qu, Y.; Shi, C.; Du, H.; Zhang, J.; Peng, F.; Wang, X.; Liu, R.; Wu, L.; et al. Oleanolic acid inhibits mesangial cell proliferation and inflammatory response in mesangial proliferative glomerulonephritis through IL-17/ERK/AKT pathway. *Int. Immunopharmacol.* **2025**, *152*, 114459. [CrossRef] [PubMed]
34. Wang, Y.N.; Miao, H.; Yu, X.Y.; Guo, Y.; Su, W.; Liu, F.; Cao, G.; Zhao, Y.Y. Oxidative stress and inflammation are mediated via aryl hydrocarbon receptor signalling in idiopathic membranous nephropathy. *Free Radic. Biol. Med.* **2023**, *207*, 89–106. [CrossRef]
35. Elahi, T.; Ahmed, S.; Mubarak, M. Short-term renal and patient outcomes of primary immunoglobulin-associated mesangiocapillary glomerulonephritis: Insights from a developing country. *World J. Nephrol.* **2024**, *13*, 98969. [CrossRef] [PubMed]
36. Hayashi, K.; Sada, K.E.; Asano, Y.; Asano, S.H.; Yamamura, Y.; Ohashi, K.; Morishita, M.; Watanabe, H.; Narazaki, M.; Matsumoto, Y.; et al. Risk of higher dose methotrexate for renal impairment in patients with rheumatoid arthritis. *Sci. Rep.* **2020**, *10*, 18715. [CrossRef]
37. Tyczynska, K.M.; Augustyniak-Bartosik, H.; Swierkot, J. Rheumatoid arthritis—Medication dosage in chronic kidney disease. *Reumatologia* **2023**, *61*, 481–491. [CrossRef]
38. Bergner, R.; Peters, L.; Schmitt, V.; Loffler, C. Leflunomide in dialysis patients with rheumatoid arthritis—A pharmacokinetic study. *Clin. Rheumatol.* **2013**, *32*, 267–270. [CrossRef] [PubMed]
39. Akiyama, Y.; Sakurai, Y.; Kato, Y.; Furuta, E.; Mimura, T. Retrospective study of salazosulfapyridine in eight patients with rheumatoid arthritis on hemodialysis. *Mod. Rheumatol.* **2014**, *24*, 285–290. [CrossRef]
40. Rao, I.R.; Kolakemar, A.; Shenoy, S.V.; Prabhu, R.A.; Nagaraju, S.P.; Rangaswamy, D.; Bhojaraja, M.V. Hydroxychloroquine in nephrology: Current status and future directions. *J. Nephrol.* **2023**, *36*, 2191–2208. [CrossRef]
41. Honda, S.; Katsumata, Y.; Karasawa, K.; Yamanaka, H.; Harigai, M. Management of End-stage Renal Disease Associated with Systemic Rheumatic Diseases. *JMA J.* **2020**, *3*, 20–28. [CrossRef]
42. Kaneko, Y.; Kawahito, Y.; Kojima, M.; Nakayama, T.; Hirata, S.; Kishimoto, M.; Endo, H.; Seto, Y.; Ito, H.; Nishida, K.; et al. Efficacy and safety of tacrolimus in patients with rheumatoid arthritis—A systematic review and meta-analysis. *Mod. Rheumatol.* **2021**, *31*, 61–69. [CrossRef] [PubMed]
43. Heerspink, H.J.L.; Stefansson, B.V.; Correa-Rotter, R.; Chertow, G.M.; Greene, T.; Hou, F.F.; Mann, J.F.E.; McMurray, J.J.V.; Lindberg, M.; Rossing, P.; et al. Dapagliflozin in Patients with Chronic Kidney Disease. *N. Engl. J. Med.* **2020**, *383*, 1436–1446. [CrossRef]
44. Chakrabarti, K.; McCune, W.J. SGLT-2 inhibitors: New horizons for rheumatologists. *Curr. Opin. Rheumatol.* **2024**, *36*, 351–359. [CrossRef]
45. Marso, S.P.; Bain, S.C.; Consoli, A.; Eliaschewitz, F.G.; Jodar, E.; Leiter, L.A.; Lingvay, I.; Rosenstock, J.; Seufert, J.; Warren, M.L.; et al. Semaglutide and Cardiovascular Outcomes in Patients with Type 2 Diabetes. *N. Engl. J. Med.* **2016**, *375*, 1834–1844. [CrossRef] [PubMed]
46. Bilgin, E.; Venerito, V.; Bogdanos, D.P. Glucagon-Like Peptide-1 (GLP-1) receptor agonists in rheumatology: A review of current evidence and future directions. *Autoimmun. Rev.* **2025**, *24*, 103864. [CrossRef] [PubMed]
47. Calvet, X.; Carpio, D.; Rodriguez-Lago, I.; Garcia-Vicuna, R.; Barreiro-de-Acosta, M.; Juanola, X.; Aguas, M.; Castillo, C.; Gratacos, J. Risk of infection associated with Janus Kinase (JAK) inhibitors and biological therapies in inflammatory intestinal disease and rheumatoid arthritis. Prevention strategies. *Gastroenterol. Hepatol.* **2021**, *44*, 587–598. [CrossRef]
48. Konzett, V.; Smolen, J.S.; Nash, P.; Aletaha, D.; Winthrop, K.; Dorner, T.; Fleischmann, R.; Tanaka, Y.; Primdahl, J.; Baraliakos, X.; et al. Efficacy of Janus kinase inhibitors in immune-mediated inflammatory diseases a systematic literature review informing the 2024 update of an international consensus statement. *Ann. Rheum. Dis.* **2025**, *84*, 680–696. [CrossRef]
49. Narbutt, J.; Zuber, Z.; Lesiak, A.; Bien, N.; Szepietowski, J.C. Vaccinations in Selected Immune-Related Diseases Treated with Biological Drugs and JAK Inhibitors-Literature Review and Statement of Experts from Polish Dermatological Society. *Vaccines* **2024**, *12*, 82. [CrossRef]
50. Fragoulis, G.E.; Nikiphorou, E.; Dey, M.; Zhao, S.S.; Courvoisier, D.S.; Arnaud, L.; Atzeni, F.; Behrens, G.M.; Bijlsma, J.W.; Bohm, P.; et al. 2022 EULAR recommendations for screening and prophylaxis of chronic and opportunistic infections in adults with autoimmune inflammatory rheumatic diseases. *Ann. Rheum. Dis.* **2023**, *82*, 742–753. [CrossRef]
51. Yoshimura, Y.; Yamanouchi, M.; Mizuno, H.; Ikuma, D.; Koizumi, R.; Kurihara, S.; Oba, Y.; Suwabe, T.; Sawada, Y.; Kamido, H.; et al. Efficacy and safety of first-line biological DMARDs in rheumatoid arthritis patients with chronic kidney disease. *Ann. Rheum. Dis.* **2024**, *83*, 1278–1287. [CrossRef]
52. Onishi, A.; Yamada, H.; Yamamoto, W.; Watanabe, R.; Hara, R.; Katayama, M.; Okita, Y.; Maeda, Y.; Amuro, H.; Son, Y.; et al. Comparative effectiveness of biological disease-modifying antirheumatic drugs and Janus kinase inhibitor monotherapy in rheumatoid arthritis. *Rheumatology* **2024**, *63*, 3065–3073. [CrossRef]
53. Nishimura, N.; Onishi, A.; Yamamoto, W.; Nagai, K.; Shiba, H.; Okita, Y.; Son, Y.; Amuro, H.; Okano, T.; Ueda, Y.; et al. Comparative effects of biological and targeted synthetic DMARDs on incident chronic kidney disease in patients with rheumatoid arthritis. *Rheumatology* **2025**, *64*, 2395–2402. [CrossRef] [PubMed]
54. Williams, E.L.; Gadola, S.; Edwards, C.J. Anti-TNF-induced lupus. *Rheumatology* **2009**, *48*, 716–720. [CrossRef] [PubMed]
55. De Bandt, M. Anti-TNF-alpha-induced lupus. *Arthritis Res. Ther.* **2019**, *21*, 235. [CrossRef] [PubMed]

 https://doi.org/10.3390/jcm15010108

56. Suh, S.H.; Jung, J.H.; Oh, T.R.; Yang, E.M.; Choi, H.S.; Kim, C.S.; Bae, E.H.; Ma, S.K.; Han, K.D.; Kim, S.W. Rheumatoid arthritis and the risk of end-stage renal disease: A nationwide, population-based study. *Front. Med.* **2023**, *10*, 1116489. [CrossRef]
57. Chiu, H.Y.; Huang, H.L.; Li, C.H.; Chen, H.A.; Yeh, C.L.; Chiu, S.H.; Lin, W.C.; Cheng, Y.P.; Tsai, T.F.; Ho, S.Y. Increased Risk of Chronic Kidney Disease in Rheumatoid Arthritis Associated with Cardiovascular Complications—A National Population-Based Cohort Study. *PLoS ONE* **2015**, *10*, e0136508. [CrossRef]

https://doi.org/10.3390/jcm15010108

Journal of
Clinical Medicine

MDPI

Article

Influence of Safety Warnings on the Prescribing Attitude of JAK Inhibitors for Rheumatoid Arthritis in Italy

Marino Paroli [1,*,†], Andrea Becciolini [2,†], Alberto Lo Gullo [3], Simone Parisi [4], Elena Bravi [5], Romina Andracco [6], Valeria Nucera [7], Francesca Ometto [8], Federica Lumetti [9], Antonella Farina [10], Patrizia Del Medico [11], Matteo Colina [12,13], Viviana Ravagnani [14], Palma Scolieri [15], Maddalena Larosa [16], Marta Priora [17], Elisa Visalli [18], Olga Addimanda [19], Rosetta Vitetta [20], Alessandro Volpe [21], Alessandra Bezzi [22], Francesco Girelli [23], Aldo Biagio Molica Colella [24], Rosalba Caccavale [1], Eleonora Di Donato [2], Giuditta Adorni [2], Daniele Santilli [2], Gianluca Lucchini [2], Eugenio Arrigoni [5], Ilaria Platè [5], Natalia Mansueto [6], Aurora Ianniello [7], Enrico Fusaro [4], Maria Chiara Ditto [4], Vincenzo Bruzzese [15], Dario Camellino [16], Gerolamo Bianchi [16], Francesca Serale [17], Rosario Foti [18], Giorgio Amato [18], Francesco De Lucia [18], Ylenia Dal Bosco [18], Roberta Foti [18], Massimo Reta [19], Alessia Fiorenza [20], Guido Rovera [20], Antonio Marchetta [21], Maria Cristina Focherini [22], Fabio Mascella [22], Simone Bernardi [23], Gilda Sandri [25], Dilia Giuggioli [25], Carlo Salvarani [25], Maria Ilenia De Andres [3], Veronica Franchina [26], Francesco Molica Colella [27], Giulio Ferrero [28], Bernd Raffeiner [29] and Alarico Ariani [2]

1 Department of Clinical, Internist, Anesthesiologic and Cardiovascular Sciences, Sapienza University of Rome, 00185 Rome, Italy; rosalba_caccavale@yahoo.it
2 Internal Medicine and Rheumatology Unit, University Hospital of Parma, 43126 Parma, Italy; beccio@yahoo.it (A.B.); eleonoradidonato@ymail.com (E.D.D.); gadorni@ao.pr.it (G.A.); dsantilli@ao.pr.it (D.S.); glucchini@ao.pr.it (G.L.); dott.alaricoariani@libero.it (A.A.)
3 Rheumatology Unit, ARNAS Garibaldi, 95124 Catania, Italy; albertologullo@virgilio.it (A.L.G.); ilenia.deandres@gmail.com (M.I.D.A.)
4 Rheumatology Department, Azienda Ospedaliero-Universitaria Città della Salute e della Scienza di Torino, 10126 Turin, Italy; simone.parisi@hotmail.it (S.P.); fusaro.reumatorino@gmail.com (E.F.)
5 Rheumatology Unit, Guglielmo da Saliceto Hospital, 29121 Piacenza, Italy; e.bravi@ausl.pc.it (E.B.); e.arrigoni@ausl.pc.it (E.A.); i.plate@ausl.pc.it (I.P.)
6 Rheumatology Unit, ASL1 Liguria, 18038 Bussana di Sanremo, Italy; r.andracco@gmail.com (R.A.); natalia.mansueto@libero.it (N.M.)
7 Rheumatology Unit, ASL Novara, 28100 Novara, Italy; v.nucera@asl.novara.it (V.N.); a.ianniello@asl.novara.it (A.I.)
8 Rheumatology Unit, Azienda ULSS 6 Euganea, 35131 Padua, Italy; f.ometto@gmail.com
9 Rheumatology Unit, Azienda USL of Modena and AOU Policlinico of Modena, 41100 Modena, Italy; fedelumetti@gmail.com
10 Internal Medicine Unit, Augusto Murri Hospital, 63900 Fermo, Italy; antonella_farina@hotmail.com
11 Internal Medicine Unit, Civitanova Marche Hospital, 62012 Civitanova Marche, Italy; patdelmedico@hotmail.com
12 Rheumatology Unit, Internal Medicine Division, Department of Medicine and Oncology, Santa Maria della Scaletta Hospital, 40026 Imola, Italy; matteo.colina2@unibo.it
13 Rheumatology Unit, Alma Mater Studiorum—University of Bologna, 40126 Bologna, Italy
14 Rheumatology Unit, Santa Chiara Hospital APSS—Trento, 38122 Trento, Italy; viviana.ravagnani@gmail.com
15 Rheumatology Unit, Nuovo Regina Margherita Hospital, 00154 Rome, Italy; palma.scolieri@gmail.com (P.S.); vinbruzzese@tiscali.it (V.B.)
16 Division of Rheumatology, Department of Medical Specialties, Azienda Sanitaria Locale 3 Genovese, 16132 Genoa, Italy; madlarosa8@gmail.com (M.L.); dario.camellino@asl3.liguria.it (D.C.); gerolamo.bianchi@asl3.liguria.it (G.B.)
17 Rheumatology Unit, ASL CN1, 12100 Cuneo, Italy; marta.priora@gmail.com (M.P.); francesca.serale@gmail.com (F.S.)
18 Rheumatology Unit, Policlinico San Marco Hospital, 95121 Catania, Italy; elivisa21@gmail.com (E.V.); rosfoti5@gmail.com (R.F.); giorgioamato@hotmail.it (G.A.); francescodelucia89@yahoo.it (F.D.L.); yleniadalbosco@gmail.com (Y.D.B.); robertafoti@hotmail.com (R.F.)
19 Rheumatology Unit, AUSL of Bologna—Policlinico Sant'Orsola—AOU—IRCCS of Bologna, 40138 Bologna, Italy; olga.addimanda@ausl.bologna.it (O.A.); massimo.reta@ausl.bologna.it (M.R.)
20 Rheumatology Unit, ASL VC Sant'Andrea Hospital, 13100 Vercelli, Italy; rosetta.vitetta@aslvc.piemonte.it (R.V.); alessia.fiorenza@aslvc.piemonte.it (A.F.); guido.rovera.gr@gmail.com (G.R.)

[21] Rheumatology Unit, IRCCS Sacro Cuore Don Calabria Hospital, 37024 Negrar di Valpolicella, Italy; avolpe127@gmail.com (A.V.); antonio.marchetta@sacrocuore.it (A.M.)
[22] Internal Medicine and Rheumatology Unit, AUSL della Romagna—Rimini, 47924 Rimini, Italy; alessandra.bezzi@auslromagna.it (A.B.); mariacristina.focherini@auslromagna.it (M.C.F.); fabio.mascella@auslromagna.it (F.M.)
[23] Rheumatology Unit, G.B. Morgagni—L. Pierantoni Hospital, 47121 Forlì, Italy; francesco.girelli@auslromagna.it (F.G.); siiberna@yahoo.it (S.B.)
[24] Departmental Unit of Rheumatology, Azienda Ospedaliera Papardo, 98158 Messina, Italy; aldomolica@alice.it
[25] Rheumatology Unit, University of Modena and Reggio Emilia, 41125 Modena, Italy; gilda.sandri@unimore.it (G.S.); dilia.giuggioli@unimore.it (D.G.); carlo.salvarani@unimore.it (C.S.)
[26] Medical Oncology Unit, Azienda Ospedaliera Papardo, 98158 Messina, Italy; verifra82@yahoo.it
[27] Medicine Unit, Milano-Bicocca University, 20126 Milan, Italy; francesco.molica3@gmail.com
[28] Unit of Diagnostic and Interventional Radiology, Santa Corona Hospital, 17027 Pietra Ligure, Italy; giulio.ferrero@gmail.com
[29] Department of Rheumatology, Bolzano Central Hospital, 39100 Bolzano, Italy; berndraffeiner@yahoo.com
* Correspondence: marino.paroli@uniroma1.it
† These authors contributed equally to this work.

Abstract: Background/Objectives: The Janus kinase inhibitors (JAKi) tofacitinib (TOFA), baricitinib (BARI), upadacitinib (UPA), and filgotinib (FILGO) are effective drugs for the treatment of rheumatoid arthritis. However, the US Food and Drug Administration (FDA) raised concerns about the safety of TOFA after its approval. This prompted the European Medicines Agency (EMA) to issue two safety warnings for limiting TOFA use, then extended a third warning to all JAKi in patients at high risk of developing serious adverse effects (SAE). These include thrombosis, major adverse cardiac events (MACE), and cancer. The purpose of this work was to analyze how the first two safety warnings from the EMA affected the prescribing of JAKi by rheumatologists in Italy. **Methods:** All patients with rheumatoid arthritis who had been prescribed JAKi for the first time in a 36-month period from 1 July 2019, to 30 June 2022 were considered. Data were obtained from the medical records of 29 Italian tertiary referral rheumatology centers. Patients were divided into three groups of 4 months each, depending on whether the JAKi prescription had occurred before the EMA's first safety alert (1 July–31 October 2019, Group 1), between the first and second alerts (1 November 2019–29 February 2020, Group 2), or between the second and third alerts (1 March 2021–30 June 2021, Group 3). The percentages and absolute changes in the patients prescribed the individual JAKi were analyzed. Differences among the three groups of patients regarding demographic and clinical characteristics were also assessed. **Results:** A total of 864 patients were prescribed a JAKi during the entire period considered. Of these, 343 were identified in Group 1, 233 in Group 2, and 288 in Group 3. An absolute reduction of 32% was observed in the number of patients prescribed a JAKi between Group 1 and Group 2 and 16% between Group 1 and Group 3. In contrast, there was a 19% increase in the prescription of a JAKi in patients between Group 2 and Group 3. In the first group, BARI was the most prescribed drug (227 prescriptions, 66.2% of the total), followed by TOFA (115, 33.5%) and UPA (1, 0.3%). In the second group, the most prescribed JAKi was BARI (147, 63.1%), followed by TOFA (65, 27.9%) and UPA (33, 11.5%). In the third group, BARI was still the most prescribed JAKi (104 prescriptions, 36.1%), followed by UPA (89, 30.9%), FILGO (89, 21.5%), and TOFA (33, 11.5%). The number of patients prescribed TOFA decreased significantly between Group 1 and Group 2 and between Group 2 and Group 3 (p < 0.01). The number of patients who were prescribed BARI decreased significantly between Group 1 and Group 2 and between Group 2 and Group 3 (p < 0.01). In contrast, the number of patients prescribed UPA increased between Group 2 and Group 3 (p < 0.01). **Conclusions**: These data suggest that the warnings issued for TOFA were followed by a reduction in total JAKi prescriptions. However, the more selective JAKi (UPA and FILGO) were perceived by prescribers as favorable in terms of the risk/benefit ratio, and their use gradually increased at the expense of the other molecules.

Keywords: janus kinase inhibitors; safety warnings; prescribing attitude; rheumatoid arthritis

1. Introduction

Rheumatoid arthritis (RA) is a chronic autoimmune disease characterized by systemic inflammation and persistent synovitis, which can lead to joint damage, disability, and significant comorbidities [1]. The pathogenesis of RA involves a complex interaction between genetic, environmental, and immunological factors that lead to the activation of the immune system against joint tissues [2]. The latest recommendations of the European Alliance of Associations for Rheumatology (EULAR) recommend adding or switching to biologic disease-modifying antirheumatic drugs (bDMARDs) or targeted synthetic DMARDs (tsDMARDs), such as JAK inhibitors (JAKi), for patients with inadequate responses to conventional synthetic DMARDs (csDMARDs) [3]. Specifically, JAKi are a class of drugs approved in recent years for the treatment of rheumatoid arthritis [4] that inhibit the JAK enzymes involved in cytokine signaling through the intracellular JAK/STAT pathway, leading in turn to the activation of intranuclear transcription factors of several genes encoding for pro-inflammatory molecules [5]. Currently, four JAKi have been approved by the European Medicines Agency (EMA). These include tofacitinib (TOFA), which mainly inhibits JAK1 and JAK2 and to a lesser extent JAK2; baricitinib (BARI), which primarily inhibits JAK 1 and JAK2; and upadacitinib (UPA) and filgotinib (FILGO), both selective for JAK1 [6]. In addition to the indication for the treatment of rheumatoid arthritis, TOFA and UPA have been approved for the treatment of psoriatic arthritis (PsA) and radiographic (TOFA and UPA) or non-radiographic (UPA) axial spondyloarthritis (axSpA) [7]. JAKi have some advantages over biologics, such as oral administration, rapid onset of action, broad mechanism of action, efficacy in treatment-resistant cases, and absence of immunogenicity, which, on the other hand, may be responsible for the formation of anti-drug antibodies (ADAs) during biologic therapy, possibly reducing its efficacy [8]. Although in registrational studies these drugs have been shown to have an acceptable safety profile, further concerns emerged in the post-marketing phase for TOFA regarding the possible increased risk of thromboembolism, major cardiovascular events (MACE), and cancer development [9–11]. This prompted the FDA to add in July of 2019 a warning (Boxed Warning) to the TOFA label and to request a phase 3b-4, a randomized, open-label, noninferiority ORAL surveillance study [12,13]. In November of that year, the EMA issued a similar notice, followed by two subsequent notices in March of 2021 and November of 2022 [14] emphasizing the increased risk of the aforementioned complications and serious and fatal infections associated with TOFA use. Therefore, in accordance with EMA recommendations, the manufacturer informed the physicians of TOFA-associated risks, recommending that a dose of 5 mg twice daily for the treatment of rheumatoid arthritis not be exceeded and treating patients older than 65 years only when alternative treatments are not available. Moreover, physicians were made aware that patients aged 50 years and older with at least one additional cardiovascular risk factor had been shown by ORAL surveillance study to have an increased incidence of myocardial infarction compared with patients treated with an anti-TNF-alpha biologic, and that there was in the treated patients an increased incidence of malignancies, including lung cancer and lymphoma. This communication was followed by a similar recommendation that TOFA should not be used in patients older than 65 years, in smokers or former smokers, and in patients with other risk factors for cardiovascular disease, unless suitable therapeutic alternatives are unavailable. In January of 2023, the EMA's Committee for Medicinal Products for Human Use (CHMP) approved the measures recommended by the Pharmacovigilance Risk Assessment Committee (PRAC). These recommendations not only confirmed that TOFA increases the risk of major cardiovascular problems, cancer, VTE, serious infections, and death from any cause compared with drugs in the TNF-alpha inhibitor class but were also extended to all other officially approved JAKi, although specific studies on these molecules had not yet been conducted [15].

The purpose of the present multicenter study was to analyze any changes in the prescribing attitude of JAKi in the treatment of rheumatoid arthritis by Italian rheumatologists over a period of 36 months, including the period before and after the first and second EMA safety warnings.

2. Material and Methods

All patients with rheumatoid arthritis who had been prescribed a specific JAK inhibitor for the first time within a 36-month period from 1 July 2019 to 30 June 2022 were considered. The patients were then divided into three groups based on the timing of their prescriptions: Group 1 included patients prescribed the JAK inhibitor before the first EMA safety alert (1 July–31 October 2019), Group 2 included those prescribed between the first and second alerts (1 November 2019–29 February 2021), and Group 3 included patients prescribed between the second and third alerts (1 March 2021–30 June 2022). The percentage and absolute changes in patients prescribed a single JAKi were analyzed. Differences in the three groups of patients, with regard to the demographics and clinical characteristics of the treated patients, were also assessed. Therefore, the differences in the prescription of JAKi in the three groups considered were analyzed in both absolute and relative terms with respect to single molecules. Any differences in the 3 groups considered with regard to the demographic and clinical data of the treated patients were also considered. Specifically, the male/female ratio, the age of the treated patients, the presence or absence of a cigarette smoking habit, and associated comorbidities were analyzed. Other parameters such as the seropositivity/seronegativity of rheumatoid arthritis, disease activity, and previous or concomitant treatments were also analyzed. Prescription data were extracted from the medical records of 29 tertiary rheumatology centers distributed in different Italian regions. This study is part of the BIologics Retention Rate Assessment (BIRRA) project, which focuses on studying the effects of current therapy in rheumatic diseases. The study was conducted according to the principles of the Declaration of Helsinki and was approved by local ethics committees, the main one being the Ethics Committee of the Emilia Vasta Nord Area, protocol code 34.713, approved on 28 August 2019. The statistical analysis was conducted by the Fisher–Yates exact test for qualitative data and the Mann–Whitney U test and the Wilcoxon Signed Rank test for quantitative data. A p value less than or equal to 0.05 or 0.01 indicated a statistically significant result. The MedCalc program, version 12.5.0.0 (MedCalc software Ltd., Ostend, Belgium), was used for statistical analysis.

3. Results

A total of 864 patients were prescribed JAKi during the entire period considered in this study. Of these, 343 were identified in Group 1, 233 in Group 2, and 288 in Group 3. An absolute reduction of 32% was observed in the number of patients prescribed JAKi between Group 1 and Group 2 and 16% between Group 1 and Group 3. In contrast, there was a 19% increase of the prescription of JAKi in patients between Group 2 and Group 3. In the first group, BARI was the most prescribed drug (227 prescriptions, 66.2% of the total), followed by TOFA (115, 33.5%) and UPA (1, 0.3%). In the second group, the most prescribed JAKi was BARI (147, 63.1%), followed by TOFA (65, 27.9%) and UPA (33, 11.5%). In the third group, BARI was still the most prescribed JAKi (104 prescriptions, 36.1%), followed by UPA (89, 30.9%), FILGO (89, 21.5%), and TOFA (33, 11.5%). However, the number of patients prescribed TOFA decreased significantly between Group 1 and Group 2 and between Group 2 and Group 3 ($p < 0.01$). The number of patients who were prescribed BARI decreased significantly between Group 1 and Group 2 and between Group 2 and Group 3 ($p < 0.01$). In contrast, the number of patients prescribed UPA increased between Group 2 and Group 3 ($p < 0.01$). The F:M ratio increased between Groups 1 and 2 (4.0 vs. 4.8; $p < 0.05$) and then decreased between Groups 2 and 3 (4.8 vs. 2.7; $p < 0.01$). A reduction in the visual analog scale of pain (VAS) 0–100 was observed in Group 2 as compared to Group 1 (median 60, IQR 40–80 vs median 70, IQR 50–80; $p < 0.05$). There was also a significant reduction in dyslipidemia and cancer cases between Group 1 and Group 2 ($p < 0.05$). Glucocorticoid use in combination with JAKi treatment increased significantly between Group 1 and Group 2 ($p < 0.05$) and between Group 2 and Group 3 ($p < 0.01$). All these data are summarized in Table 1 and Figure 1.

Table 1. Demographic and clinical characteristics of patients.

Characteristic		Group 1	Group 2	Group 3
N		343	233	288
M:F		68:275	40:193 *	78–210 *
Age, yrs [IQR]		61 54–70	58 48–66	58 50–67
BMI, kg/m^2 [IQR]		24.6 22.7–27.0	24.7 23.0–27.0	25 22.8–27.9
Smokers, n yes:no:former		52:198:63	51:130:32	48:176:49
Disease duration, yrs [IQR]		6.3 1.8–13.5	6.5 3.2–12.8	6.7 2.6–12.8
RF presence, %		63.4	61.2	59.3
ACPA presence, %		59.5	58.4	54.9
Comorbidities, %	Diabetes Arterial hypertension Hypercholesterolemia MACE Cancer	9.3 37.0 26.5 5.2 6.4	5.2 30.9 18.0 3.4 2.1 *	9.0 35.7 21.9 6.6 5.2
Tender Joints, n [IQR]		8 4–12	8 4–12	8 4–12
Swollen Joints, n [IQR]		5 2–8	5 3–8	4 3–8
ESR, mm/h [IQR]		32 19–46	34 20–46	31 18–48
PCR, mg/dL [IQR]		1.3 0.5–3.0	1.3 0.6–2.6	1.2 0.5–3.8
VAS, 0–100 * [IQR]		60 40–80	70 50–80	70 50–80
PGA-Med, 0–10 [IQR]		7 5–8	5 5–8	7 5–7
DAS28 [IQR]		5.4 4.8–6.1	5.4 4.8–6.0	5.3 4.7–5.9
DAS28-CRP [IQR]		4.9 4.3–5.6	5.0 4.2–5.4	5.0 4.3–5.6
JAKi; %	Baricitinib Filgotinib Tofacitinib Upadacitinib	66.2 0 33.5 0.3	63.1 * 0 27.9 * 9.0	36.1 * 21.5 11.5 * 30.9 *
JAKi naive; %	None One Two	74.6 25.1 0.3	71.2 27.9 0.9	65.3 30.9 3.8
Treatment line after csDMARD-IR [IQR]		2 1–4	2 2–4	2 2–4
csDMARDs concomitant, %		49.0	45.5	43.4
Glucocorticoid *, %		32.7	42.0 *	43.8 *
Glucocorticoid, mg/day (PDN-eq) [IQR]		5 4–5	5 5–5	5 4–6

RF = rheumatoid factor; ACPA = anti-citrullinated peptide antibody; ESR = erythrocyte sedimentation rate; CRP = C-reactive protein; VAS = visual analog scale; PGA = global physical assessment; DAS = disease activity score; JAKi = JAK inhibitor; csDMARDs-IR = inadequate response to treatment with conventional synthetic DMARDs; PDN-eq = Prednisone-equivalent; * = statistically significant (see results sections for details).

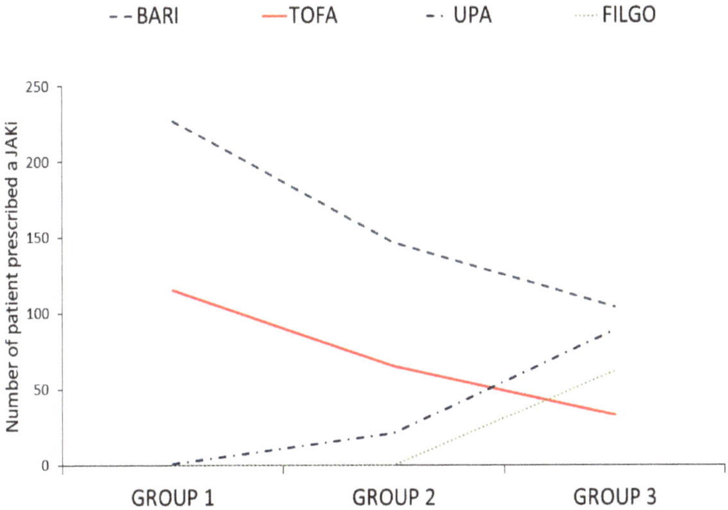

Figure 1. Variation over time in the number of patients prescribed a given JAKi.

4. Discussion

In this multicenter retrospective observational study, we analyzed how the first two safety warnings issued by the EMA on the use of TOFA influenced the attitudes of Italian rheumatologists in prescribing TOFA and the other JAKi approved for rheumatoid arthritis.

The first observed finding is that the total number of patients prescribed JAKi decreased after the first and second safety alerts as compared to the previous period over a comparable time frame. Because we did not consider the total number of patients treated with other second-line drugs such as biologics during the periods covered by our study, we cannot demonstrate that the observed absolute reduction in the number of JAKi prescriptions is statistically significant. However, assuming with good probability that the total number of patients treated with any type of second-line drug was constant throughout the duration of the study, our results suggest that JAKI prescribing actually decreased after the safety alerts.

We found that the percentage of patients treated with the individual JAKi changed significantly over the different periods considered. Specifically, the relative percentage of prescriptions of non-selective JAKi and, in particular, the pan-JAK inhibitor TOFA and the selective JAK1/JAK2 inhibitor BARI, decreased significantly both in the comparison between Group 1 and Group 2 and in the comparison between Group 2 and Group 3.

In the pre-alert period, BARI was the most prescribed JAKi. This is probably due to some features of BARI, including its once-daily administration and the possibility of reducing the dosage in elderly subjects, making its use more flexible than TOFA [16]. BARI remained the most prescribed JAKi even in the later periods considered in this study, although its prescriptions decreased significantly along with those of TOFA despite the fact that the safety warning referred only to TOFA. This may be explained assuming that BARI was perceived to be just as risky as TOFA because it belongs to the same class of drugs.

On the other hand, we observed a gradual increase in prescriptions of the JAK1-selective inhibitor UPA throughout the period examined and a significant number of prescriptions of the JAK1-selective inhibitor FILGO in Group 3. It should be noted that UPA was approved and made reimbursable by the Italian Drug Agency (AIFA) after the start of the first study period considered. A portion of the UPA prescriptions in Group 1 were therefore allowed through a limited number of free samples provided by the manufacturer.

Therefore, it was not possible to fairly compare UPA prescriptions in Group 1 with those in the subsequent groups. In addition, the statistical analysis of FILGO prescriptions was not possible because FILGO was approved only in the third period of our study.

It is likely that the reduction in prescriptions of non-selective or partially selective JAKi compared with second-generation JAK1-selective molecules was influenced by the perception that safety problems mainly affected older molecules. This probably favored the progressive prescriptions of UPA and FILGO over TOFA and BARI. It should be noted that this study was conducted prior to the EMA's third warning of November 2022, which extended the alert to all JAKi molecules. However, data from another study indicate that even after this third alert, the prescriptions of JAK-1 selective inhibitors, and in particular UPA, continued to increase, even though selectivity is more a concept based on theory than on actual data [17].

The renal elimination of UPA has been shown to be minimal, with only about 20 percent of the dose eliminated in the urine as unchanged drug. This reduces the risk of drug accumulation in patients with impaired renal function, contributing to the safety of the treatment. Although data on the renal function of patients included in this study are not available, it cannot be ruled out that part of the increase in UPA prescriptions is due to this pharmacokinetic peculiarity of the drug [18]. In this regard, it has been reported that the co-occurrence of RA with end-stage renal disease (ESRD) is greater than 1%, probably due to the impact of diabetes and hypertension, comorbidities often associated with this rheumatic disease [19].

An unexpected result of our study was the relative decrease in the ratio of females to males treated with JAKi between Group 1 and Group 3. One possible explanation is the different risk perception of the therapy between the two genders, which consequently favored prescribing JAKi in males after receiving information about the potential risks from the physician [20]. A statistically significant reduction in cancer cases was also observed between Groups 1 and 2 ($p < 0.05$). We do not have detailed information on the nature of the cancer cases reported during the study. However, all cases were incidental and led to the discontinuation of treatment with JAKi. Non-melanoma skin cancers (NMSCs) were excluded from the calculation. The reduction in cancer cases could be due to more careful patient selection following EMA warnings.

Finally, an interesting finding was the statistically significant increase in glucocorticoid use expressed as a prednisone-equivalent (PDN-eq) dose in combination with JAKi in Groups 2 and 3 as compared to the initial group ($p < 0.01$), respectively. This could reflect an increasing confidence in the safety of JAKi due to actual experience in the use of these molecules, with a reduction in prescribers' fear of possible cardiovascular and infectious adverse effects after combination with glucocorticoids [21,22]. In addition, the increased glucocorticoid use expressed as prednisone-equivalent doses in Groups 2 and 3 could be related to the higher severity of disease in these patients, who had already failed other therapies.

The limitations of the study are that the periods between the groups were not contiguous, and this could have introduced bias related to seasonal variations or other uncontrolled external factors. The periods were also not directly comparable because of different drug availability. In addition, the retrospective nature of the study could have introduced selection and information bias. An additional limitation is that the second period analyzed in this study coincided with the peak of COVID-19 cases. In this regard, a three-month observational study conducted in the United States showed that patients taking biologic DMARDs (bDMARDs) and JAKi were more likely to discontinue or delay drug use than those taking conventional synthetic DMARDs (csDMARDs). The main reason was concern about possible increased susceptibility or the severity of COVID-19, as well as the cancellation or postponement of appointments [23].

In conclusion, the data reported by this Italian multicenter study underscore that the first two EMA safety warnings negatively affected the use of JAKi but at the same time promoted a shift toward the use of more selective molecules in this class, and in particular the JAK1-selective molecules. Further studies are needed to clarify how JAKi prescribing might be affected in the future as more data on its safety become available. It will also be necessary to clarify whether safety issues will affect other indications of JAKi besides rheumatic diseases, such as chronic inflammatory bowel disease, psoriasis and atopic dermatitis. In this way, it will be possible to refine patient selection criteria, ensuring a balanced approach that maximizes therapeutic efficacy and minimizes potential adverse effects without depriving those who might benefit from JAKi therapy in view of the high disabling potential of immune-mediated inflammatory diseases.

Author Contributions: M.P. (Marino Paroli), A.B. (Andrea Becciolini) and A.A. were involved in the conception and design of this study and the interpretation of results; A.B. (Andrea Becciolini) and A.A. performed statistical analysis; A.L.G., S.P., E.B., R.A., V.N., F.O., F.L., A.F. (Antonella Farina), P.D.M., M.C., V.R., P.S., M.L., M.P. (Marta Priora), E.V., O.A., R.V., A.V., A.B. (Alessandra Bezzi), F.G., A.B.M.C., R.C., E.D.D., G.A. (Giuditta Adorni), D.S., G.L., E.A., I.P., N.M., A.I., E.F., M.C.D., V.B., D.C., G.B., F.S., R.F. (Rosario Foti), G.A. (Giorgio Amato), F.D.L., Y.D.B., R.F. (Roberta Foti), M.R., A.F. (Alessia Fiorenza), G.R., A.M., M.C.F., F.M., S.B., G.S., D.G., C.S., M.I.D.A., V.F., F.M.C., G.F., B.R. and A.A. were involved in recruitment of patients, contributed to participating in the discussion of the final draft and revised it critically for intellectual content; M.P. (Marino Paroli) prepared the first draft of the paper. All authors have read and agreed to the published version of the manuscript.

Funding: This research received no external funding.

Institutional Review Board Statement: As a part of the BIRRA (Biologics Retention Rate Assessment) project, this study was performed according to the Declaration of Helsinki's principles, and it was approved by the local Ethics Committees (the main is the Comitato Etico dell'Area Vasta Emilia Nord, protocol code 34713, approved on 28 August 2019).

Informed Consent Statement: Written informed consent for the use of clinical data was obtained from all subjects in accordance with the Helsinki declaration.

Data Availability Statement: All data generated or analyzed during the study are included in this published article.

Conflicts of Interest: The authors declare no conflicts of interest.

References

1. Smolen, J.S.; Aletaha, D.; McInnes, I.B. Rheumatoid arthritis. *Lancet* **2016**, *388*, 2023–2038. [CrossRef] [PubMed]
2. Firestein, G.S.; McInnes, I.B. Immunopathogenesis of Rheumatoid Arthritis. *Immunity* **2017**, *46*, 183–196. [CrossRef] [PubMed]
3. Smolen, J.S.; Landewe, R.B.M.; Bergstra, S.A.; Kerschbaumer, A.; Sepriano, A.; Aletaha, D.; Caporali, R.; Edwards, C.J.; Hyrich, K.L.; Pope, J.E.; et al. EULAR recommendations for the management of rheumatoid arthritis with synthetic and biological disease-modifying antirheumatic drugs: 2022 update. *Ann. Rheum. Dis.* **2023**, *82*, 3–18. [CrossRef] [PubMed]
4. Kubo, S.; Nakayamada, S.; Tanaka, Y. JAK inhibitors for rheumatoid arthritis. *Expert. Opin. Investig. Drugs* **2023**, *32*, 333–344. [CrossRef] [PubMed]
5. Yamaoka, K.; Oku, K. JAK inhibitors in rheumatology. *Immunol. Med.* **2023**, *46*, 143–152. [CrossRef] [PubMed]
6. Langbour, C.; Rene, J.; Goupille, P.; Carvajal Alegria, G. Efficacy of Janus kinase inhibitors in rheumatoid arthritis. *Inflamm. Res.* **2023**, *72*, 1121–1132. [CrossRef]
7. Benucci, M.; Bernardini, P.; Coccia, C.; De Luca, R.; Levani, J.; Economou, A.; Damiani, A.; Russo, E.; Amedei, A.; Guiducci, S.; et al. JAK inhibitors and autoimmune rheumatic diseases. *Autoimmun. Rev.* **2023**, *22*, 103276. [CrossRef] [PubMed]
8. Caporali, R.; Germinario, S.; Kacsandi, D.; Choy, E.; Szekanecz, Z. Start RA treatment-Biologics or JAK-inhibitors? *Autoimmun. Rev.* **2024**, *23*, 103429. [CrossRef] [PubMed]
9. Mease, P.; Charles-Schoeman, C.; Cohen, S.; Fallon, L.; Woolcott, J.; Yun, H.; Kremer, J.; Greenberg, J.; Malley, W.; Onofrei, A.; et al. Incidence of venous and arterial thromboembolic events reported in the tofacitinib rheumatoid arthritis, psoriasis and psoriatic arthritis development programmes and from real-world data. *Ann. Rheum. Dis.* **2020**, *79*, 1400–1413. [CrossRef]
10. Taylor, P.C.; Weinblatt, M.E.; Burmester, G.R.; Rooney, T.P.; Witt, S.; Walls, C.D.; Issa, M.; Salinas, C.A.; Saifan, C.; Zhang, X.; et al. Cardiovascular Safety during Treatment with Baricitinib in Rheumatoid Arthritis. *Arthritis Rheumatol.* **2019**, *71*, 1042–1055. [CrossRef]
11. Olivera, P.A.; Lasa, J.S.; Bonovas, S.; Danese, S.; Peyrin-Biroulet, L. Safety of Janus Kinase Inhibitors in Patients with Inflammatory Bowel Diseases or Other Immune-mediated Diseases: A Systematic Review and Meta-Analysis. *Gastroenterology* **2020**, *158*, 1554–1573.e12. [CrossRef]

12. Ytterberg, S.R.; Bhatt, D.L.; Connell, C.A. Cardiovascular and Cancer Risk with Tofacitinib in Rheumatoid Arthritis. Reply. *N. Engl. J. Med.* **2022**, *386*, 1768. [CrossRef]
13. Winthrop, K.L.; Cohen, S.B. Oral surveillance and JAK inhibitor safety: The theory of relativity. *Nat. Rev. Rheumatol.* **2022**, *18*, 301–304. [CrossRef]
14. Russell, M.D.; Yang, Z.; Walter, B.; Alveyn, E.; Bechman, K.; Miracle, A.; Nagra, D.; Adas, M.A.; Norton, S.; Cope, A.P.; et al. The influence of safety warnings on the prescribing of JAK inhibitors. *Lancet Rheumatol.* **2024**, *6*, e138–e139. [CrossRef]
15. Solitano, V.; Facheris, P.; Petersen, M.; D'Amico, F.; Ortoncelli, M.; Aletaha, D.; Olivera, P.A.; Bieber, T.; Ramiro, S.; Ghosh, S.; et al. Implementation of regulatory guidance for JAK inhibitors use in patients with immune-mediated inflammatory diseases: An international appropriateness study. *Autoimmun. Rev.* **2024**, *23*, 103504. [CrossRef]
16. Mogul, A.; Corsi, K.; McAuliffe, L. Baricitinib: The Second FDA-Approved JAK Inhibitor for the Treatment of Rheumatoid Arthritis. *Ann. Pharmacother.* **2019**, *53*, 947–953. [CrossRef]
17. Traves, P.G.; Murray, B.; Campigotto, F.; Galien, R.; Meng, A.; Di Paolo, J.A. JAK selectivity and the implications for clinical inhibition of pharmacodynamic cytokine signalling by filgotinib, upadacitinib, tofacitinib and baricitinib. *Ann. Rheum. Dis.* **2021**, *80*, 865–875. [CrossRef]
18. Mohamed, M.F.; Trueman, S.; Feng, T.; Anderson, J.; Marbury, T.C.; Othman, A.A. Characterization of the Effect of Renal Impairment on Upadacitinib Pharmacokinetics. *J. Clin. Pharmacol.* **2019**, *59*, 856–862. [CrossRef]
19. Paudyal, S.; Yang, F.M.; Rice, C.; Chen, C.C.; Skelton, M.; Bethel, M.; Brown, S.; Nahman, N.S., Jr.; Carbone, L. End-stage renal disease in patients with rheumatoid arthritis. *Semin. Arthritis Rheum.* **2017**, *46*, 418–422. [CrossRef]
20. Rolnick, S.J.; Pawloski, P.A.; Hedblom, B.D.; Asche, S.E.; Bruzek, R.J. Patient characteristics associated with medication adherence. *Clin. Med. Res.* **2013**, *11*, 54–65. [CrossRef]
21. Paroli, M.; Becciolini, A.; Bravi, E.; Andracco, R.; Nucera, V.; Parisi, S.; Ometto, F.; Lumetti, F.; Farina, A.; Del Medico, P.; et al. Long-Term Retention Rate of Tofacitinib in Rheumatoid Arthritis: An Italian Multicenter Retrospective Cohort Study. *Medicina* **2023**, *59*, 1480. [CrossRef] [PubMed]
22. Parisi, S.; Andrea, B.; Chiara, D.M.; Alberto, L.G.; Maddalena, L.; Palma, S.; Olga, A.; Massimo, R.; Marino, P.; Rosalba, C.; et al. Analysis of survival rate and persistence predictors of baricitinib in real-world data from a large cohort of rheumatoid arthritis patients. *Curr. Res. Pharmacol. Drug Discov.* **2024**, *6*, 100178. [CrossRef] [PubMed]
23. Michaud, K.; Pedro, S.; Wipfler, K.; Agarwal, E.; Katz, P. Changes in Disease-Modifying Antirheumatic Drug Treatment for Patients with Rheumatoid Arthritis in the US during the COVID-19 Pandemic: A Three-Month Observational Study. *Arthritis Care Res.* **2021**, *73*, 1322–1331. [CrossRef] [PubMed]

Journal of
Clinical Medicine

MDPI

Article

Serum Anti-Aminoacyl-Transfer Ribonucleic Acid Synthetase Antibody Levels Are Involved in Rheumatoid Arthritis Complicated with Interstitial Lung Disease

Shomi Oka [1,2], Takashi Higuchi [1], Hiroshi Furukawa [1,2,*], Kota Shimada [3,4], Akira Okamoto [5,†], Misuzu Fujimori [5], Atsushi Hashimoto [3,6], Akiko Komiya [2,7], Koichiro Saisho [8,9], Norie Yoshikawa [8], Masao Katayama [10,†], Toshihiro Matsui [2,3], Naoshi Fukui [2,11], Kiyoshi Migita [12,13] and Shigeto Tohma [1,2]

1 Department of Rheumatology, NHO Tokyo National Hospital, Kiyose 204-8585, Japan; oka-tkb@umin.org (S.O.); takashi.qef@ac.auone-net.jp (T.H.); touma.shigeto.jy@mail.hosp.go.jp (S.T.)
2 Clinical Research Center for Allergy and Rheumatology, NHO Sagamihara National Hospital, Sagamihara 252-0392, Japan; komiya.akiko.zy@mail.hosp.go.jp (A.K.); ninja02matsui@gmail.com (T.M.); n-fukui@idaten.c.u-tokyo.ac.jp (N.F.)
3 Department of Rheumatology, NHO Sagamihara National Hospital, Sagamihara 252-0392, Japan; kouta_shimada@tmhp.jp (K.S.); hako@happy.email.ne.jp (A.H.)
4 Department of Rheumatic Diseases, Tokyo Metropolitan Tama Medical Center, Fuchu 183-8524, Japan
5 Department of Rheumatology, NHO Himeji Medical Center, Himeji 670-8520, Japan; misuzufujimori@yahoo.co.jp (M.F.)
6 Department of Internal Medicine, Sagami Seikyou Hospital, Sagamihara 252-0303, Japan
7 Department of Clinical Laboratory, NHO Sagamihara National Hospital, Sagamihara 252-0392, Japan
8 Department of Orthopedics/Rheumatology, NHO Miyakonojo Medical Center, Miyakonojo 885-0014, Japan; saisho889@miyazaki-catv.ne.jp (K.S.); nori1004@me.com (N.Y.)
9 Tanimura Hospital, Nobeoka 882-0041, Japan
10 Department of Internal Medicine, NHO Nagoya Medical Center, Nagoya 460-0001, Japan
11 Department of Life Sciences, Graduate School of Arts and Sciences, The University of Tokyo, Tokyo 153-890, Japan
12 Clinical Research Center, NHO Nagasaki Medical Center, Omura 856-8562, Japan; k-migita@sfh.or.jp
13 Department of Gastroenterology and Rheumatology, Fukushima Medical University School of Medicine, Fukushima 960-1295, Japan
* Correspondence: furukawa-tky@umin.org; Tel.: +81-42-491-2111; Fax: +81-42-494-2168
† Deceased.

Abstract: Objectives: A common complication in patients with rheumatoid arthritis (RA) is interstitial lung disease (ILD). Antibodies (Abs) to anti-aminoacyl-transfer ribonucleic acid synthetase (ARS) are linked to ILD in patients with idiopathic inflammatory myopathies (IIM). There have been limited studies of anti-ARS Abs in RA. In this study, we examined anti-ARS Abs in ILD in patients with RA. **Methods:** Anti-ARS Abs in serum from patients with RA were measured. **Results:** There were higher anti-ARS Ab levels in RA patients with ILD (mean ± SDM, 16.3 ± 32.3 vs. 7.4 ± 7.0 (Index), $p = 5.58 \times 10^{-12}$), usual interstitial pneumonia (14.4 ± 24.4 vs. 7.4 ± 7.0 [Index], $p = 3.14 \times 10^{-12}$), and nonspecific interstitial pneumonia (17.9 ± 37.7 vs. 7.4 ± 7.0 (Index), $p = 5.07 \times 10^{-5}$) compared with patients without chronic lung disease. The area under the curve (AUC) of the receiver operating characteristic curve for anti-ARS Ab was too low to allow for discrimination among RA patients with/without chronic lung disease (0.608, 95% confidence interval (CI) 0.560–0.655, $p = 8.69 \times 10^{-6}$). Multiple logistic regression analyses of age, smoking status, anti-ARS Abs, as well as Steinbrocker stage generated an ARS-index with a high AUC value (0.707, 95%CI 0.662–0.752, $p = 2.20 \times 10^{-19}$). **Conclusions:** Anti-ARS Abs are related to ILD pathogenesis in RA and may be a biomarker for ILD.

Keywords: rheumatoid arthritis; anti-aminoacyl-transfer ribonucleic acid synthetase antibodies; interstitial lung disease

1. Introduction

Rheumatoid arthritis (RA), characterized by synovial joint destruction, is a representative systemic inflammatory disease [1]. It can be complicated with extra-articular manifestations such as chronic lung diseases (CLD), including interstitial lung disease (ILD), emphysema, and airway disease (AD) [2]. Unfortunately, patients with RA complicated with ILD or AD often have a prognosis that is poor [3–7]. The usual interstitial pneumonia (UIP) pattern of ILD confers a poor prognosis in patients with RA [8]. Thus, the pathogenesis of ILD and AD in RA should be elucidated. The term acute-onset diffuse ILD (AoDILD) covers a broad range of disorders that frequently occur in RA patients, including drug-induced ILD, acute exacerbation of ILD, and pneumocystis pneumonia, which confer a poor prognosis [9,10].

Antibodies (Abs) that recognize the Fc of immunoglobulin G are designated as rheumatoid factors (RFs), and Abs against citrullinated peptides are termed anti-citrullinated peptide antibodies (ACPAs). ACPA and RF are specific for RA and, therefore, can aid the diagnosis of RA [11]. RF and ACPA were reported to be involved in ILD in RA [12–15] and are considered auto-Ab biomarkers of ILD in RA [16]. The production of Abs to anti-melanoma differentiation-associated gene 5, which recognizes RNA helicase, was linked to clinically amyopathic dermatomyositis with rapidly progressive ILD [17]. However, it was reported that these auto-Abs were present in RA patients with AD [18]. Auto-Abs against enzymes that attach specific amino acids to transfer ribonucleic acid (tRNA) present in idiopathic inflammatory myopathies (IIM) are designated anti-aminoacyl-tRNA synthetase (ARS) Abs. Anti-ARS Abs include antibodies against eight antigens (Jo1 [histidyl tRNA synthetases], PL-7 [threonyl tRNA synthetases], PL-12 [alanyl tRNA synthetases], EJ [glycyl tRNA synthetases], OJ [isoleucyl tRNA synthetases], KS [asparaginyl tRNA synthetases], Zo [phenylalanyl tRNA synthetases], and Ha [tyrosyl tRNA synthetases]) and were specifically detected as myositis-specific Abs in patients with IIM [19,20]. ILD is frequently complicated in patients with IIM who also have anti-ARS Abs [20]. Anti-synthetase syndrome, a clinical subset of IIM, is categorized by mechanic's hands, ILD, myositis, arthritis, the production of anti-ARS Abs, fever, and Raynaud's phenomenon [21]. ILD in IIM patients with anti-ARS Abs was reported to progress slowly but did not confer a poor prognosis in patients [22]. Anti-ARS Abs were also detected in idiopathic interstitial pneumonia [23–27], but not RA [19,27,28]. Another study analyzed anti-ARS Abs qualitatively and showed they were involved in ILD with RA [29]. Limited studies have examined anti-ARS Abs in RA or other autoimmune diseases. Here, anti-ARS Abs were quantitated and their association with ILD was investigated in patients with RA.

2. Materials and Methods

2.1. Patients

Five hundred and fifty-eight RA patients with chest computed tomography findings and fifty-two healthy controls were recruited at Tokyo Hospital, Sagamihara Hospital, Nagoya Medical Center, Miyakonojo Medical Center, Nagasaki Medical Center, and Himeji Medical Center. All patients with RA fulfilled the American College of Rheumatology criteria for RA [30] or rheumatoid arthritis classification criteria [11]. Predominant chest computed tomography findings of RA patients [31] were used to diagnose emphysema, nonspecific interstitial pneumonia (NSIP), AD, no CLD, or UIP (Supplementary Figure S1). The ILD groups included UIP and NSIP patients and the CLD (+) group included NSIP, emphysema, AD, and UIP. The production of anti-ARS Abs was analyzed using serum collected from patients with RA and controls. The 558 RA patients included 1 case complicated with polymyositis, 1 with dermatomyositis, 1 with scleroderma, and 1 with systemic lupus erythematosus.

Eleven RA patients with AoDILD were treated with corticosteroid pulse therapy at Sagamihara Hospital (mean age at admission ± standard deviation [SD], 65.9 ± 8.1 years, five male patients). These patients fulfilled the American College of Rheumatology RA criteria 30. Five had an acute exacerbation of ILD and six had drug-induced ILD; the definitions of these cases were previously described [10]. Sera from patients with RA with

AoDILD were obtained at admission and under stable conditions at least three months before admission.

This study was reviewed and approved by the Research Ethics Committees of Tokyo Hospital (190010, 29 May 2019), Sagamihara Hospital, and the Central Institutional Review Board of the National Hospital Organization. Written informed consent was obtained from all study participants except for those who were deceased before the initiation of the study. Any serum samples obtained before this study were anonymized to prevent identifying participants and analyses were only approved by the Sagamihara National Hospital Research Ethics Committee based on this condition. This study was conducted in accordance with the principles of the Declaration of Helsinki.

2.2. Detection of Anti-ARS Abs

Serum anti-ARS Abs were measured by enzyme-linked immunosorbent assay (ELISA, Mesacup anti-ARS tests, Medical & Biological Laboratories, Tokyo, Japan) according to the manufacturer's instructions. Index values = (sample absorbance—negative control absorbance)/(positive control absorbance—negative control absorbance) $\times$ 100. The cut-off value was 11.374 based on the 98th percentile of healthy controls (n = 52), although the cut-off level recommended by the kit manufacturer was 25. To discriminate between anti-Jo1 Abs, anti-PL7 Abs, anti-PL12 Abs, anti-EJ Abs, and anti-OJ Abs, anti-ARS Abs were also detected by a line blot assay (Euroline Myositis Profile 3, Euroimmun AG, Lübeck, Germany) using patient sera positive for anti-ARS Abs as determined by ELISA. Clinical information of some RA patients was previously described [18]. Steinbrocker stages were assessed as previously reported [32].

2.3. Statistical Analysis

Anti-ARS Abs titers between RA patients without CLD or controls were compared by the Mann–Whitney U-test. Fisher's exact test with 2 $\times$ 2 contingency tables was used to compare the presence of anti-ARS Abs in RA patients without CLD. Multiple logistic regression analyses were used to generate an ARS-index from anti-ARS Ab, smoking status [never smoker: 0; past smoker: 1; current smoker: 2], Steinbrocker stage [1–4], and age [years]. To compare RA patients with/without CLD, receiver operating characteristic (ROC) curves for anti-ARS Abs or the ARS-index were used. The area under the curve (AUC) values of ROC curves were compared by the chi-squared test. Cut-off levels were optimized on the basis of the highest Youden's index. Anti-ARS Ab levels in serum from RA patients with stable lung disease and AoDILD conditions were tested by the Wilcoxon signed-rank test.

3. Results

3.1. Comparisons of Anti-ARS Abs in RA Subsets with CLD (−) RA Patients

Anti-ARS Abs in RA patient sera detected by ELISA and Ab levels in subsets underwent a comparison with those in the CLD (−) group (Supplementary Figure S2 and Table 1). Anti-ARS Ab levels were increased in RA with ILD (mean $\pm$ SD, 16.3 $\pm$ 32.3 vs. 7.4 $\pm$ 7.0 [Index], $p = 5.58 \times 10^{-12}$), UIP (14.4 $\pm$ 24.4 vs. 7.4 $\pm$ 7.0 [Index], $p = 3.14 \times 10^{-12}$), and NSIP (17.9 $\pm$ 37.7 vs. 7.4 $\pm$ 7.0 [Index], $p = 5.07 \times 10^{-5}$). Anti-ARS Ab levels were also increased in RA and CLD (11.2 $\pm$ 21.4 vs. 7.4 $\pm$ 7.0 [Index], $p = 1.77 \times 10^{-5}$). This indicated that anti-ARS Ab titers were linked with ILD, UIP, NSIP, and CLD in RA.

Table 1. Anti-ARS Ab levels in RA patients.

	n	Anti-ARS Ab, Index (SD)	p
ILD	138	16.3 (32.3)	5.58×10^{-12}
UIP	63	14.4 (24.4)	3.14×10^{-12}
NSIP	75	17.9 (37.7)	5.07×10^{-5}
Airway disease	166	7.1 (3.5)	0.3559
Emphysema	39	10.4 (12.7)	0.2131
CLD (+)	343	11.2 (21.4)	1.77×10^{-5}
CLD (−)	215	7.4 (7.0)	

RA: rheumatoid arthritis; ARS: aminoacyl-transfer ribonucleic acid synthetase; UIP: usual interstitial pneumonia; NSIP: nonspecific interstitial pneumonia; ILD: interstitial lung disease; AD: airway disease; CLD: chronic lung disease; Ab: antibody. ILD group includes UIP and NSIP groups. The CLD (+) group includes UIP, NSIP, AD, and emphysema patients. The average values for each group are shown. Standard deviations are shown in parentheses. Differences compared with the CLD (−) population were tested using the Mann–Whitney U-test.

Evaluations of RA patients that might have been positive for anti-ARS Abs used a cut-off value based on the results from healthy controls (Table 2). Anti-ARS Ab positivity was associated with ILD (n [%], 47 [34.1%] vs. 18 [8.4%], $p = 1.08 \times 10^{-13}$), UIP (25 [39.7%] vs. 18 [8.4%], $p = 1.15 \times 10^{-11}$), NSIP (22 [29.3%] vs. 18 [8.4%], $p = 2.63 \times 10^{-8}$), and emphysema (9 [23.1%] vs. 18 [8.4%], $p = 0.0003$) in RA. Anti-ARS Ab positivity was also increased in RA with CLD (70 [20.4%] vs. 18 [8.4%], $p = 1.73 \times 10^{-8}$). Evaluations of anti-ARS Abs positivity in RA patients used the recommended cut-off value (Supplementary Table S2). Anti-ARS Ab positivity was associated with ILD (n [%], 10 [7.2%] vs. 3 [1.4%], $p = 0.0070$) and NSIP (7 [9.3%] vs. 3 [1.4%], $p = 0.0037$) in RA. The precise profiles of anti-ARS Abs were analyzed by line blot assay in 16 RA patient sera positive for anti-ARS Abs by ELISA (Supplementary Table S2); these RA patients included 1 with polymyositis, 1 with dermatomyositis, and 1 with scleroderma. Anti-ARS Abs were detected in 12 patients (75.0%) by line blot assays of samples from 16 patients. The sera from two RA patients with UIP and one with NSIP were positive for two or more anti-ARS Abs by line blot assay. Anti-PL7 Abs were found in all RA patients with UIP.

Table 2. The positivity of anti-ARS Ab in RA patients.

	Anti-ARS Ab Positive, n (%)	p
ILD	47 (34.1)	1.08×10^{-13}
UIP	25 (39.7)	1.15×10^{-11}
NSIP	22 (29.3)	2.63×10^{-8}
AD	14 (8.4)	0.1272
Emphysema	9 (23.1)	0.0003
CLD (+)	70 (20.4)	1.73×10^{-8}
CLD (−)	18 (8.4)	

RA: rheumatoid arthritis; ARS: aminoacyl-transfer ribonucleic acid synthetase; ILD: interstitial lung disease; UIP: usual interstitial pneumonia; NSIP: nonspecific interstitial pneumonia; AD: airway disease; CLD: chronic lung disease; Ab: antibody. ILD group includes UIP and NSIP groups. The CLD (+) group includes UIP, NSIP, AD, and emphysema patients. The cut-off value was set to 11.374 based on the 98th percentile of 52 healthy controls. The value for each group is shown. Percentages are shown in parentheses. Differences compared with the CLD (−) population were tested using Fisher's exact test using 2×2 contingency tables.

3.2. Comparison of Anti-ARS Abs Between RA Patients and Healthy Controls

A comparison of anti-ARS Ab levels demonstrated increased levels in all RA subsets and RA, per se, compared with healthy controls ($n = 52$, 5.3 ± 2.1 [Index], Supplementary Figure S2 and Table 3).

Table 3. The anti-ARS Ab levels in RA subsets or overall RA patients were compared with healthy controls.

	p
ILD	3.83×10^{-12}
UIP	3.85×10^{-13}
NSIP	2.34×10^{-7}
AD	9.12×10^{-6}
Emphysema	0.0002
CLD (+)	2.58×10^{-9}
CLD (−)	0.0007
RA	2.61×10^{-7}

RA: rheumatoid arthritis; ARS: aminoacyl-transfer ribonucleic acid synthetase; UIP: usual interstitial pneumonia; NSIP: nonspecific interstitial pneumonia; ILD: interstitial lung disease; AD: airway disease; CLD: chronic lung disease; Ab: antibody. Differences compared with the healthy control group were tested using the Mann–Whitney *U*-test.

3.3. Multiple Logistic Regression Analysis of Anti-ARS Ab

Multiple logistic regression analyses were performed to eliminate the effects of clinical manifestation on the association of anti-ARS Abs with CLD (Supplementary Table S3). The association of anti-ARS Abs with CLD was observed in univariate analysis (p = 0.0241, odds ratio [OR] 1.04, 95% confidence interval [CI] 1.01–1.08), and it remained significant ($P_{adjusted}$ = 0.0204, $OR_{adjusted}$ 1.04, 95% CI 1.01–1.08),when conditioned on age, Steinbrocker stage, and smoking status. Thus, these data suggested the independent association of anti-ARS Abs with CLD in RA.

Multiple logistic regression analyses were also conducted to eliminate the possibility of confounding the association of anti-ARS Abs between RA and healthy controls (Supplementary Table S4). The association was revealed to be independent of age and sex.

3.4. ROC Analyses

A ROC curve of anti-ARS Ab was used for comparisons between RA with/without CLD (Figure 1A). The AUC of the ROC curve for anti-ARS Ab (0.608, 95% confidence interval [CI] 0.560–0.655, $p = 8.69 \times 10^{-6}$) was not high enough for clinical use as a biomarker. Multiple logistic regression analysis of age, anti-ARS Abs, smoking status, and Steinbrocker stage was performed to generate an ARS-index: 0.0415 × (anti-ARS Abs) + 0.0565 × (age)—0.1917 × (Steinbrocker stage) + 0.4560 × (smoking status) − 3.3217. The AUC of the ROC curve was 0.707 (95% CI 0.662–0.752, $p = 2.20 \times 10^{-19}$, Figure 1B) and was significantly greater than that for anti-ARS Abs (p = 0.0024). An ARS-index with a greater AUC value was generated by multiple logistic regression analysis of age, anti-ARS Abs, smoking status, and Steinbrocker stage.

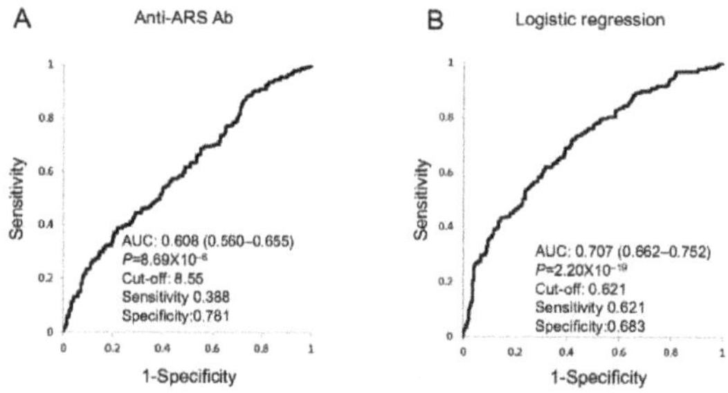

Figure 1. ROC curves using anti-ARS Abs and multiple logistic regression analysis to compare CLD (+) and CLD (−) RA. ROC curves for anti-ARS Abs (**A**) and multiple logistic regression analysis (**B**) with anti-ARS Abs (Index), Steinbrocker stage (1–4), age (years), and smoking status (never smoker: 0; past smoker: 1; current smoker: 2) were calculated. The AUC values of the ROC curves with 95% CIs and the cut-off levels are shown. RA: rheumatoid arthritis; ARS: aminoacyl-transfer ribonucleic acid synthetase; CLD: chronic lung disease; Ab: antibody; ROC: receiver operating characteristic; AUC: area under the curve; CI: confidence interval.

3.5. Detection of Anti-ARS Abs in RA Patients with AoDILD

Anti-ARS Abs measured in sera from patients with RA and AoDILD indicated that two RA patients were positive (Figure 2). No difference was found between RA patients under stable or AoDILD conditions. Anti-ARS Abs in two RA patients with AoDILD were analyzed by line blot assay; one patient had anti-PL7 Abs, anti-PL12 Abs, and anti-Jo1Abs, and the other had anti-Jo1Abs. The Ab profiles of the two patients under stable conditions were the same as those in patients with RA and AoDILD.

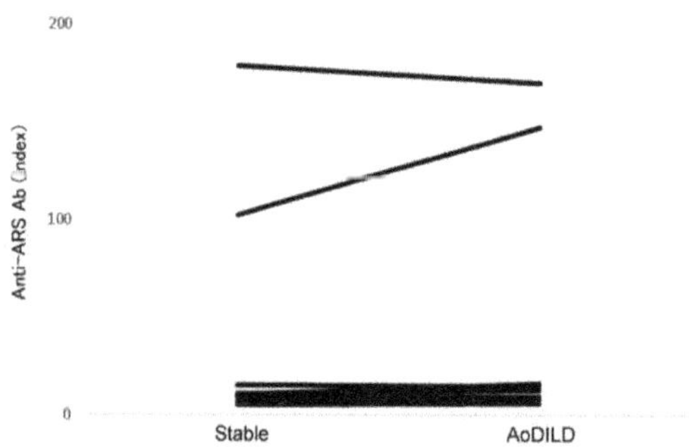

Figure 2. Anti-ARS Ab levels in sera from RA patients with AoDILD. Anti-ARS Ab levels in sera from RA patients under stable and AoDILD conditions are shown. Differences were tested using the Wilcoxon signed-rank test. AoDILD: acute-onset diffuse interstitial lung disease; RA: rheumatoid arthritis; ARS: aminoacyl-transfer ribonucleic acid synthetase; Ab: antibody.

4. Discussion

The current study showed that anti-ARS Abs were involved in ILD, NSIP, and UIP in patients with RA. The AUC value of ROC curves for anti-ARS Abs was not sufficiently high for clinical use as a biomarker for the comparison between RA with/without CLD. An ARS-index was generated using age, anti-ARS Abs, smoking status, and Steinbrocker stage, and the AUC value of the ROC curve for the ARS-index was higher than that for anti-ARS Ab alone.

A correlation between several auto-Abs and ILD was previously reported for RA [12–15]. We noted that anti-ARS Abs were associated with ILD in RA. A relationship between anti-ARS Abs and UIP and NSIP was demonstrated in this study, suggesting the participation of anti-ARS Abs in the common pathogenesis of UIP and NSIP in RA.

The functions of individual ACPA, RF, and anti-ARS Abs in the pathogenesis of ILD in RA might be revealed in the future.

Anti-ARS Abs were reported in idiopathic interstitial pneumonia patients without myopathy [23–27], but not in RA patients [19,27,28]. Anti-ARS Abs were reportedly present in 6.1% of RA patients by a line blot assay and these were related to ILD RA [29]. We observed that 15.8% of RA patients developed anti-ARS Abs as measured by ELISA using our cut-off level, which confirmed an association between anti-ARS Abs and ILD. Our findings suggest that ELISA has higher sensitivities than the line blot assay.

Multiple logistic regression analysis showed the independent association of anti-ARS Abs from age, Steinbrocker stage, and smoking status. However, it is still possible that other clinical factors would influence the associations.

An ARS index was generated by multiple logistic regression analysis using age, smoking status, anti-ARS Abs, and Steinbrocker stage. The AUC value of the ROC curve of the ARS-index was greater than that for anti-ARS Abs, suggesting anti-ARS Abs might be useful complex biomarkers for CLD in patients with RA. Since ILD is heterogeneous, other antibodies could be involved in the pathogenesis of other subsets of ILD in RA. Thus, other antibodies should be investigated to improve the index for clinical use.

The cut-off level in this study was set for anti-ARS Ab positivity (11.374) and it was lower than the recommended cut-off level (25). However, our cut-off level was better for the discrimination of ILD in RA patients. Anti-ARS Ab levels $\geq$ 25 were observed in 16 RA patients in the ELISA; each anti-ARS Ab was detected in 12 of these RA patients in the line blot assay. Anti-PL-7 Abs were detected in all RA patients with UIP. The 16 RA patients included 1 with polymyositis, 1 with dermatomyositis, and 1 with scleroderma. The distribution patterns of anti-ARS Abs in RA differed from those in IIM [33], suggesting different pathogenesis of ILD between patients with RA and IIM. Thus, anti-ARS Abs might be useful biomarkers for ILD or CLD in RA.

Anti-ARS Abs were present in RA with AoDILD although ILD in IIM patients with anti-ARS Abs progressed slowly [22]. These results suggested different functions of anti-ARS Abs in RA and IIM.

Because a modest sample size was used, large-scale replicating studies of anti-ARS Abs in patients with RA should be conducted on multi-ethnic populations. Since anti-ARS Abs were analyzed in only patients with RA in the present study, anti-ARS Ab profiles also should be analyzed in other autoimmune disease patients. Because the information on the prognosis of RA patients with ILD was not available, we were not able to evaluate whether the disease progression of ILD in RA patients with anti-ARS Abs was slow or rapid.

5. Conclusions

This quantitative analysis of anti-ARS Abs in RA suggests an association between anti-ARS Abs and ILD.

Supplementary Materials: The following supporting information can be downloaded at: https://www.mdpi.com/article/10.3390/jcm13226761/s1, Table S1: Clinical manifestations of patients with rheumatoid arthritis. Table S2: The positivity of anti-ARS Ab in RA patients determined by ELISA or line blot assay. Table S3: Multiple logistic regression analysis of anti-ARS Ab levels and clinical manifestations of CLD in RA. Table S4. Multiple logistic regression analysis of anti-ARS Ab levels between RA patients and healthy controls. Figure S1: Flow chart depicting rheumatoid arthritis patients examined with chest computed tomography. Figure S2: Evaluation of anti-ARS Abs in patients with RA and controls.

Author Contributions: H.F. and S.T. conceived and designed all experiments. S.O., T.H. and H.F. performed all experiments. S.O. and H.F. analyzed the data. H.F., K.S. (Kota Shimada), A.O., M.F., A.H., A.K., K.S. (Koichiro Saisho), N.Y., M.K., T.M., N.F., K.M. and S.T. contributed reagents, materials, and tools for analyses. S.O., H.F. and S.T. contributed to the writing of the manuscript. All authors have read and agreed to the published version of the manuscript.

Funding: Research grants were received from the following pharmaceutical companies: Teijin Pharma Limited, Takeda Pharmaceutical Company Limited, Pfizer Japan Inc., Merck Sharp and Dohme Inc., Mitsubishi Tanabe Pharma Corporation, Eisai Co., Ltd., Chugai Pharmaceutical Co., Ltd., Astellas Pharma Inc., and Abbott Japan Co., Ltd. This work was also supported by Bristol-Myers K.K. RA Clinical Investigation Grant from Bristol-Myers Squibb Co., Research Grants from the Mitsui Sumitomo Insurance Welfare Foundation, Research Grants from The Nakatomi Foundation, Research Grants from the Japan Research Foundation for Clinical Pharmacology, Research Grants from the Takeda Science Foundation, Grants-in-Aid for Clinical Research from the National Hospital Organization, Research Grants from the Daiwa Securities Health Foundation, Grants-in-Aid of the Practical Research Project for Allergic Diseases and Immunology (Research on Allergic Diseases and Immunology) from the Japan Agency for Medical Research and Development, Grants-in-Aid for Young Scientists (B) (24791018) and Scientific Research (B, C) (22591090, 26293123, 15K09543, 18K08402) from the Japan Society for the Promotion of Science, and Health and Labour Science Research Grants from the Ministry of Health, Labour, and Welfare of Japan.

Institutional Review Board Statement: The study was approved by the NHO Central Institutional Review Board and Research Ethics Committees of Sagamihara National Hospital and Tokyo National Hospital (190010, 29 May 2019). This study was conducted in accordance with the principles of the Declaration of Helsinki.

Informed Consent Statement: Written informed consent was obtained from all study participants except for those who were deceased before the initiation of the study. Any serum samples obtained before this study were anonymized to prevent identifying participants and analyses were only approved by the Sagamihara National Hospital Research Ethics Committee based on this condition.

Data Availability Statement: The data that support the findings of this study are available in the paper and the Supplementary File. Other data are available from the authors upon reasonable request. However, the clinical information and antibody data of each participant are not available under the condition of informed consent acquisition, which was mandated by the Act on the Protection of Personal Information.

Conflicts of Interest: H.F. has the following conflicts of interest and the following funders are supported wholly or in part by the indicated pharmaceutical companies. The Japan Research Foundation for Clinical Pharmacology is run by Daiichi Sankyo, the Takeda Science Foundation is supported by an endowment from Takeda Pharmaceutical Company, and the Nakatomi Foundation was established by Hisamitsu Pharmaceutical Co. The Daiwa Securities Health Foundation was established by Daiwa Securities Group Inc. and Mitsui Sumitomo Insurance Welfare Foundation was established by Mitsui Sumitomo Insurance Co., Ltd. HF was supported by research grants from Bristol-Myers Squibb Co. H.F. received honoraria from Ajinomoto Co., Inc., Daiichi Sankyo Co., Ltd., Dainippon Sumitomo Pharma Co., Ltd., Pfizer Japan Inc., and Takeda Pharmaceutical Company, Luminex Japan Corporation Ltd., and Ayumi Pharmaceutical Corporation. S.T. was supported by research grants from the following pharmaceutical companies: Abbott Japan Co., Ltd., Astellas Pharma Inc., Chugai Pharmaceutical Co., Ltd., Eisai Co., Ltd., Mitsubishi Tanabe Pharma Corporation, Merck Sharp and Dohme Inc., Pfizer Japan Inc., Takeda Pharmaceutical Company Limited, and Teijin Pharma Limited. S.T. received honoraria from Asahi Kasei Pharma Corporation, Astellas Pharma Inc., AbbVie GK., Chugai Pharmaceutical Co., Ltd., Ono Pharmaceutical Co., Ltd., Mitsubishi Tanabe Pharma Corporation, and Pfizer Japan Inc. The other authors have no financial or commercial conflicts of interest to declare.

References

1. Smolen, J.S.; Aletaha, D.; McInnes, I.B. Rheumatoid arthritis. *Lancet* **2016**, *388*, 2023–2038. [CrossRef] [PubMed]
2. Stainer, A.; Tonutti, A.; De Santis, M.; Amati, F.; Ceribelli, A.; Bongiovanni, G.; Torrisi, C.; Iacopino, A.; Mangiameli, G.; Aliberti, S.; et al. Unmet needs and perspectives in rheumatoid arthritis-associated interstitial lung disease: A critical review. *Front. Med.* **2023**, *10*, 1129939. [CrossRef] [PubMed]
3. Hakala, M. Poor prognosis in patients with rheumatoid arthritis hospitalized for interstitial lung fibrosis. *Chest* **1988**, *93*, 114–118. [CrossRef]
4. Turesson, C.; Jacobsson, L.T. Epidemiology of extra-articular manifestations in rheumatoid arthritis. *Scand. J. Rheumatol.* **2004**, *33*, 65–72. [CrossRef]

5. Koduri, G.; Norton, S.; Young, A.; Cox, N.; Davies, P.; Devlin, J.; Dixey, J.; Gough, A.; Prouse, P.; Winfield, J.; et al. Interstitial lung disease has a poor prognosis in rheumatoid arthritis: Results from an inception cohort. *Rheumatology* **2010**, *49*, 1483–1489. [CrossRef]
6. Vergnenegre, A.; Pugnere, N.; Antonini, M.T.; Arnaud, M.; Melloni, B.; Treves, R.; Bonnaud, F. Airway obstruction and rheumatoid arthritis. *Eur. Respir. J.* **1997**, *10*, 1072–1078. [CrossRef] [PubMed]
7. Swinson, D.R.; Symmons, D.; Suresh, U.; Jones, M.; Booth, J. Decreased survival in patients with co-existent rheumatoid arthritis and bronchiectasis. *Br. J. Rheumatol.* **1997**, *36*, 689–691. [CrossRef]
8. Kim, E.J.; Elicker, B.M.; Maldonado, F.; Webb, W.R.; Ryu, J.H.; Van Uden, J.H.; Lee, J.S.; King, T.E.; Collard, H.R. Usual interstitial pneumonia in rheumatoid arthritis-associated interstitial lung disease. *Eur. Respir. J.* **2010**, *35*, 1322–1328. [CrossRef]
9. Kameda, H.; Tokuda, H.; Sakai, F.; Johkoh, T.; Mori, S.; Yoshida, Y.; Takayanagi, N.; Taki, H.; Hasegawa, Y.; Hatta, K.; et al. Clinical and radiological features of acute-onset diffuse interstitial lung diseases in patients with rheumatoid arthritis receiving treatment with biological agents: Importance of Pneumocystis pneumonia in Japan revealed by a multicenter study. *Intern. Med.* **2011**, *50*, 305–313. [CrossRef]
10. Oka, S.; Furukawa, H.; Shimada, K.; Hayakawa, H.; Fukui, N.; Tsuchiya, N.; Tohma, S. Serum biomarker analysis of collagen disease patients with acute-onset diffuse interstitial lung disease. *BMC Immunol.* **2013**, *14*, 9. [CrossRef]
11. Aletaha, D.; Neogi, T.; Silman, A.J.; Funovits, J.; Felson, D.T.; Bingham, C.O., III; Birnbaum, N.S.; Burmester, G.R.; Bykerk, V.P.; Cohen, M.D.; et al. 2010 Rheumatoid arthritis classification criteria: An American College of Rheumatology/European League Against Rheumatism collaborative initiative. *Arthritis Rheum.* **2010**, *62*, 2569–2581. [CrossRef]
12. Mori, S.; Koga, Y.; Sugimoto, M. Different risk factors between interstitial lung disease and airway disease in rheumatoid arthritis. *Respir. Med.* **2012**, *106*, 1591–1599. [CrossRef]
13. Kakutani, T.; Hashimoto, A.; Tominaga, A.; Kodama, K.; Nogi, S.; Tsuno, H.; Ogihara, H.; Nunokawa, T.; Komiya, A.; Furukawa, H.; et al. Related factors, increased mortality and causes of death in patients with rheumatoid arthritis-associated interstitial lung disease. *Mod. Rheumatol.* **2020**, *30*, 458–464. [CrossRef]
14. Zhu, J.; Zhou, Y.; Chen, X.; Li, J. A metaanalysis of the increased risk of rheumatoid arthritis-related pulmonary disease as a result of serum anticitrullinated protein antibody positivity. *J. Rheumatol.* **2014**, *41*, 1282–1289. [CrossRef]
15. Joshua, V.; Hensvold, A.H.; Reynisdottir, G.; Hansson, M.; Cornillet, M.; Nogueira, L.; Serre, G.; Nyren, S.; Karimi, R.; Eklund, A.; et al. Association between number and type of different ACPA fine specificities with lung abnormalities in early, untreated rheumatoid arthritis. *RMD Open* **2020**, *6*, e001278. [CrossRef]
16. Doyle, T.J.; Patel, A.S.; Hatabu, H.; Nishino, M.; Wu, G.; Osorio, J.C.; Golzarri, M.F.; Traslosheros, A.; Chu, S.G.; Frits, M.L.; et al. Detection of Rheumatoid Arthritis-Interstitial Lung Disease Is Enhanced by Serum Biomarkers. *Am. J. Respir. Crit. Care Med.* **2015**, *191*, 1403–1412. [CrossRef]
17. Sato, S.; Hoshino, K.; Satoh, T.; Fujita, T.; Kawakami, Y.; Fujita, T.; Kuwana, M. RNA helicase encoded by melanoma differentiation-associated gene 5 is a major autoantigen in patients with clinically amyopathic dermatomyositis: Association with rapidly progressive interstitial lung disease. *Arthritis Rheum.* **2009**, *60*, 2193–2200. [CrossRef]
18. Oka, S.; Higuchi, T.; Furukawa, H.; Shimada, K.; Okamoto, A.; Hashimoto, A.; Komiya, A.; Saisho, K.; Yoshikawa, N.; Katayama, M.; et al. Antibodies against Serum Anti-Melanoma Differentiation-Associated Gene 5 in Rheumatoid Arthritis Patients with Chronic Lung Diseases. *Medicina* **2023**, *59*, 363. [CrossRef]
19. Nishikai, M.; Reichlin, M. Heterogeneity of precipitating antibodies in polymyositis and dermatomyositis. Characterization of the Jo-1 antibody system. *Arthritis Rheum.* **1980**, *23*, 881–888. [CrossRef] [PubMed]
20. Satoh, M.; Tanaka, S.; Ceribelli, A.; Calise, S.J.; Chan, E.K.L. A Comprehensive Overview on Myositis-Specific Antibodies: New and Old Biomarkers in Idiopathic Inflammatory Myopathy. *Clin. Rev. Allergy Immunol.* **2017**, *52*, 1–19. [CrossRef] [PubMed]
21. Solomon, J.; Swigris, J.J.; Brown, K.K. Myositis-related interstitial lung disease and antisynthetase syndrome. *J. Bras. Pneumol.* **2011**, *37*, 100–109. [CrossRef] [PubMed]
22. Hirakata, M.; Nagai, S. Interstitial lung disease in polymyositis and dermatomyositis. *Curr. Opin. Rheumatol.* **2000**, *12*, 501–508. [CrossRef] [PubMed]
23. Targoff, I.N.; Arnett, F.C. Clinical manifestations in patients with antibody to PL-12 antigen (alanyl-tRNA synthetase). *Am. J. Med.* **1990**, *88*, 241–251. [CrossRef] [PubMed]
24. Hirakata, M.; Suwa, A.; Nagai, S.; Kron, M.A.; Trieu, E.P.; Mimori, T.; Akizuki, M.; Targoff, I.N. Anti-KS: Identification of autoantibodies to asparaginyl-transfer RNA synthetase associated with interstitial lung disease. *J. Immunol.* **1999**, *162*, 2315–2320. [CrossRef]
25. Friedman, A.W.; Targoff, I.N.; Arnett, F.C. Interstitial lung disease with autoantibodies against aminoacyl-tRNA synthetases in the absence of clinically apparent myositis. *Semin. Arthritis Rheum.* **1996**, *26*, 459–467. [CrossRef]
26. Okayasu, K.; Ohtani, Y.; Takemura, T.; Uchibori, K.; Tamaoka, M.; Furuiye, M.; Miyazaki, Y.; Inase, N.; Yoshizawa, Y. Nonspecific interstitial pneumonia (NSIP) associated with anti-KS antibody: Differentiation from idiopathic NSIP. *Intern. Med.* **2009**, *48*, 1301–1306. [CrossRef]
27. Matsushita, T.; Hasegawa, M.; Fujimoto, M.; Hamaguchi, Y.; Komura, K.; Hirano, T.; Horikawa, M.; Kondo, M.; Orito, H.; Kaji, K.; et al. Clinical evaluation of anti-aminoacyl tRNA synthetase antibodies in Japanese patients with dermatomyositis. *J. Rheumatol.* **2007**, *34*, 1012–1018.

28. Yoshida, S.; Akizuki, M.; Mimori, T.; Yamagat, H.; Inada, S.; Homma, M. The precipitating antibody to an acidic nuclear protein antigen, the Jo-1, in connective tissue diseases. A marker for a subset of polymyositis with interstitial pulmonary fibrosis. *Arthritis Rheum.* **1983**, *26*, 604–611. [CrossRef]
29. Matsushita, M.; Tamura, N.; Ogasawara, M.; Tada, K.; Yamaji, K.; Takasaki, Y. The Association of Anti-Aminoacyl-Transfer Ribonucleic Acid Synthetase Antibodies in Patients With Rheumatoid Arthritis and Interstitial Lung Disease. *Arch. Rheumatol.* **2018**, *33*, 26–32. [CrossRef]
30. Arnett, F.C.; Edworthy, S.M.; Bloch, D.A.; Mcshane, D.J.; Fries, J.F.; Cooper, N.S.; Healey, L.A.; Kaplan, S.R.; Liang, M.H.; Luthra, H.S.; et al. The American Rheumatism Association 1987 revised criteria for the classification of rheumatoid arthritis. *Arthritis Rheum.* **1988**, *31*, 315–324. [CrossRef]
31. Oka, S.; Furukawa, H.; Shimada, K.; Sugii, S.; Hashimoto, A.; Komiya, A.; Fukui, N.; Suda, A.; Tsunoda, S.; Ito, S.; et al. Association of Human Leukocyte Antigen Alleles with Chronic Lung Diseases in Rheumatoid Arthritis. *Rheumatology* **2016**, *55*, 1301–1307. [CrossRef] [PubMed]
32. Steinbrocker, O.; Traeger, C.H.; Batterman, R.C. Therapeutic criteria in rheumatoid arthritis. *J. Am. Med. Assoc.* **1949**, *140*, 659–662. [CrossRef] [PubMed]
33. Noguchi, E.; Uruha, A.; Suzuki, S.; Hamanaka, K.; Ohnuki, Y.; Tsugawa, J.; Watanabe, Y.; Nakahara, J.; Shiina, T.; Suzuki, N.; et al. Skeletal Muscle Involvement in Antisynthetase Syndrome. *JAMA Neurol.* **2017**, *74*, 992–999. [CrossRef]

Journal of
Clinical Medicine

MDPI

Article

Real-World Clinical Effectiveness and Safety of Antifibrotics in Progressive Pulmonary Fibrosis Associated with Rheumatoid Arthritis

Javier Narváez [1,*,†], Martí Aguilar-Coll [1,†], Vanesa Vicens-Zygmunt [2], Juan José Alegre [3], Guadalupe Bermudo [2] and María Molina-Molina [2]

1 Department of Rheumatology, Hospital Universitario de Bellvitge, Bellvitge Biomedical Research Institute (IDIBELL), 08907 Barcelona, Spain; maguilarco@bellvitgehospital.cat
2 Interstitial Lung Disease Unit, Department of Pneumology, Hospital Universitario de Bellvitge, Bellvitge Biomedical Research Institute (IDIBELL), 08907 Barcelona, Spain; vvicens@bellvitgehospital.cat (V.V.-Z.); mbermudo@bellvitgehospital.cat (G.B.); mariamolinamolina@hotmail.com (M.M.-M.)
3 Department of Rheumatology, Hospital Universitario Dr. Peset, 46017 Valencia, Spain; txantxo@gmail.com
* Correspondence: fjnarvaez@bellvitgehospital.cat
† These authors contributed equally to this work.

Abstract: Background/Objectives: Interstitial lung disease (ILD) is one of the most severe complications of rheumatoid arthritis (RA). Real-world data on antifibrotic treatment are needed. Our objective was to evaluate the real-world effectiveness and tolerability of antifibrotic agents in patients with progressive fibrosing RA-ILD. **Methods:** A longitudinal, retrospective, observational study was conducted on a cohort of RA-ILD patients treated with either nintedanib or pirfenidone. The data collected included pulmonary function test (PFT) results, adverse events (AEs), tolerability, and drug retention. **Results:** Twenty-seven patients were included; 25 (92.5%) initiated nintedanib, while two initiated pirfenidone. The median follow-up duration was 25 months (IQR 7–27). The mean decline in %pFVC and %pDLCO from ILD diagnosis to the initiation of antifibrotic therapy were −8.9% and −14.8%, respectively. After 6 months of treatment, most patients achieved stabilization in PFT: a Δ%pFVC of +1.2% ($p = 0.611$ compared with baseline) and a Δ%pDLCO of +3.9% ($p = 0.400$). Eighteen patients completed one year of therapy, with a modest improvement in %pFVC (+4.7%; $p = 0.023$) and stabilization in %pDLCO (−3.8%; $p = 0.175$). This trend persisted among the nine patients who completed 2 years of treatment (%pFVC +7.7%; $p = 0.037$ and %pDLCO −2.2%; $p = 0.621$). During the follow-up period, 15% of patients died, and 4% underwent lung transplantation. Adverse events occurred in 81% of patients, leading to discontinuation in 18.5% of cases. The most frequent adverse events were gastrointestinal events and hepatitis, leading to a permanent dose reduction of 40% for nintedanib and 14% for pirfenidone. A second antifibrotic agent was prescribed for 18.5% of the patients. At the end of the follow-up period, 63% of the total cohort remained on antifibrotic therapy. **Conclusions:** According to our results, antifibrotic initiation was associated with a modest improvement in the trajectory of %pFVC and stabilization in %pDLCO. The discontinuation rate in our cohort (37%) was higher than that reported in clinical trials but similar to that reported in previously published real-world studies.

Keywords: rheumatoid arthritis; interstitial lung diseases; antifibrotics; nintedanib; pirfenidone

1. Introduction

Interstitial lung disease (ILD) is one of the most common and severe extra-articular manifestations of rheumatoid arthritis (RA) and significantly contributes to both morbidity and mortality [1–7]. The most prevalent ILD subtypes among RA patients are usual interstitial pneumonia (UIP) and nonspecific interstitial pneumonia (NSIP). The UIP pattern observed in RA-ILD closely resembles idiopathic pulmonary fibrosis (IPF), and both are associated with a high risk of progressive pulmonary fibrosis (PPF) and increased short-term mortality. Additionally, some RA patients with NSIP-type ILD may also develop progressive fibrosing patterns [7].

The clinical trajectory of RA-ILD varies widely. Approximately 55% of RA-ILD patients experience disease progression [8,9], with an estimated 40% meeting the criteria for PPF within 5 years of onset, characterized by a rapid decline in lung function, progression to chronic respiratory failure, and an increased risk of premature mortality [10,11]. In patients with a fibrosing phenotype, the same profibrotic pathways that lead to pulmonary fibrosis in IPF are activated [12,13]. Once these pathways are triggered, they follow an autonomous and self-perpetuating clinical course [12,13]. Inhibiting these activated profibrotic pathways with antifibrotic agents, such as nintedanib or pirfenidone, remains the only strategy to slow or potentially stop fibrosis progression.

Nintedanib has been formally approved by health authorities for the treatment of progressive fibrosing ILD, regardless of its underlying cause, based on the INBUILD trial, which demonstrated a significantly reduced annual rate of forced vital capacity (FVC) decline in these patients [14]. In a focused evaluation of the INBUILD study comparing the rate of decline in % FVC over 52 weeks among patients with autoimmune-related ILD, no significant differences were observed based on the HRCT pattern. The adjusted difference for the UIP-like fibrotic pattern was 124.2 (95% CI: 31.1 to 217.4), compared to 41.7 (95% CI: −112.2 to 195.5) for other fibrotic patterns ($p = 0.37$) [15]. Subanalyses of the 89 patients with RA-ILD in the INBUILD trial revealed similar efficacy to that observed in other causes of PF-ILD [16].

Pirfenidone was evaluated in RA-ILD patients in the TRAIL1 trial, a placebo-controlled study with limited statistical power [17]. Although the primary endpoint (a composite of ≥10% decline in percent predicted FVC (%pFVC) or death within one year) was not met, pirfenidone was associated with a significantly slower rate of FVC decline compared to placebo. Post hoc analyses revealed that the effect of pirfenidone on the decline in FVC was more significant in patients with a UIP pattern [17]. Based on these findings, the 2023 guidelines from the American College of Rheumatology (ACR) and the American College of Chest Physicians (CHEST) for the management of ILD in systemic autoimmune rheumatic diseases conditionally recommend adding pirfenidone as a treatment option for RA-ILD patients with progression despite first-line treatment [18].

Although nintedanib and pirfenidone are effective in slowing the progression of ILD, both drugs are associated with adverse events (AEs) that may restrict their use, often resulting in dose adjustments or discontinuation. While clinical trials provide valuable insights, real-world studies are particularly important because they reflect a broader and more representative patient population typically encountered in clinical practice. Clinical trials frequently exclude patients with advanced disease stages or prevalent comorbidities, while real-world studies not only encompass these individuals but also offer the opportunity for extended follow-up periods.

This study aims to bridge this gap by evaluating the effectiveness and tolerability of antifibrotic therapy in a real-world cohort of patients with RA-ILD PFF.

2. Methods

2.1. Study Sample

We conducted a review of medical records and hospital pharmacy-prescribing databases to identify all RA patients who initiated nintedanib or pirfenidone as part of routine clinical care at two tertiary referral hospitals (Bellvitge University Hospital and Dr. Peset University Hospital, Spain). Antifibrotic therapies were prescribed in all cases due to progressive fibrosing RA-associated interstitial lung disease (RA-ILD), and no patients were excluded based on poor outcomes or early death.

In line with previous studies from our group [19–21], progressive ILD was defined by one or more of the following criteria during follow-up: a relative decline of ≥10% in the %pFVC or ≥15% in the predicted diffusing capacity for carbon monoxide, corrected for hemoglobin (%pDLCO) during follow-up, or a relative decline of 5–10% in %pFVC accompanied by a reduction of less than 15% in %pDLCO, together with worsening respiratory symptoms and increased fibrosis as assessed by thoracic high-resolution computed tomography (HRCT) [14,22]. These changes occurred within 2 years of ILD diagnosis [14].

RA was diagnosed according to the ACR 1987 classification criteria [23] or the ACR/EULAR 2010 criteria [24], depending on the year of diagnosis. ILD was identified using HRCT of the chest, with experienced thoracic radiologists classifying cases into three main radiologic patterns based on the American Thoracic Society (ATS)/European Respiratory Society (ERS) International Multidisciplinary Consensus Classification of Idiopathic Interstitial Pneumonias [25]: (1) UIP; (2) NSIP, and (3) other patterns. The final diagnosis of progressive fibrosing RA-ILD was confirmed in all patients through a multidisciplinary approach.

Patients were managed according to a standardized protocol within a specialized multidisciplinary unit, overseen jointly by a pulmonologist and a rheumatologist. Pre-existing treatments, including glucocorticoids (GCs), conventional synthetic disease-modifying antirheumatic drugs (csDMARDs), immunosuppressants (ISs), and biologic DMARDs (bDMARDs) initially remained unchanged in all patients. However, adjustments to GC dosages were made as needed after the initiation of antifibrotic therapy, at the discretion of the treating physician.

Pulmonary function tests (PFTs) were conducted every 6 months following the initiation of treatment. All tests were performed in a standardized manner, following the 2002 recommendations of the Spanish Society of Pneumology and Thoracic Surgery [26]. Both %pFVC and %pDLCO were measured simultaneously for each patient.

2.2. Clinical Assessments and Outcome Variables

The effectiveness of antifibrotic therapies was assessed by evaluating changes in %pFVC and %pDLCO before and after treatment initiation. The progression of PFTs was categorized according to the definitions established by the ATS as worsening (a decrease in %pFVC > 10% or %pDLCO > 15%), stabilization (changes in %pFVC < 10% or %pDLCO < 15%), or improvement (an increase in %pFVC > 10% or %pDLCO > 15%) [27,28].

Data regarding antifibrotic therapies included the specific drug used, dosage, duration of follow-up from the first dose, treatment status at the endpoint (continuation or discontinuation), reasons for discontinuation (if applicable), tolerability, and side effect profile. Additional information on lung transplants and deaths (including causes of death) was also collected. The endpoint for follow-up was defined as the date of the last clinic visit, death, or lung transplant. A retrospective analysis of prospectively collected data was performed.

2.3. Statistical Analysis

The results are expressed as the mean ± standard deviation (SD) or as the median (interquartile range [IQR], 25th–75th) as appropriate for continuous data, whereas categorical variables are presented as the number of cases and percentages.

The Kolmogorov–Smirnov test was employed to determine whether numerical variables followed a normal distribution. Depending on the distribution, numerical variables were compared using either the Student's t-test or the Mann–Whitney U test. For categorical variables, the chi-squared test or Fisher's exact test was applied, as appropriate.

Pulmonary function trends were quantified as a percentage change (delta) from the time of diagnosis of RA-ILD to the time of initiation of antifibrotic treatment (T0) and in relation to T0 for all subsequent evaluations after starting therapy. The paired sample t-test was used to compare pre- and post- antifibrotic treatment means of the main outcome efficacy measures evaluated. Statistical significance was defined as $p < 0.05$.

3. Results

3.1. Patient Characteristics

To date, antifibrotic therapies have been administered to 27 patients with ongoing progressive fibrosing RA-ILD despite prior immunosuppressive treatment. The key baseline characteristics of this cohort are summarized in Table 1. The mean age at the start of antifibrotic therapy was 67 ± 10 years. At that time, the median duration of RA was 70.5 months (interquartile range [IQR], 25th–75th percentile: 27.5–114 months), while the median time since ILD diagnosis was 29 months (IQR: 20–50 months).

Table 1. Characteristics of patients with RA-ILD at the initiation of initial antifibrotic medication.

Demographics and RA Characteristics	N = 27
Age at age at initiation of antifibrotic treatment, years (mean ± SD)	67 ± 10
Sex, woman/man	12 (44.5%)/15 (55.5%)
Body mass index (BMI), missing data = 4 (mean ± SD)	28.3 ± 5.3
Smoker or ex-smoker	18 (67%) Current: 1 (4%)
Positive rheumatoid factor	23 (85%)
Positive ACPA	22 (81.5%)
Median duration of RA, months (IQR 25th–75th)	70.5 (27.5–114)
DAS28-ESR at initiation of antifibrotic treatment	
Remission or low activity	17 (63%)
Moderate or high activity	10 (37%)
ILD characteristics	
Median duration of ILD, months (IQR 25th–75th)	29 (20–50)
HRCT pattern of ILD	
Usual interstitial pneumonia (definite or probable)	21 (78%)
Fibrotic non-specific interstitial pneumonia	5 (18%)
Combined pulmonary fibrosis and emphysema	1 (4%)
%pFVC at initiation of initial antifibrotic medication	86.6 ± 15
%pDLCO at initiation of initial antifibrotic medication	54.3 ± 14.8
Prior treatments	
Glucocorticoids	26 (96%)
Mean dose (± SD), mg/day (IQR 25th–75th)	8.3 ± 5.4 (5–10)
csDMARDs or immunosuppressants *	22 (81.5%)
Number of previous csDMARDs or immunosuppressants	1.4 (minimum 1, maximum 2)
Methotrexate	7 (26%)
Leflunomide	18 (67%)
Sulfasalazine	2 (8%)
Mycophenolate mofetil	2 (8%)
bDMARD *	20 (74%)
Number of previous bDMARD	1.5 (minimum 1, maximum 6)
Rituximab	10 (37%)
Number of cycles	4.4 (minimum 1, maximum 10)
Abatacept	11 (41%)
TNFi	4 (15%)
Tocilizumab	1 (4%)
Antifibrotic medication	
Nintedanib	25 (92%)
Pirfenidone	
As initial antifibrotic medication/After nintedanib	2 (8%)/5 (18.5%)
Concomitant medication	
Glucocorticoids	25 (93%)

Table 1. *Cont.*

Dose of prednisone at initiation of initial antifibrotic medication, (mean ± SD)	7.9 ± 5
csDMARDs or immunosuppressants	21 (78%)
Leflunomide	16 (59%)
Mycophenolate mofetil	4 (15%)
Methotrexate	1 (4%)
bDMARD or JAKi *	22 (81.5%)
Abatacept	13 (48%)
Rituximab	10 (37%)
TNFi	1 (4%)
JAKi	2 (8%)
Need for oxygen therapy at initiation of initial antifibrotic medication	7 (26%)

* Some patients received more than one. Abbreviations ACPA: anticitrullinated protein autoantibodies; bDMARD: biologic disease-modifying antirheumatic drugs; csDMARDs: conventional synthetic disease-modifying antirheumatic drugs; DAS28-ESR: Disease Activity Score in 28 joints using Erythrocyte Sedimentation Rate; HRCT: high-resolution computed tomography; ILD: interstitial lung disease; IQR: interquartile range; JAKi: Janus kinase inhibitors; %pDLCO: percent predicted diffusing capacity for carbon monoxide corrected for hemoglobin; %pFVC: percent predicted forced vital capacity; RA: rheumatoid arthritis; SD: standard deviation; TNFi: tumor necrosis factor inhibitor.

Anticitrullinated protein antibodies (ACPA) were positive in 81.5% of patients, and rheumatoid factor (RF) in 85%. Radiologically, 21 patients (78%) were classified as having UIP, five (18%) as fibrotic NSIP, and one (4%) as combined pulmonary fibrosis and emphysema (CPFE). A smoking history was reported in 18 patients (67%).

With respect to antifibrotic treatment, 25 (92.5%) patients initiated therapy with nintedanib, while two started therapy with pirfenidone due to concurrent anticoagulant use. During follow-up, nintedanib was switched to pirfenidone in five patients because of adverse effects; thus, seven (26%) patients received pirfenidone at some point during the follow-up period.

At the onset of antifibrotic therapy, 10 (37%) patients exhibited moderate to high RA activity according to the DAS28 ESR score (>3.2). The mean %pFVC was 86.6 ± 15 (IQR 25th–75th percentile, 73–97.1), and the mean %pDLCO was 54.3 ± 14.8 (IQR 44–66). Fourteen (52%) patients presented a decline of ≥10% in %pFVC.

3.2. Treatment Characteristics

Prior to the initiation of antifibrotic therapy (see Table 1), 26 (96%) patients had been treated with GCs, 22 (82%) had received at least one csDMARD or IS, and 20 (74%) had been treated with one or more bDMARDs.

Previous csDMARDs and IS included leflunomide (LEF) in 18 (67%) patients, methotrexate (MTX) in seven (26%), sulfasalazine in two (8%), and mycophenolate mofetil (MMF) in two (8%). The previous bDMARDs administered were rituximab (RTX) in 10 (37%), abatacept (ABA) in 11 (41%), anti-tumor necrosis factor (TNF) alpha agents in four (15%), and tocilizumab in one (4%).

All patients received antifibrotic therapy combined with either a bDMARD, a csDMARD/IS, or both: 17 (63%) received a bDMARD plus a csDMARD/IS, 5 (19%) received only a csDMARD/IS, and five (19%) were on bDMARD monotherapy. Additionally, 25 (93%) patients also received GC at a mean dose of 8.3 ± 5.4 mg/day (IQR 5–10).

The biologic agents initially administered at the start of antifibrotic therapy were ABA in 11 (41%), RTX in 8 (30%), JAK inhibitors (JAKis) in one (4%), and adalimumab in one (4%). During follow-up, ABA was replaced by a JAKi in one patient, and RTX was exchanged with ABA or vice versa in three patients (two initially treated with ABA were switched to RTX, and one initially treated with RTX to ABA). The immunosuppressive treatments used were LEF in 16 patients (59%), MMF in four (15%), and MTX in one (4%).

Two patients (7.4%) had type 3 pulmonary hypertension confirmed by right heart catheterization and seven patients (26%) required oxygen therapy at the start of antifibrotic therapy. The median follow-up period after initiating antifibrotic agents was 25 months (IQR 7–27), with a total follow-up of 48.7 patient years.

3.3. *Efficacy Endpoints*

Changes in the primary efficacy outcome measures assessed at 6 months and 1 year following the initiation of antifibrotic therapy are presented in Tables 2 and 3 and illustrated in Figure 1. Across the entire study population, prior to starting therapy, the mean decline in %pFVC and %pDLCO from the time of ILD diagnosis to the initiation of antifibrotic treatment (T0) was −8.9% (95% CI: 7.81 to 16.02; $p = 0.0001$) and −14.8% (95% CI: 9.53 to 20.16; $p = 0.0001$), respectively.

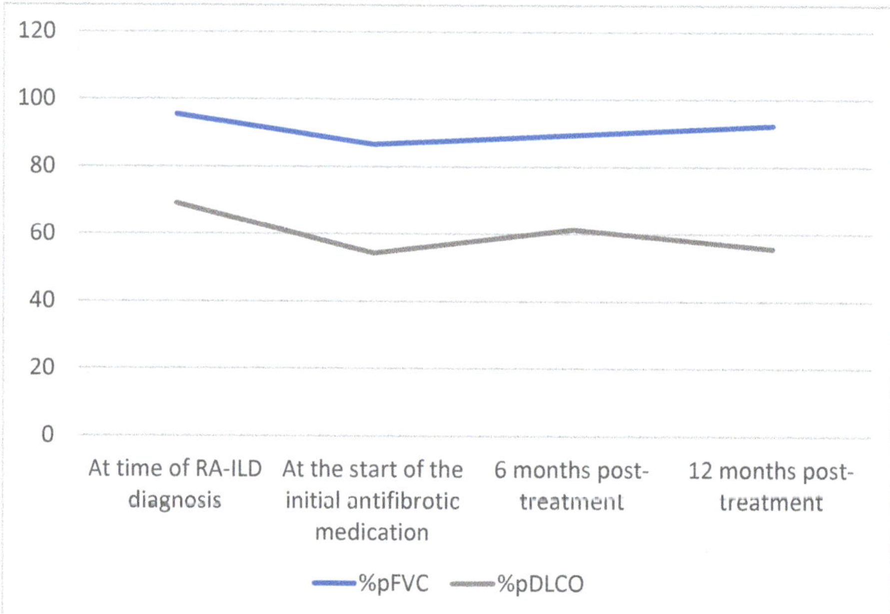

Figure 1. Evolution of the predicted forced vital capacity (%pFVC) and the predicted diffusing capacity for carbon monoxide corrected for hemoglobin (%pDLCO) before initiation of antifibrotic therapy and after 1 year of treatment.

In three patients, antifibrotic therapy was discontinued due to adverse effects before completing 6 months of treatment. In the remaining 24 patients (twenty-one UIP and three non-UIP patterns), a slower decline in PFT parameters was observed after 6 months of therapy (delta: percentage change from baseline): Δ%pFVC + 1.2% (95% CI: −5.67 to 3.41; $p = 0.611$ compared with T0) and Δ%pDLCO + 3.9% (95% CI: −13.51 to 5.63; $p = 0.400$).

At 1 year of treatment, data were unavailable for nine patients: three had died due to ILD progression, four had discontinued treatment due to adverse effects, and two had not yet completed 12 months of therapy. Among the 18 patients who completed one year of therapy (15 UIP and three NSIP patterns), a modest improvement in %pFVC was observed (Δ + 4.7%, 95% CI: −8.66 to −0.74; $p = 0.023$), along with a slowing in %pDLCO decline (Δ − 3.8%, 95% CI: −1.82 to −9.25; $p = 0.175$).

Nine of the 24 patients completed 2 years of treatment (seven UIP and two NSIP), maintaining a response in PFTs: Δ%pFVC: +7.7% (95% CI: −16.07 to −0.66; $p = 0.037$) and Δ%pDLCO: −2.2% (95% CI: −7.67 to −12.07; $p = 0.621$).

Table 2. Changes before and after 6 months and after 1 and 2 years of treatment with antifibrotic medication.

	Before Antifibrotics			
	At Time of RA-ILD Diagnosis Mean ± SD (IQR, 25th–75th)	**At Time of Initiation of Initial Antifibrotic Medication Mean ± SD (IQR, 25th–75th)**	**Delta (Mean)**	***p* Value (95% CI)**
Total sample (N = 27)				
%FVC predicted	95.5 ± 14.6 (88.1–107.5)	86.6 ± 15 (73–97.1)	−8.9%	0.0001 (7.81 to 16.02)
%DLCO predicted	69.1 ± 18.8 (55.4–79.5)	54.3 ± 14.8 (44–66)	−14.8%	0.0001 (9.53 to 20.16)
	After 6 months of treatment			
	At time ofinitiation of initial antifibrotic medication mean ± SD (IQR, 25th–75th)	**6 months post-treatment mean ± SD (IQR, 25th–75th)**	**Delta (mean)**	***p* value (95% CI)**
Total sample (N = 24)				
UIP: 21/Non-UIP: 3				
%FVC predicted	88.2 ± 19 (73.7–102.7)	89.4 ± 22.7 (74.4–105.5)	+1.2%	0.611 (−5.67 to 3.41)
%DLCO predicted	57.4 ± 16.6 (46.2–68.1)	61.3 ± 24.9 (40.5–79.6)	+3.9%	0.400 (−13.51 to 5.63)
	After 1 year of treatment			
	At time ofinitiation of initial antifibrotic medication mean ± SD (IQR, 25th–75th)	**12 months post-treatment mean ± SD (IQR, 25th–75th)**	**Delta (mean)**	***p* value (95% CI)**
Total sample (N = 18)				
UIP: 15/NSIP: 3				
%FVC predicted	87.5 ± 20.7 (71.8–108.6)	92.2 ± 24.8 (76–115.8)	+4.7%	0.023 (−8.66 to 0.74)
%DLCO predicted	58.2 ± 17.9 (45.7–69.9)	54.4 ± 16.7 (42.7–67)	−3.8%	0.175 (−1.82 to −9.25)
	After 2 years of treatment			
	At time ofinitiation of initial antifibrotic medication mean ± SD (IQR, 25th–75th)	**24 months post-treatment mean ± SD (IQR, 25th–75th)**	**Delta (mean)**	***p* value (95% CI)**
Total sample (N = 9)				
UIP: 7/NSIP: 2				
%FVC predicted	89.1 ± 19.7 (71.6–111.4)	97.4 ± 19.7 (84.3–120.1)	+7.7%	0.037 (−16.07 to 0.66)
%DLCO predicted	60.8 ± 20.3 (43.8–81.9)	58.6 ± 15.1 (45.5–73.1)	−2.2%	0.621 (−7.67 to −12.07)

%pFVC = predicted forced vital capacity; %pDLCO = predicted diffusing capacity for carbon monoxide, corrected for hemoglobin; UIP: usual interstitial pneumonia and NSIP: fibrotic non-specific interstitial pneumonia.

A comparison of pre- and post-treatment pulmonary variables revealed that PFT deterioration either slowed or stabilized in approximately three quarters of the patients (Table 3 and Figure 2). Additionally, prednisone doses were reduced in 10 out of 25 patients (40%) following the initiation of antifibrotic therapy, with a mean reduction of −5.8 mg/day (SD: 3.5 mg; 95% CI: 7.73 to 15.62; $p < 0.046$). Efficacy comparisons between radiological patterns could not be performed due to the low number of non-UIP patterns.

3.4. Antifibrotic Tolerability and Retention

Seventeen patients (63%) continued treatment after a median follow-up period of 25 months (IQR 7–27) following the initiation of antifibrotic therapy. Among the 10 patients who discontinued treatment, the reasons were death due to ILD progression and infectious complications in four patients (15%), lung transplantation in one patient (4%), and adverse events leading to treatment discontinuation in five patients (18.5%). The retention rate of patients initially treated with nintedanib was 52% (13/25).

Table 3. Lung function test results according to the definitions of ATS after antifibrotic therapy.

After 6 Months of Treatment **N = 24**			
	Improvement	**Stabilization**	**Worsening**
%FVC predicted	12.5% (3)	75% (18)	12.5% (3)
%DLCO predicted	21% (5)	58% (14)	21% (5)
After 12 months of treatment N = 18			
%FVC predicted	22.2% (4)	66.7% (12)	11.1% (2)
%DLCO predicted	11.1% (2)	61.2% (11)	27.7% (5)
After 24 months of treatment N = 9			
%FVC predicted	44.5% (4)	55.5% (5)	0
%DLCO predicted	22.2% (2)	44.5% (4)	33.3% (3)

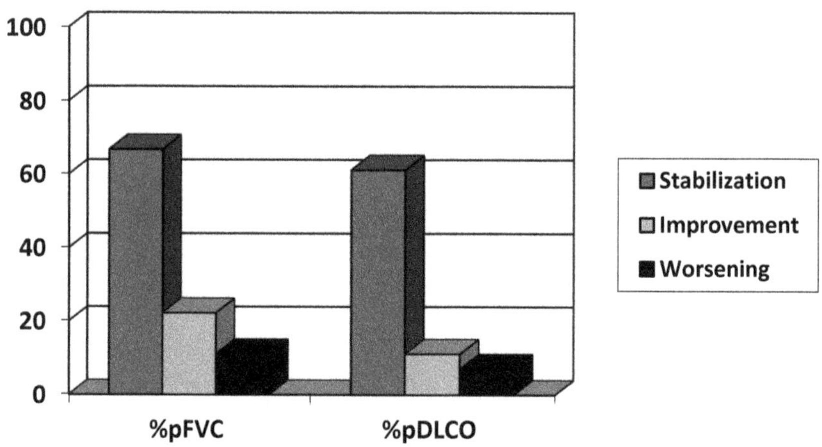

Figure 2. Lung function test results (as defined by the ATS) after 12 months of antifibrotic therapy.

A total of 81.5% (22/27) of patients experienced adverse events (AEs) attributed to antifibrotic treatment. Their frequency and types are detailed in Table 4. As expected, the most common events were gastrointestinal events and hepatitis.

In 48.1% (13/27) of patients, antifibrotic therapy was temporarily suspended (mean number of suspensions: 1.38 ± 0.5; range: 1–2), and in 63% (17/27) of patients, the recommended dosage was temporarily reduced (mean number of dose reductions: 1.53 ± 0.5; range: 1–3).

The most frequent AEs leading to treatment discontinuation or permanent dose reduction were diarrhea and hepatitis.

As previously reported, a second antifibrotic agent was prescribed for five (18.5%) patients; all were initially treated with nintedanib and were switched to pirfenidone due to adverse events. Among these five patients, three (60%) remained on pirfenidone after a median follow-up of 13 months.

Table 4. Adverse events associated with antifibrotic therapy.

	N = 27
Any adverse event	22 (81.5%)
Most frequent adverse events	
Diarrhea	17 (63%)
Nausea/Vomiting	9 (33%)
ALT o AST increased	7 (26%)
Decreased appetite/weight loss	10 (37%)
Asthenia	2 (7.4%)
Abdominal pain	3 (11%)
Adverse event leading to permanent dose reduction	
Nintedanib (N = 25)/Pirfenidone (N = 7)	10 (40%)/1 (14%)
Adverse event leading to treatment discontinuation	5 (18.5%)

4. Discussion

To date, the effectiveness and tolerability of antifibrotics in RA-ILD have been evaluated in two randomized controlled trials (INBUILD and TRAIL1) [16,17], three observational studies [29–31], and several case reports and case series [32–36]. Our study is among the few real-world analyses assessing antifibrotic effectiveness and drug retention in RA-ILD patients. Real-world data enable the inclusion of a more diverse patient population, making the findings more reflective of daily clinical practice. Additionally, real-world studies offer valuable insights into long-term safety, especially concerning rare adverse events.

In both clinical trials (INBUILD with nintedanib and TRAIL1 with pirfenidone), antifibrotic treatment demonstrated only a significant reduction in the rate of FVC decline, without stopping or improving its value [16,17]. In contrast, real-world studies appear to demonstrate either stabilization or a modestly improved trajectory in %pFVC [29–31].

In our cohort, the initiation of antifibrotics was associated with an initial stabilization in %pFVC at 6 months, followed by a gradual, modest improvement (+4.7%; $p = 0.023$) after the first year of therapy, whereas %pDLCO showed a mild, non-significant decline (−3.8%; $p = 0.175$), indicating stabilization. The discrepancy between our results and those of the clinical trials may be explained by selection bias, as all our patients were worsening prior to starting antifibrotic treatment, which may bias outcomes toward improvement or stabilization after this time point.

Duarte et al. [30] also reported that antifibrotic therapy interrupted the decline in FVC, shifting from a pre-treatment decrease of 300 ± 500 mL per year to an improvement of 200 ± 400 mL in the year following treatment initiation ($p = 0.336$), whereas %pDLCO continued to decline slightly (3% pre-treatment vs. 2.9% post-treatment, $p = 0.75$). In Juge et al.'s study, both nintedanib and pirfenidone were associated with a reduced decline in the FVC and DLCO trajectories over 18 months [29]. This trajectory change was significant for %pFVC (0.3% per year post-initiation compared with 6.2% per year pre-initiation, $p = 0.03$) but not for absolute FVC or DLCO. In Behera's study, after 6 months of antifibrotic treatment, the lung function values stabilized, with the %FVC from 62.5 ± 20.04 at baseline to 63.2 ± 18.2 ($p = 0.3$) and the %DLCO increasing from 70.1 ± 15.2 to 72.1 ± 12.4 ($p = 0.15$) [31].

Recently, Ushio et al. have further demonstrated that nintedanib combined with ISs significantly improves %FVC in patients with connective tissue disease-associated progressive fibrosing ILD, including cases with RA-ILD. Before treatment, the mean monthly decline in FVC was −0.70%/month. After therapy, this shifted to a mean increase of +0.54%/month ($p < 0.001$), with greater improvements observed in the nintedanib+IS group (+1.71%/month) compared to the nintedanib monotherapy group (+0.34%/month). Additionally, serum KL-6 levels, a biomarker of fibrosis, decreased significantly. The authors concluded that nintedanib improves %FVC in connective tissue disease-associated PF-ILD, with the combination of nintedanib plus ISs proving more effective than nintedanib monotherapy in stabilizing pulmonary function [32].

Despite the apparent beneficial effect of antifibrotic therapy, 15% of our patients died, and 4% underwent lung transplantation during the follow-up period. In other observational studies, mortality rates ranged from 22% to 35% [29,30], whereas Juge's study reported a lung transplant rate of 5% [29], which closely aligns with our findings. Given the persistently high rates of lung transplant and mortality, it may be worth reconsidering whether antifibrotics are being introduced too late in clinical practice and assessing the potential benefit of initiating them earlier in patients with fibrotic ILD patterns.

Real-world data confirm the safety of antifibrotic treatments combined with glucocorticoids, csDMARDs/ISs (LEF, MTX, and MMF), with or without biologic agents (particularly ABA and RTX) or JAK inhibitors, without any observed increase in serious infection risk [29–36]. AEs occurred in 81% of our patients, which is higher than the 25% to 55.4% reported in other observational studies [29–31], but lower than the 100% reported in the INBUILD and TRAIL 1 trials [16,17]. As in other studies, the most common AEs were gastrointestinal events and hepatitis.

In our series, adverse events resulted in a permanent dose reduction for 40% of patients on nintedanib and 14% on pirfenidone and led to the discontinuation of antifibrotic therapy in 18.5% of patients (compared with 21.4% of RA-ILD patients treated with nintedanib in the INBUILD trial [16] and 24% of patients treated with pirfenidone in the TRAIL1 trial [17]).

However, owing to this and other factors (such as death from ILD progression and infectious complications, or the need for lung transplantation), the retention rate at the end of the follow-up period was only 63% (52% for nintedanib). The discontinuation rate in our cohort was 37% overall and 48% among those initially treated with nintedanib, which was higher than that reported in clinical trials (INBUILD: 23.8%, TRAIL1: 24%), but similar to that reported in previously published real-world studies (30% to 46%) [29,30].

Finally, on the basis of our experience with both RA-ILD and systemic sclerosis-associated ILD, switching to pirfenidone may be a successful alternative for patients intolerant to nintedanib. In our series, efficacy comparisons between radiological patterns could not be performed due to the low number of non-UIP patterns. However, in the study by Juge et al. [29], both nintedanib and pirfenidone demonstrated similar changes in FVCpp trajectory, with no statistically significant differences.

When interpreting our study's results, it is crucial to acknowledge several limitations inherent to its retrospective observational design. These include the small sample size, selection bias (as all patients had experienced ILD worsening prior to initiating antifibrotic therapy), the absence of post-treatment HRCT, the concomitant use of oral GCs, csDMARDs/ISs, and/or biologics in all patients, and the lack of a control group. While the effects on lung progression cannot be definitively attributed solely to antifibrotics, the study specifically included patients with progressive RA-ILD who had not responded to conventional therapies. Furthermore, the baseline regimens of csDMARDs, ISs, and/or biologic agents were maintained without de-escalation throughout the follow-up period after antifibrotic initiation, allowing patients to serve as their own controls. Pre- and post-treatment lung function trends provided compelling evidence of treatment effects attributable to antifibrotic rescue therapy, a conclusion further supported by the use of objective outcome measures, which minimized examiner bias. Nonetheless, we cannot rule out other residual confounders affecting associations between antifibrotics use and outcomes, since no adjusted analysis could be performed due to the small sample size.

However, our data reflect outcomes from real-world clinical practice in managing refractory cases of this severe complication, with the added strength that our study was conducted independently of corporate sponsorship. Additionally, patients were followed in a structured, protocolized manner with standardized data collection, and the duration of antifibrotic exposure was relatively prolonged.

In conclusion, our real-world data indicate that antifibrotic therapy stabilizes lung function in most patients with progressive fibrosing RA-ILD. Adverse events are frequent, particularly gastrointestinal events, which impact treatment survival and lead to a nonnegligible rate of permanent dose reduction and treatment discontinuation. Further studies with larger sample sizes are necessary to strengthen these findings, particularly regarding effectiveness analysis, and to better establish the optimal therapeutic window for their use.

Author Contributions: Conceptualization, J.N., M.A.-C. and M.M.-M.; methodology, J.N., M.A.-C. and M.M.-M.; software, J.N.; validation, J.N., M.A.-C., V.V.-Z., J.J.A., G.B. and M.M.-M. formal analysis, J.N. and M.A.-C.; investigation, J.N., M.A.-C., V.V.-Z., J.J.A., G.B. and M.M.-M.; data curation, J.N., M.A.-C., V.V.-Z., J.J.A., G.B. and M.M.-M.; writing—original draft preparation, J.N.; writing—review and editing, J.N., M.A.-C., V.V.-Z., J.J.A., G.B. and M.M.-M. All authors have read and agreed to the published version of the manuscript.

Funding: This research received no external funding.

Institutional Review Board Statement: This study was approved by our institutional ethics committee (Clinical Research Ethics Committee of Bellvitge University Hospital-IDIBELL, PR391/23, 12 January 2024). This study was conducted in accordance with the principles of the Declaration of Helsinki and the International Conference for Harmonization.

Informed Consent Statement: Not applicable.

Data Availability Statement: The authors confirm that all data underlying the findings are fully available without restriction. All relevant data are included in the paper.

Conflicts of Interest: The authors declare that they have no competing interests related to the preparation of this manuscript.

References

1. Farquhar, H.; Vassallo, R.; Edwards, A.L.; Matteson, E.L. Pulmonary Complications of Rheumatoid Arthritis. *Semin. Respir. Crit. Care Med.* **2019**, *40*, 194–207. [CrossRef] [PubMed]
2. Yunt, Z.X.; Solomon, J.J. Lung disease in rheumatoid arthritis. *Rheum. Dis. Clin. North Am.* **2015**, *41*, 225–236. [CrossRef] [PubMed]
3. Spagnolo, P.; Lee, J.S.; Sverzellati, N.; Rossi, G.; Cottin, V. The lung in rheumatoid arthritis: Focus on interstitial lung disease. *Arthritis Rheumatol.* **2018**, *70*, 1544–1554. [CrossRef] [PubMed]
4. Bongartz, T.; Nannini, C.; Medina-Velasquez, Y.F.; Achenbach, S.J.; Crowson, C.S.; Ryu, J.H.; Vassallo, R.; Gabriel, S.E.; Matteson, E.L. Incidence and mortality of interstitial lung disease in rheumatoid arthritis: A population-based study. *Arthritis Rheum.* **2010**, *62*, 1583–1591. [CrossRef] [PubMed]
5. Assayag, D.; Lubin, M.; Lee, J.S.; King, T.E.; Collard, H.R.; Ryerson, C.J. Predictors of mortality in rheumatoid arthritis-related interstitial lung disease. *Respirology* **2014**, *19*, 493–500. [CrossRef]
6. Hyldgaard, C.; Hilberg, O.; Pedersen, A.B.; Ulrichsen, S.P.; Løkke, A.; Bendstrup, E.; Ellingsen, T. A population-based cohort study of rheumatoid arthritis-associated interstitial lung disease: Comorbidity and mortality. *Ann. Rheum. Dis.* **2017**, *76*, 1700–1706. [CrossRef]
7. Koduri, G.; Solomon, J.J. Identification, monitoring, and management of rheumatoid arthritis-associated interstitial lung disease. *Arthritis Rheumatol.* **2023**, *75*, 2067–2077. [CrossRef]
8. Zamora-Legoff, J.A.; Krause, M.L.; Crowson, C.S.; Ryu, J.H.; Matteson, E.L. Progressive Decline of Lung Function in Rheumatoid Arthritis–Associated Interstitial Lung Disease. *Arthritis Rheumatol.* **2017**, *69*, 542–549. [CrossRef]
9. Hyldgaard, C.; Ellingsen, T.; Hilberg, O.; Bendstrup, E. Rheumatoid arthritis-associated interstitial lung disease: Clinical characteristics and predictors of mortality. *Respiration* **2019**, *98*, 455–460. [CrossRef]
10. Spagnolo, P.; Distler, O.; Ryerson, C.J.; Tzouvelekis, A.; Lee, J.S.; Bonella, F.; Bouros, D.; Hiffman-Vold, A.-M.; Crestani, B.; Matteson, E.L. Mechanisms of progressive fibrosis in connective tissue disease (CTD)-associated interstitial lung diseases (ILDs). *Ann. Rheum. Dis.* **2021**, *80*, 143–150. [CrossRef]
11. Olson, A.; Hartmann, N.; Patnaik, P.; Wallace, L.; Schlenker-Herceg, R.; Nasser, M.; Richeldi, L.; Hoffmann-Vold, A.-M.; Cottin, V. Estimation of the Prevalence of Progressive Fibrosing Interstitial Lung Diseases: Systematic Literature Review and Data from a Physician Survey. *Adv. Ther.* **2021**, *38*, 854–867. [CrossRef] [PubMed]
12. Wijsenbeek, M.; Cottin, V. Spectrum of Fibrotic Lung Diseases. *New Engl. J. Med.* **2020**, *383*, 958–968. [CrossRef] [PubMed]

13. Liang, M.; Matteson, E.L.; Abril, A.; Distler, J.H. The role of antifibrotics in the treatment of rheumatoid arthritis–associated interstitial lung disease. *Ther. Adv. Musculoskelet. Dis.* **2022**, *14*, 1759720X221074457. [CrossRef] [PubMed]
14. Flaherty, K.R.; Wells, A.U.; Cottin, V.; Devaraj, A.; Walsh, S.L.; Inoue, Y.; Richeldi, L.; Kolb, M.; Tetzlaff, K.; Stowasser, S.; et al. Nintedanib in Progressive Fibrosing Interstitial Lung Diseases. *N. Engl. J. Med.* **2019**, *381*, 1718–1727. [CrossRef]
15. Matteson, E.L.; Kelly, C.; Distler, J.H.W.; Hoffmann-Vold, A.; Seibold, J.R.; Mittoo, S.; Dellaripa, P.F.; Aringer, M.; Pope, J.; Distler, O.; et al. Nintedanib in Patients with Autoimmune Disease–Related Progressive Fibrosing Interstitial Lung Diseases: Subgroup Analysis of the INBUILD Trial. *Arthritis Rheumatol.* **2022**, *74*, 1039–1047. [CrossRef]
16. Matteson, E.L.; Aringer, M.; Burmester, G.R.; Mueller, H.; Moros, L.; Kolb, M. Effect of nintedanib in patients with progressive pulmonary fibrosis associated with rheumatoid arthritis: Data from the INBUILD trial. *Clin. Rheumatol.* **2023**, *42*, 2311–2319. [CrossRef]
17. Solomon, J.J.; Danoff, S.K.; Woodhead, F.A.; Hurwitz, S.; Maurer, R.; Glaspole, I.; Dellaripa, P.F.; Gooptu, B.; Vassallo, R.; Cox, P.G.; et al. Safety, tolerability, and efficacy of pirfenidone in patients with rheumatoid arthritis-associated interstitial lung disease: A randomized, double-blind, placebo-controlled, phase 2 study. *Lancet Respir. Med.* **2023**, *11*, 87–96. [CrossRef]
18. Johnson, S.R.; Bernstein, E.J.; Bolster, M.B.; Chung, J.H.; Danoff, S.K.; George, M.D.; Khanna, D.; Guyatt, G.; Mirza, R.D.; Aggarwal, R.; et al. 2023 American College of Rheumatology (ACR)/American College of Chest Physicians (CHEST) Guideline for the Treatment of Interstitial Lung Disease in People with Systemic Autoimmune Rheumatic Diseases. *Arthritis Rheumatol.* **2024**, *76*, 1182–1200. [CrossRef]
19. Narváez, J.; Cañadillas, E.; Castellví, I.; Alegre, J.J.; Vincens-Zygmunt, V.; Bermudo, G.; Vidal-Montal, P.; Molina, M.M.; Nolla, J.M. Rituximab in the treatment of progressive interstitial lung disease associated with the antisynthetase syndrome. *Arthritis Res. Ther.* **2024**, *26*, 1–12. [CrossRef]
20. Narváez, J.; Lluch, J.; Molina-Molina, M.; Vicens-Zygmunt, V.; Luburich, P.; Yañez, M.A.; Nolla, J.M. Rituximab as a rescue treatment added on mycophenolate mofetil background therapy in progressive systemic sclerosis associated interstitial lung disease unrespon-sive to conventional immunosuppression. *Semin. Arthritis Rheum.* **2020**, *50*, 977–987. [CrossRef]
21. Narváez, J.; Robles-Pérez, A.; Molina-Molina, M.; Vicens-Zygmunt, V.; Luburich, P.; Yañez, M.A.; Alegre, J.J.; Nolla, J.M. Real-world clinical effectiveness of rituximab rescue therapy in patients with progressive rheumatoid arthritis-related interstitial lung disease. *Semin. Arthritis Rheum.* **2020**, *50*, 902–910. [CrossRef] [PubMed]
22. George, P.M.; Spagnolo, P.; Kreuter, M.; Altinisik, G.; Bonifazi, M.; Martinez, F.J.; Molyneaux, P.L.; A Renzoni, E.; Richeldi, L.; Tomassetti, S.; et al. Progressive fibrosing interstitial lung disease: Clinical uncertainties, consensus recommendations, and research priorities. *Lancet Respir. Med.* **2020**, *8*, 925–934. [CrossRef] [PubMed]
23. Arnett, F.C.; Edworthy, S.M.; Bloch, D.A.; Mcshane, D.J.; Fries, J.F.; Cooper, N.S.; Healey, L.A.; Kaplan, S.R.; Liang, M.H.; Luthra, H.S.; et al. The american rheumatism association 1987 revised criteria for the classification of rheumatoid arthritis. *Arthritis Rheum.* **1988**, *31*, 315–324. [CrossRef] [PubMed]
24. Aletaha, D.; Neogi, T.; Silman, A.J.; Funovits, J.; Felson, D.T.; Bingham, C.O.; Birnbaum, N.S.; Burmester, G.R.; Bykerk, V.P.; Cohen, M.D.; et al. 2010 Rheumatoid artritis classification criteria:an American College of Rheumatology/European League Against Rheumatism collaborative initiative. *Arthritis Rheum.* **2010**, *62*, 2569–2581. [CrossRef] [PubMed]
25. American Thoracic Society. European Respiratory Society. American Thoracic Society/European Respiratory Society international multidisciplinary consensus classification of the idiopathic interstitial pneumonias. *Am. J. Respir. Crit. Care Med.* **2002**, *15*, 277–304, *Erratum in Am. J. Respir. Crit. Care Med.* **2002**, *166*, 426.
26. García-Río, F.; Calle, M.; Burgos, F.; Casan, P.; Del Campo, F.; Galdiz, J.B.; Giner, J.; González-Mangado, N.; Ortega, F.; Maestu, L.P.; et al. Spirometry. Spanish Society of Pulmonology and Thoracic Surgery (SEPAR). *Arch Bronconeumol.* **2013**, *49*, 388–401. [CrossRef]
27. Raghu, G.; Collard, H.R.; Egan, J.J.; Martinez, F.J.; Behr, J.; Brown, K.K.; Colby, T.V.; Cordier, J.-F.; Flaherty, K.R.; Lasky, J.A.; et al. An official ATS/ERS/JRS/ALAT statement: Idiopathic pulmonary fibrosis: Evidence-based guidelines for diagnosis and Management Committee on Idiopathic Pulmonary Fibrosis. *Am. J. Respir. Crit. Care Med.* **2011**, *15*, 788–824. [CrossRef]
28. Raghu, G.; Rochwerg, B.; Zhang, Y.; Cuello-Garcia, C.; Azuma, A.; Behr, J.; Brozek, J.L.; Collard, H.R.; Cunningham, W.; Homma, S.; et al. An Official ATS/ERS/JRS/ALAT Clinical Practice Guideline: Treatment of Idiopathic Pulmonary Fibrosis. An Update of the 2011 Clinical Practice Guideline. *Am. J. Respir. Crit. Care Med.* **2015**, *192*, e3–e19. [CrossRef]
29. Juge, P.-A.; Hayashi, K.; McDermott, G.C.; Vanni, K.M.; Kowalski, E.; Qian, G.; Bade, K.; Saavedra, A.; Dieudé, P.; Dellaripa, P.F.; et al. Effectiveness and tolerability of antifibrotics in rheumatoid arthritis-associated interstitial lung disease. *Semin. Arthritis Rheum.* **2023**, *64*, 152312. [CrossRef]
30. Duarte, A.C.; Marques Gomes, C.; Correia, M.; Mendes, B.; Mazeda, C.; Guimarães, F.; Abelha-Aleixo, J.; Guerra, M.; da Costa, R.B.; Meirinhos, T.; et al. Antifibrotics in rheumatoid arthri-tis-associated interstitial lung disease - real-world data from a nationwide cohort. *ARP Rheumatol.* **2024**, *3*, 182–188. [CrossRef]
31. Behera, A.K.; Kumar, V.; Sharma, P.; Ganga, R.; Meher, J.; Pati, S.; Sinha, K. Antifibrotics in the Management of Rheumatoid Arthri-tis-Associated Interstitial Lung Disease: Prospective Real-World Experience from an Interstitial Lung Disease Clinic in India. *Cureus* **2024**, *16*, e63518. [PubMed]
32. Ushio, Y.; Wakiya, R.; Kameda, T.; Nakashima, S.; Shimada, H.; Miyagi, T.; Sugihara, K.; Mino, R.; Mizusaki, M.; Chujo, K.; et al. Nintedanib combined with immunosuppressive agents improves forced vital capacity in connective tissue disease-associated PF-ILD: A single-center study. *BMC Rheumatol.* **2024**, *8*, 1–9. [CrossRef] [PubMed]

33. Cassone, G.; Sebastiani, M.; Vacchi, C.; Cerri, S.; Salvarani, C.; Manfredi, A. Pirfenidone for the treatment of interstitial lung disease associated to rheumatoid arthritis: A new scenario is coming? *Respir. Med. Case Rep.* **2020**, *30*, 101051. [CrossRef] [PubMed]
34. Vacchi, C.; Manfredi, A.; Cassone, G.; Salvarani, C.; Cerri, S.; Sebastiani, M. Combination Therapy with Nintedanib and Sarilumab for the Management of Rheumatoid Arthritis Related Interstitial Lung Disease. *Case Rep. Med.* **2020**, *2020*, 1–4. [CrossRef] [PubMed]
35. Mochizuki, T.; Yano, K.; Ikari, K.; Okazaki, K. Combination treatment with Janus kinase inhibitor and nintedanib for rheumatoid arthritis with progressive interstitial lung disease: A case report. *Mod. Rheumatol. Case Rep.* **2023**, *7*, 350–353. [CrossRef]
36. Narváez, J.; Vicens-Zygmunt, V.; Alegre, J.-J.; Herrera-Lara, S.; Nolla, J.-M.; Molina-Molina, M. Nintedanib for the treatment of refractory progressive rheumatoid arthritis–related interstitial lung disease: A real-life case series. *Rheumatology* **2020**, *59*, 3983–3986. [CrossRef]

Journal of
Clinical Medicine

MDPI

Article

Asymmetrical Damage of the Wrist Joint Induces Lateralized Cortical Bone Loss in the Metacarpal Diaphysis in Patients with Rheumatoid Arthritis

Akikatsu Nakashima [1,2], Hiroshi Fujii [2], Masahiro Kuroda [1], Takeshi Zoshima [3], Ichiro Mizushima [3], Hideki Nomura [4] and Mitsuhiro Kawano [5,*]

1 Department of Internal Medicine, Asanagi Hospital, 1-8 Gofuku-machi, Takaoka 933-0906, Japan; nakashima_skh@yahoo.co.jp (A.N.)
2 Division of Nephrology and Rheumatology, Ishikawa Prefectural Central Hospital, 2-1 Kuratsukihigashi, Kanazawa 920-8530, Japan
3 Department of Nephrology and Laboratory Medicine, Graduate School of Medical Science, Kanazawa University, 13-1 Takara-Machi, Kanazawa 920-8640, Japan
4 Department of General Medicine, Kanazawa University Hospital, 13-1 Takara-Machi, Kanazawa 920-8640, Japan
5 Department of Hematology and Immunology, Kanazawa Medical University, 1-1 Daigaku, Uchinada, Kahoku-gun 920-0293, Japan
* Correspondence: sk33166@gmail.com

Abstract: Background/Objectives: Osteoporosis is common in rheumatoid arthritis (RA), occurring either systemically or locally around inflamed joints. Decreased metacarpal bone density is a known marker of RA progression and hand function impairment. Although RA is generally characterized by symmetrical arthritis, some patients exhibit asymmetrical joint involvement. This study investigates the frequency of unilateral metacarpal bone density reduction in RA patients and aims to identify associated factors. **Methods**: This study included 143 RA patients (107 females, mean age 62.4 yrs., mean disease duration 11.1 yrs.). Bilateral hand X-rays were used to measure the cortical thickness rate (CTR) of the 2nd to 4th metacarpals. Unilateral bone density reduction was defined as a thin-to-thick-side CTR ratio (CTRR) < 0.8. Associations between CTR reduction and unilateral wrist joint damage (WJD) were analyzed. **Results**: Unilateral CTR reduction (CTRR < 0.8) was observed in 16.8% of patients, significantly associated with unilateral WJD. Among patients with unilateral WJD, 50.0% showed CTRR lateral (+) compared to 10.1% without unilateral WJD ($p < 0.01$). ANCOVA revealed significant effects of WJD laterality on CTRR, with an interaction effect showing greater CTRR laterality when thin-side WJD was present without thick-side WJD. Post-biologic treatment, CTR values decreased in both hands, indicating no improvement in bone density reduction. **Conclusions**: Approximately 17% of RA patients exhibited unilateral relative metacarpal bone density reduction, closely associated with unilateral WJD. This first detailed report on bone density laterality in RA underscores the need for early intervention and rehabilitation strategies in RA patients with hand involvement.

Keywords: rheumatoid arthritis; metacarpal bone density laterality; asymmetric wrist joint damage

1. Introduction

Rheumatoid arthritis (RA) is a chronic inflammatory systemic autoimmune disease characterized by the inflammation of the synovial membrane. While the etiology of RA is unclear, environmental factors, genetic susceptibility, and interactions among multiple immune cells are assumed to be involved in RA pathogenesis [1].

In this era of biological agents, the prognosis of patients with RA has improved. However, the prevalence of osteoporosis in RA patients remains high. Osteoporosis in RA patients likely occurs through two mechanisms: generalized osteoporosis, observed as axial skeletal osteoporosis associated with factors such as immobility, glucocorticoid use, and other comorbidities [2,3]; and localized osteoporosis that develops around the joints due to inflammation and inflammatory mediators, which is observed as cortical bone loss in the diaphysis [4,5]. Research on osteoporosis in RA has mainly focused on generalized bone loss, with less attention to localized loss, seen as cortical reduction around the joints [6,7].

Periarticular osteoporosis, a form of localized osteoporosis, has been identified as one of the characteristics of RA [8,9]. Evidence suggests periarticular osteoporosis occurs early in the course of RA [10] and has been suggested to precede bone erosion [11]. Periarticular osteoporosis is thought to be directly influenced by inflammation, primarily driven by the local release of inflammatory cytokines [12]. Cross-sectional studies showed that bone loss in the diaphysis regions of hand cortical bones was associated with joint damage, suggesting a relationship between these processes. Therefore, periarticular osteoporosis has distinct risk factors compared to systemic osteoporosis, which is primarily induced by immobility and treatments such as glucocorticoids [13–15].

Regarding inflammatory bone loss in the hands, osteoporosis occurs not only in periarticular regions directly affected by arthritis but in the cortical bone of the metacarpal diaphysis. This suggests that inflammation-induced bone loss may extend to adjacent cortical bones even without direct synovial contact [16–18]. Furthermore, decreased bone density in the metacarpals has been reported as a surrogate marker for disease progression [19–21], morbidity [22,23], comorbidity [24,25], and impaired hand function [26], highlighting the importance of its assessment.

Symmetrical arthritis is characteristic of RA and was included in the 1987 Rheumatoid Arthritis Classification criteria [27]. It is defined as simultaneous involvement of the same joint areas on both sides of the body, where bilateral involvement of one or more proximal interphalangeal, metacarpophalangeal, and metatarsophalangeal joints is acknowledged without requiring absolute symmetry. However, studies show that some patients exhibit asymmetrical arthritis [28,29].

We encountered a case of asymmetrical osteoporosis in the metacarpals of a patient presenting with asymmetrical lesions in carpal bones (Figure 1). While decreased bone density in the metacarpal diaphysis is characteristic of RA-associated osteoporosis, whether or not asymmetrical hand arthritis leads to unilateral reduction in hand bone density remains unclear. Based on previously reported methods to evaluate the thickness of metacarpal cortical bone [25,30], we examined the frequency of unilateral cortical bone density reduction in the metacarpal diaphysis. We aimed to determine the frequency of unilateral bone density reduction in RA patients with asymmetrical hand arthritis and to identify contributing factors beyond joint damage that may underlie these differences.

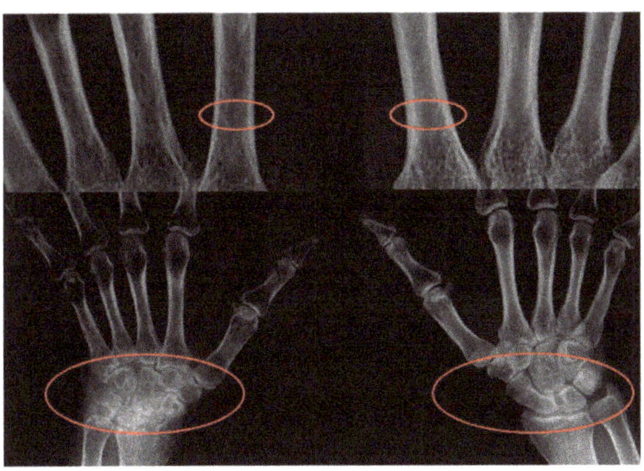

Figure 1. Rheumatoid arthritis patients typically exhibit symmetrical arthritis, though some are known to show asymmetric arthritis. We encountered a patient with asymmetrical osteoporosis of

the metacarpal bones and asymmetrical carpal lesions, which inspired this study. Upper Red Circled Regions: These focus on the cortical bone of the metacarpal diaphysis, showing differences in cortical thickness. The thinning of the cortical bone in these areas is more pronounced on one side, suggesting localized bone loss, often associated with periarticular osteoporosis in rheumatoid arthritis. Lower Red Circled Regions: These highlight the wrist joint areas, illustrating bone erosion, joint space narrowing, or other joint damage. A clear asymmetry between the left and right wrist joints is observed, indicating more severe joint damage on one side, likely due to localized inflammation and progressive joint damage.

2. Materials and Methods

2.1. Subjects

The study participants comprised 143 RA patients (107 females) diagnosed according to 1987 American College of Rheumatology classification criteria for RA [27] and/or 2010 ACR/EULAR classification criteria for RA [31] and treated at Ishikawa Prefectural Central Hospital or Kanazawa University Hospital. Although patients diagnosed before 2010 were initially classified using the 1987 criteria due to the unavailability of the 2010 criteria at that time, all patients met the 2010 ACR/EULAR classification criteria at the time of this investigation.

2.2. Methods

C-reactive protein (CRP), rheumatoid factor (RF), anti-cyclic citrullinated peptide antibodies (anti-CCP), and erythrocyte sedimentation rate were measured from patient serum samples. Swollen and tender joints, patient visual analogue score (VAS), and physician VAS were assessed during physical examinations. Based on these assessments, disease activity indices such as the Clinical Disease Activity Index, Simplified Disease Activity Index, Disease Activity Score in 28 joints with Erythrocyte Sedimentation Rate, and Disease Activity Score in 28 joints with CRP were calculated. In some patients, the Health Assessment Questionnaire was also evaluated. Smoking status, alcohol consumption, and comorbidities, including diabetes mellitus and chronic kidney disease (CKD), were assessed from medical records. Diabetes was defined as its diagnosis prior to or at baseline, or use of oral antidiabetic medications. CKD was defined as estimated glomerular filtration rate < 60 mL/min/1.73 m^2, or persistent kidney abnormalities, such as proteinuria, $\geq$3-months [32]. Dominant hand, and history of hand surgery, were also evaluated in medical records. Regarding medications, the use of nonsteroidal anti-inflammatory drugs, disease-modifying antirheumatic drugs, prednisolone, methotrexate, bisphosphonates, vitamin D supplements, and other anti-osteoporosis drugs was investigated. For patients taking prednisolone or methotrexate, the dosage was recorded. The use of biological agents (infliximab, etanercept, adalimumab, tocilizumab, abatacept, golimumab, and certolizumab pegol) was also evaluated. Additionally, Steinbrocker's staging and functional classification were assessed from medical records [33].

2.3. Radiological Examinations

X-rays of both hands were obtained using Fuji computed radiography (FCR 9000C, Fujifilm Corporation, Tokyo, Japan). Radiographs were examined in the electronic medical record system by one of two blinded readers. The method for evaluating cortical thickness rate (CTR) was based on the techniques described by Roldan et al. [30] and Haara et al. [25]. The outer (periosteal) diameter and inner (endosteal) diameter were measured at the midpoint of the diaphysis in the 2nd to 4th metacarpal bones of both hands. The CTR for each metacarpal was calculated as the thickness of the cortical bone (difference between outer and inner diameters) divided by the outer diameter (Figure 2). The average CTR across the 2nd to 4th metacarpals was then calculated and defined as the CTR for this study. Based on the report by Vehmas et al. [34], CTR < 0.50 was defined as low. CTR was evaluated in both hands and the metacarpal with lower CTR was designated "thin-side" while that with higher was designated "thick-side." The ratio of thin- to thick-side

CTRs was termed CTRR. In the absence of studies on CTRR laterality, from osteoporosis diagnostic criteria [35], we defined CTRR < 0.8 as CTRR lateral (+). Bone damage was classified as Stage II per Steinbrocker's criteria [33]. Wrist joint damage (WJD), including damage of the wrist, carpal bones, and metacarpophalangeal (MP) joints of the 2nd to 4th fingers, was assessed in both hands. For WJD, patients with findings on only one side were classified as WJD lateral (+) and on both or neither side as WJD lateral (−).

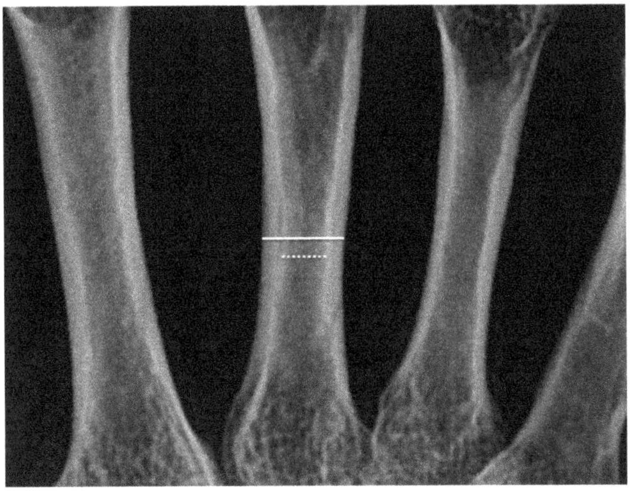

Figure 2. In this radiographic image of the metacarpal bone, the solid white line (upper line in the figure) represents the periosteal (outer) diameter, and the dotted white line (lower line in the figure) represents the endosteal (inner) diameter. These measurements are taken at the midpoint of the diaphysis. Cortical thickness is calculated as the difference between the outer and inner diameters, and the cortical thickness rate (CTR) is calculated by dividing the cortical thickness by the outer diameter.

The formula for CTR is as follows:

$$\text{CTR} = (\text{outer diameter} - \text{inner diameter})/\text{outer diameter}$$

2.4. Statistical Analyses

Results are expressed as mean ± standard deviation for normally distributed data, while non-normally distributed data are presented as median with interquartile ranges (25th percentile [Q1] to 75th percentile [Q3]). For univariate analyses, differences in means between two groups were evaluated using the Mann–Whitney U test for continuous variables. For categorical data, Chi-square or Fisher's exact test was applied. For nonparametric paired data, the Wilcoxon test was used. To evaluate correlations between continuous parametric data, Pearson's correlation test was used. Multivariate analysis was performed using analysis of covariance (ANCOVA). Explanatory variables included those with significant correlations in univariate analysis as well as clinically relevant variables. Variables that did not have a normal distribution were logit-transformed to meet the normality assumption required for statistical analysis. SPSS version 26.0 was used for all statistical analyses with two-tailed $p < 0.05$ deemed statistically significant.

3. Results

3.1. Study Participants

This study included 143 RA patients (107 females, 36 males, mean ± SD: age 62.4 ± 12.1 yrs, disease duration 11.1 ± 9.3 yrs). Demographic data are shown in Table 1. Smoking was reported in 25 patients (17.5%), alcohol consumption in 23 (16.1%), and

126 (88.1%) were right-handed. A history of hand surgery was reported in seven (4.9%), diabetes mellitus in eighteen (12.6%), and chronic kidney disease in six (4.2%) patients. As most study participants were outpatients, disease activity indices indicated remission or low activity (Table 1). Regarding medication, 4.8 ± 4.1 mg/week methotrexate was administered to 95 (66.4%), 1.8 ± 2.3 mg/day prednisolone to 73 (51.0%) and disease-modifying antirheumatic drugs to 47 patients (32.8%). Biologic agents were administered to 56 patients (39.2%). Bisphosphonates were used by forty-three (30.1%), vitamin D supplements by twenty-five (17.3%), and other anti-osteoporosis drugs by three patients (2.1%) (Table 1).

Table 1. Characteristics of study participants.

Variable	Values (n = 143)
Age (yrs.)	Median (IQR): 64 (54–71)
Sex (female/male)	107/36
Disease duration (yrs)	Median (IQR): 8 (4–14)
Height (cm)	156.9 ± 9.4
Weight (kg)	Median (IQR): 52.3 (46.2–61.4)
Body mass index	22.0 ± 3.1
Smoking, n (%)	25 (17.5%)
Alcohol drinking, n (%)	23 (16.1%)
Right-handedness, n (%)	126 (88.1%)
Operation (hand), n (%)	7 (4.9%)
Diabetes mellitus, n (%)	18 (12.6%)
Chronic kidney disease, n (%)	6 (4.2%)
CRP (mg/dL)	Median (IQR): 0.10 (0.00–0.30)
ESR (mm/1 h)	Median (IQR): 16 (9–29)
DAS28-CRP	Median (IQR): 1.73 (1.24–2.40)
DAS28-ESR	2.79 ± 1.10
CDAI	Median (IQR): 2.2 (0–5.16)
SDAI	Median (IQR): 2.4 (0.3–5.5)
RF positive, n (%)	92/113 (81.4%)
ACPA positive, n (%)	53/71 (74.6%)
Methotrexate, n (%)	95 (66.4%)
Dose (mg/week)	4.8 ± 4.1
Prednisolone, n (%)	73 (51.0%)
Dose (mg/day)	1.8 ± 2.5
DMARDs, n (%)	47 (32.8%)
Biologic therapy, n (%)	56 (39.2%)
Bisphosphonate, n (%)	43 (30.1%)
Vitamin D, n (%)	25 (17.5%)
Other anti-osteoporosis drug, n (%)	3 (2.1%)

Median (Q1–Q3): The median value is presented with the interquartile range (25th percentile [Q1] to 75th percentile [Q3]). Mean ± SD: The mean value is presented with its standard deviation (SD). Age (yrs.): Age in years. Sex (female/male): Number of female and male participants. Disease duration (yrs.): Duration of disease in years. Height (cm): Participant height in centimeters. Weight (kg): Participant weight in kilograms. Body mass index: Body mass index calculated as weight (kg) divided by height squared (m^2). Smoking, n (%): Number and percentage of participants who smoke. Alcohol drinking, n (%): Number and percentage of participants who consume alcohol. Right-handedness, n (%): Number and percentage of participants with right-handed dominance. Operation (hand), n (%): Number and percentage of participants who underwent hand surgery. Diabetes mellitus, n (%): Number and percentage of participants with diabetes. Chronic kidney disease, n (%): Number and percentage of participants with chronic kidney disease. CRP (mg/dL): C-reactive protein levels in milligrams per deciliter. ESR (mm/1 h): Erythrocyte sedimentation rate in millimeters per hour. DAS28-CRP: Disease Activity Score in 28 joints with CRP. DAS28-ESR: Disease Activity Score in 28 joints with Erythrocyte Sedimentation Rate. CDAI: Clinical Disease Activity Index. SDAI: Simplified Disease Activity Index. RF positive, n (%): Number and percentage of participants testing positive for rheumatoid factor. ACPA positive, n (%): Number and percentage of participants testing positive for anti-citrullinated protein antibody. Methotrexate, n (%): Number and percentage of participants treated with methotrexate. Dose (mg/week): Weekly dose of methotrexate in milligrams. Prednisolone, n (%): Number and percentage of participants treated with prednisolone. Dose (mg/day): Daily dose of prednisolone in milligrams. DMARDs, n (%): Number and percentage of participants treated with disease-modifying antirheumatic drugs (DMARDs). Biologic therapy, n (%): Number and percentage of participants receiving biologic therapies. Bisphosphonate, n (%): Number and percentage of participants treated with bisphosphonates f. Vitamin D, n (%): Number and percentage of participants treated with vitamin D. Other anti-osteoporosis drug, n (%): Number and percentage of participants treated with non-bisphosphonate anti-osteoporosis drugs.

3.2. Metacarpal CTR

The mean bilateral CTR of the 2nd to 4th metacarpals was 0.423 ± 0.123, with the thin-side being 0.399 ± 0.125 and the thick-side 0.446 ± 0.124, making CTRR 0.890 ± 0.088. CTR < 0.500 was observed in 114 patients (79.7%) on the thin-side and 95 (66.4%) on the thick-side. In total, 19 patients (13.2%) showed CTR < 0.500 exclusively on the thin-side and 29 (20.3%) $\geq$ 0.500 on both sides (Table 2).

Table 2. Characteristics of study participants.

	Values (*n* = 143)
Thin-side CTR	0.399 ± 0.125
Thick-side CTR	0.446 ± 0.124
Mean of thin- and thick-side CTRs	0.423 ± 0.123
Low CTR (thin-side), n (%)	114 (79.7%)
Low CTR (thick-side), n (%)	95 (66.4%)
Low CTR (only thin-side), n (%)	19 (13.2%)
Normal CTR (both thin- and thick-sides), n (%)	29 (20.3%)
Joint damage	
Wrist joint: none, n (%)	77 (53.8%)
Wrist joint: unilateral, n (%)	24 (16.7%)
Wrist joint: bilateral, n (%)	42 (29.4%)
2nd MP joint: none, n (%)	113 (79.0%)
2nd MP joint: unilateral, n (%)	8 (5.6%)
2nd MP joint: bilateral, n (%)	22 (15.4%)
3rd MP joint: none, n (%)	117 (81.8%)
3rd MP joint: unilateral, n (%)	12 (8.4%)
3rd MP joint: bilateral, n (%)	14 (9.8)
4th MP joint: none, n (%)	122 (85.3%)
4th MP joint: unilateral, n (%)	12 (8.4%)
4th MP joint: bilateral, n (%)	8 (5.6%)

Mean ± SD: The mean value is presented with its standard deviation (SD). CTR: cortical thickness rate. In each patient, the side with the lower cortical thickness rate (CTR) of the metacarpals was designated the "thin-side" and that with the higher CTR the "thick-side". Low CTR (thin-side), n (%): proportion of cases with CTR < 0.50 on the thin-side. Low CTR (thick-side), n (%): proportion of cases with CTR < 0.50 on the thick-side. Low CTR (only thin-side), n (%): proportion of cases with CTR < 0.50 on thin-side only. Normal CTR (both thin- and thick-side), n (%): proportion of cases with CTR > 0.50 on both sides. Wrist joint/2nd–4th MP joint: none, n (%): No lesions detected. Wrist joint/2nd–4th MP joint: unilateral, n (%): Lesions present on one side (right or left). Wrist joint/2nd–4th MP joint: bilateral, n (%): Lesions present on both sides (right and left). MP joint: Metacarpophalangeal joint.

3.3. Damage to Wrist and Metacarpophalangeal Joints

Regarding WJD, 77 patients (53.8%) showed none, 24 (16.8%) showed unilateral and 42 (29.4%) bilateral damage. For MP joints, the figures were as follows: 2nd MP joint—one hundred and thirteen (79.0%), eight (5.6%), and twenty-two (15.4%) patients; 3rd MP joint—one hundred and seventeen (81.8%), twelve (8.4%), and fourteen (9.8%); and 4th MP joint—one hundred and twenty-two (85.9%), twelve (8.5%), and eight patients (5.6%), respectively (Table 2).

3.4. Unilateral Reduction of Metacarpal CTR

CTRR lateral (+) was observed in 24 patients (16.8%). Among the 20 patients with known hand dominance, 10 showed reduced cortical thickness on the dominant side, and

10 on the non-dominant side. A total of 119 patients (83.2%) had CTRR $\geq$ 0.8, classified as CTRR lateral (−). CTRR showed a non-normal distribution; therefore, a logit transformation was applied to approximate normality. This approximation was confirmed by examining the histogram of the transformed data (Figure 3).

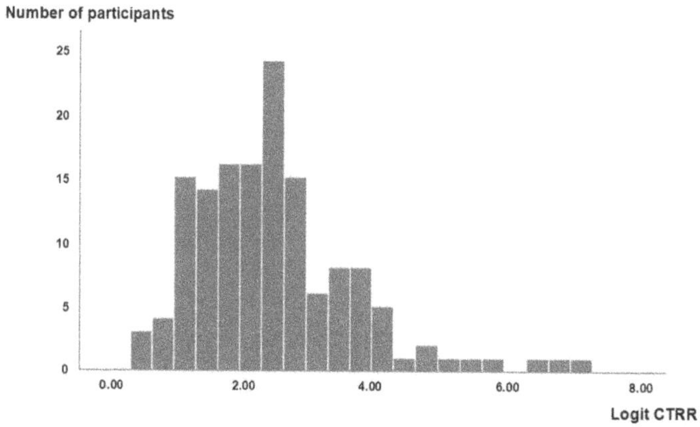

Figure 3. Histogram of Logit CTRR values. This histogram shows the distribution of Logit CTRR values. The x-axis represents Logit CTRR values, ranging from approximately 0 to 8, and the y-axis indicates the frequency of occurrences in each range. The distribution of this histogram closely approximates a normal distribution.

3.5. Comparative Analysis of Laterality in Metacarpal CTR and WJD

In patients with WJD, a Chi-square test revealed a significant association between WJD and metacarpal CTR laterality where 50.0% of patients classified as WJD lateral (+) were also CTRR lateral (+), compared to only 10.1% of those classified as WJD lateral (−). Thus, unilateral WJD was associated with an almost 5-fold higher frequency of laterality in metacarpal cortical thickness. While this strong association was observed between CTR and WJD laterality ($p < 0.01$, Table 3), no significant association was found between WJD laterality and hand dominance, nor between WJD laterality and other parameters. In additional analysis, we compared 102 patients diagnosed with the 1987 criteria and later meeting the 2010 criteria (Old group), with 41 patients meeting the 2010 criteria from the start (New group). CTR lateral (+) was observed in twenty of the Old group and four of the New group with no significant difference between these groups (Chi-square test, $p = 0.24$). These findings suggest that the diagnostic criteria did not influence CTRR laterality (Supplementary Data, Table S1).

Table 3. Comparison of laterality in wrist joint damage and cortical thickness rate ratio (CTRR) in RA Patients.

	WJD Lateral (+)	WJD Lateral (−)	
CTRR lateral (+)	12	12	24
CTRR lateral (−)	12	107	119
	24	119	143

CTRR: cortical thickness rate ratio = CTR (thin-side)/CTR (thick-side). CTRR lateral (+) = CTRR < 0.8. CTRR lateral (−) = CTRR $\geq$ 0.8. WJD: wrist joint damage. WJD lateral (+) = WJD in one hand. WJD lateral (−) = WJD in both hands or no hand. WJD lateral (+) and CTRR lateral (+) were significantly related: χ^2 test ($p < 0.001$).

3.6. Relationship Between Thin- and Thick-Side CTRs, Logit CTRR, and Various Parameters (ANCOVA)

ANCOVA were conducted using thin- and thick-side CTRs as dependent variables to assess the effects of wrist joint lesions, sex (female), handedness, age, and interactions between thin- and thick-side WJDs. No significant interaction between thin- and thick-side WJDs was observed. Age was significant in both analyses ($p < 0.001$), whereas high p-values for sex and handedness indicated adjustment was unnecessary (Analysis 1, Table 4). ANCOVA was repeated with thin- and thick-side CTRs as dependent variables adjusted for age, excluding sex and handedness as parameters. Consistently, no significant interaction effect between thin- and thick-side WJDs was observed (Analysis 2, Table 4). Additional analyses were conducted excluding the interaction between thin- and thick-side WJDs. For thin-side CTR, significant effects were observed for thin-side WJD (p = 0.004), thick-side WJD (p = 0.005), and age ($p < 0.001$). For thick-side CTR, significant effects were found for thick-side WJD ($p < 0.001$) and age ($p < 0.001$), while no significant effect for thin-side WJD was observed (p = 0.627) (Analysis 3, Table 4). Further multiple comparisons were performed. For thin-side CTR, a significant difference was observed based on presence or absence of thin-side WJD (main effect test: p = 0.005, estimated marginal mean CTR difference of 0.05637) and thick-side WJD (main effect test: p = 0.004, estimated marginal mean CTR difference of 0.06035) (Table 5). For thick-side CTR, no significant difference was found based on presence or absence of thin-side WJD (main effect test: p = 0.627, mean CTR difference of 0.00956); however, a significant difference was observed for presence or absence of thick-side WJD (main effect test: $p < 0.001$, estimated marginal mean CTR difference of 0.093) (Table 5). ANCOVA was conducted with Logit CTRR as the dependent variable. Following the approach used in Analysis 2 for thin- and thick-side CTRs, adjustments were made for age, and the effects of thin-side WJD, thick-side WJD, and their interaction were examined. Neither age, thin-side WJD, nor thick-side WJD showed statistical significance, whereas interaction between thin- and thick-side WJDs was significant (Table 4). Further multiple comparisons were performed. In the simple main effects test, when thick-side WJD was absent, Logit CTRR was significantly lower in the presence of thin-side WJD compared to its absence (mean difference: −1.461, OR: 0.232, $p < 0.001$). When thin-side WJD was present, Logit CTRR was significantly higher in the presence of thick-side WJD compared to its absence (mean difference: 0.833, OR: 2.300, p = 0.014). In contrast, no significant difference in Logit CTRR was observed between the presence and absence of thin-side WJD when thick-side WJD was present or between presence and absence of thick-side WJD when thin-side WJD was absent (Table 5). Additional analyses revealed that neither rheumatoid factor (RF) and/or anti-CCP Ab nor prednisolone use had a significant impact on thin-CTR, thick-CTR or CTRR (Supplementary Data, Tables S2 and S3). Prednisolone use had also no significant impact on the laterality of joint damage (Supplementary Data, Table S4).

Table 4. Analysis of covariance between thin-side CTR, thick-side CTR, Logit CTRR, and associated parameters.

		Analysis 1			Analysis 2			Analysis 3		
		F	df	p-value	F	df	p-value	F	df	p-value
Thin-side CTR	Age	63.54	1, 125	<0.001 **	72.18	1, 138	<0.001 **	72.78	1, 139	<0.001 **
	Sex (Female)	0.99	1, 125	0.32		not included			not included	
	Dominant hand	0.00	1, 125	0.95		not included			not included	
	Thin-side WJD	334.40	1, 8.041	<0.001 **	33.60	1, 1.060	0.10	8.00	1, 136	0.005 **
	Thick-side WJD	114.22	1, 8.041	<0.001 **	46.58	1, 1.030	0.09	8.69	1, 139	0.004 **
	Interaction †	0.01	1, 125	0.92	0.19	1, 138	0.67		not included	
		Analysis 1			Analysis 2			Analysis 3		
		F	df	p-value	F	df	p-value	F	df	p-value
Thick-side CTR	Age	72.78	1, 125	<0.001 **	86.36	1, 138	<0.001 **	86.22	1, 139	<0.001 **
	Sex (Female)	0.91	1, 125	0.34		not included			not included	
	Dominant hand	0.00	1, 125	0.96		not included			not included	
	Thin-side WJD	1.83	1, 1.028	0.40	0.72	1, 1.014	0.55	0.24	1, 139	0.63
	Thick-side WJD	6.64	1, 1.023	0.23	23.74	1, 1.007	0.13	21.10	1, 139	<0.001 **
	Interaction †	1.28	1, 125	0.26	0.77	1, 138	0.38		not included	

Table 4. *Cont.*

		Analysis 2		
		F	df	p-value
Logit CTRR	Age	0.41	1, 138	0.52
	Thin-side WJD	2.95	1, 1.003	0.34
	Thick-side WJD	0.30	1, 1.001	0.68
	Interaction †	3.94	1, 138	<0.05 *

CTR: cortical thickness rate. In each patient, the side with the lower cortical thickness rate (CTR) of the metacarpals was designated the "thin-side" and that with the higher CTR the "thick-side". WJD: wrist joint damage. CTRR: cortical thickness rate ratio = CTR (thin-side)/CTR (thick-side). Logit CTRR = ln {CTRR/(1-CTRR)}. To approximate a normal distribution for analysis of covariance (ANCOVA), CTRR was transformed using logit transformation. This involved applying the logit function to CTRR values, defined as: Logit CTRR = ln {CTRR/(1-CTRR)}. Interaction †: interaction between thin- and thick-side WJDs. Analysis 1: ANCOVA with the following dependent variable and factors: age, sex (female), dominant hand, WJD thin-side, WJD thick-side, and interaction between thin- and thick-side WJDs. Analysis 2: ANCOVA with the following dependent variable and factors: age, WJD thin-side, WJD thick-side, and interaction between thin- and thick-side WJDs. (excluding sex (female) and dominant hand in Analysis 1). Analysis 3: ANCOVA with the following dependent variable and factors: age, WJD thin-side, WJD thick-side (excluding interaction between thin- and thick-side WJDs in Analysis 2). F: F-value. df: degrees of freedom, expressed as F (df1, df2), where df1 is df for the factor between-groups and df2 is df for the error within-groups. *: significant, p-value < 0.05. **: significant, p-value < 0.01.

Table 5. Effect of WJD on thin-side CTR, thick-side CTR, and CTRR: post-hoc analysis of ANCOVA.

	Thinner side CTR, Analysis 3					
	Thick-side WJD (−)	Thick-side WJD (+)	EM mean	Main effect		p-value
Thin-side WJD (−)	0.443	0.383	0.413	−0.056		0.005 **
Thin-side WJD (+)	0.387	0.326	0.356			
EM mean	0.415	0.354				
Main effect	−0.060					
p-value	0.004 **					
	Thicker side CTR, Analysis 3					
	Thick-side WJD (−)	Thick-side WJD (+)	EM mean	Main effect		p-value
Thin-side WJD (−)	0.482	0.390	0.436	−0.010		0.63
Thin-side WJD (+)	0.473	0.380	0.426			
EM mean	0.477	0.385				
Main effect	−0.093					
p-value	<0.001 **					
	Logit CTRR, Analysis 2					
	Thick-side WJD (−)	Thick-side WJD (+)		Simple main effect	OR	p-value
Thin-side WJD (−)	2.883 a	2.642 b	b-a	−0.242	0.785	0.57
Thin-side WJD(+)	1.423 c	2.255 d	d-c	0.833	2.300	0.014 *
	c-a	d-b				
Simple main effect	−1.461	−0.386				
OR	0.232	0.680				
p-value	<0.001 **	0.38				

In each patient, the side with the lower cortical thickness rate (CTR) of the metacarpals was designated the "thin-side" and that with the higher CTR the "thick-side". WJD: wrist joint damage. CTRR: cortical thickness rate ratio = CTR (thin-side)/CTR (thick-side). Logit CTRR = ln {CTRR/(1-CTRR)}. To ensure normality of variables for the analysis of covariance (ANCOVA), the variable CTRR was transformed using a logit transformation. This process involved applying the logit function to CTRR values, defined as: Logit CTRR = ln {CTRR/(1-CTRR)}. Analysis 1: ANCOVA with the following dependent variable and factors: age, sex (female), dominant hand, WJD thin-side, WJD thick-side, and interaction between thin- and thick-side WJDs. Analysis 2: ANCOVA with the following dependent variable and factors: age, WJD thin-side, WJD thick-side, and interaction between thin- and thick-side WJDs. (excluding sex (female) and dominant hand in Analysis 1). Analysis 3: ANCOVA with the following dependent variable and factors: age, WJD thin-side, WJD thick-side (excluding interaction between thin- and thick-side WJDs in Analysis 2). EM = estimated marginal mean, the adjusted mean accounting for covariates in the ANCOVA model. OD: odds ratio. *: significant, p-value < 0.05. **: significant, p-value < 0.01.

3.7. CTR Evaluation in Right and Left Hands Pre- and Post-Biologic Therapy in 30 Patients

In 30 patients, CTR was evaluated in both hands pre- and post-biologic therapy. CTR significantly decreased from 0.460 ± 0.105 to 0.413 ± 0.107 in the right hand and from 0.457 ± 0.106 to 0.423 ± 0.113 in the left hand (Table 6). Among patients with CTR ≥ 0.50 at baseline, significant reductions were also observed: right hand from 0.569 ± 0.275 to

0.497 ± 0.0855 and left hand from 0.567 ± 0.390 to 0.506 ± 0.102 (Table 6). Analysis of 30 cases revealed that the duration of biologic agent administration had no significant effect on CTRs (Supplementary Data, Table S5), and differences in effects among agents could not be evaluated due to small sample sizes.

Table 6. CTR of right and left hands pre- and post-biologic therapy.

	Pre-Biologics	Post-Biologics	Number	*p*-Value
CTR (right)	0.460 ± 0.105	0.413 ± 0.107	30	<0.001 **
CTR (left)	0.457 ± 0.106	0.423 ± 0.113	30	0.029 *
CTR (right) #	0.569 ± 0.275	0.497 ± 0.855	11	0.018 *
CTR (left) #	0.567 ± 0.390	0.506 ± 0.102	10	0.041 *

#: CTR ≥ 0.50 at baseline. *: significant, p-value < 0.05. **: significant, p-value < 0.01.

4. Discussion

Metacarpal bone density decrease was bilateral in 66.4% and relatively unilateral in 16.8% of the RA patients studied. The latter was closely associated with ipsilateral WJD, suggesting asymmetrical WJD is involved in unilateral decreased metacarpal bone density.

Roldan et al. [30] reported that cortical bone loss in the metacarpals of RA patients correlated with the length of the observation period, identifying erythrocyte sedimentation rate and total steroid dosage as independent factors in multivariate analysis. This demonstrated an association between systemic inflammation and decreased metacarpal bone density. In our study, Logit CTRR was analyzed as the dependent variable using ANCOVA, adjusted for age and including thin-side WJD, thick-side WJD, and their interaction. Age, thin-side WJD, and thick-side WJD were not significant factors, whereas the interaction was. Further multiple comparisons showed that under conditions without thick-side WJD, Logit CTRR was significantly lower when thin-side WJD was present than when absent (mean difference: −1.461, OR: 0.232, $p < 0.001$). With thin-side WJD present, Logit CTRR was significantly higher when thick-side WJD was also present (mean difference: 0.833, OR: 2.300, $p = 0.014$). The lowest Logit CTRR, indicating the greatest laterality in CTR, was observed when thick-side WJD was absent and thin-side WJD was present. This suggests unilateral WJD is reflected in the laterality of CTR. Previous research has shown that inflammatory bone loss in periarticular osteoporosis of the hand affects not only periarticular regions but the cortical bone of the metacarpal diaphysis, independent of direct synovial contact [15,17,18]. Our findings suggest inflammation in the hand joints, likely through localized cytokine release, contributed to reduction in cortical bone density of the ipsilateral metacarpal diaphysis.

RA is generally characterized by symmetrical joint involvement [36], but asymmetrical arthritis has been reported in some patients [28,29,37]. Halla et al. [37] examined small joints of the hands and feet and found asymmetrical involvement was common, with 90% of wrist joints showing symmetrical involvement and 10% asymmetry. Similarly, Zangger et al. [29] found asymmetrical joint involvement in small joints of the hands and feet in 13–16% of cases. In our study, unilateral WJD was observed in 24 patients (16.8%), consistent with previous reports, suggesting that localized factors such as cytokine release may contribute to asymmetrical metacarpal bone density reduction. Koh JH [38] and Yaku A [39] reported faster bone destruction progression in the dominant hand. However, in our study, we observed no significant difference between right and left sides nor any effect by hand dominance. This may be due to the use of different radiographic methods or that only six of the one hundred and thirty-two patients with hand dominance recorded were left-handed, preventing reliable statistical analysis of handedness. The potential contribution of repetitive manual tasks to localized joint stress and asymmetry has been reported previously [40]. Although we did not collect detailed occupational data in our cohort, this hypothesis may provide a possible explanation for the risk of asymmetric joint damage and bone density reduction. Genetic predispositions—such as the involvement of HLA-DR4 in rheumatoid arthritis [41] and WNT16 in cortical bone thickness [42]—may contribute to asymmetric joint damage and bone density reduction. However, genetic marker data were not collected in this study, representing a limitation for future investigation.

CTR values for both right and left hands were evaluated pre- and post-administration of biologic agents in 30 patients. CTR was significantly decreased post-treatment even in patients with baseline CTR $\geq$ 50 (Table 6). Hoff et al. [43] evaluated the effect of adalimumab on metacarpal bone loss, finding a significant reduction in bone loss rate in their adalimumab + MTX treatment group compared to MTX monotherapy, though without improvement in bone density. Bone loss rates of 1.15%, 2.16%, and 3.03% were observed at 26, 52, and 104 weeks, respectively. Their results match our finding of no improvement in metacarpal bone density by biologic treatment, suggesting that systemic effects beyond local joint inflammation were not fully suppressed, leading to continued CTR decrease. CTR evaluation should consider both local and systemic effects. Aggressive RA treatment with biologic agents may be necessary to suppress cytokine release from wrist joints before CTR decline begins. Additionally, Baker et al. [44] reported that muscle loss contributes to cortical bone density reduction, suggesting that rehabilitation interventions could also be beneficial. The early detection of unilateral bone erosions using MRI, followed by intensive treatment, may offer a viable strategy for managing asymmetric joint damage. While biological agents were ineffective in preventing cortical bone loss in this study, the potential of JAK inhibitors to suppress early arthritis and mitigate asymmetric joint damage deserves further exploration in future studies.

This study has several limitations. First, it involved a relatively small sample size from two institutions. Second, as the study focused on outpatients with relatively stable disease, the findings may not apply to all RA patients in terms of disease control. These factors may limit the generalizability of the results. Third, the single time-point analysis prevented assessment of longitudinal change in cortical bone or wrist joint damage. Fourth, image evaluation was performed manually using Fuji computed radiography, rather than computer-assisted digital X-ray radiogram (DXR), which may have introduced observer bias. Fifth, the lack of detailed occupational data may have limited a deeper understanding of the potential influence of repetitive manual tasks on joint stress and asymmetry. Future studies should include larger more diverse populations, use technologies such as DXR, and include longitudinal assessments to strengthen the findings.

5. Conclusions

This study is the first to report that a substantial number of RA patients exhibited decreased metacarpal bone density, with a subset displaying unilateral bone loss. Additionally, the relationship between unilateral bone loss and wrist joint damage was identified for the first time. Wrist joint inflammation was found to be associated with cortical bone loss in the metacarpals, suggesting that local cytokine release contributed to this reduction. Despite biologic treatment, no improvement in metacarpal bone loss was observed. Although previous reports have discussed reduced metacarpal bone density in RA patients, no detailed studies had focused on laterality or asymmetry until this report.

Supplementary Materials: The following supporting information can be downloaded at: https://www.mdpi.com/article/10.3390/jcm13247652/s1, Table S1: Comparison of CTRR Laterality (+/−) and Grouping by Old/New Classification in RA Patients; Table S2: Analysis of covariance between thin-side CTR, thick-side CTR, Logit CTRR and associated parameters including RF and/or CCP; Table S3: Analysis of covariance between Logit CTRR and associated parameters including prednisolone; Table S4: Comparison of Laterality in Wrist Joint Damage and Prednisolone administration in RA Patients; Table S5: Analysis of covariance between differences of thin-side CTR and thick-side CTR and duration of treatment with biologic agents.

Author Contributions: Conceptualization: T.Z. and M.K. (Mitsuhiro Kawano); methodology: A.N. and T.Z.; formal analysis: A.N.; investigation: A.N. and T.Z.; writing—original draft preparation: A.N.; writing—review and editing: I.M., H.F., M.K. (Masahiro Kuroda), and M.K. (Mitsuhiro Kawano);

supervision: H.N. and M.K (Mitsuhiro Kawano). All authors have read and agreed to the published version of the manuscript.

Funding: This research received no external funding.

Institutional Review Board Statement: The study was conducted in accordance with the Declaration of Helsinki and was approved by the Ethics Committee of Kanazawa University Hospital (approval number: 3440-1, approved on 13 August 2020) and the Ethics Committee of Ishikawa Prefectural Central Hospital (approval number: 1330, approved on 28 May 2019).

Informed Consent Statement: Informed consent was obtained using an opt-out approach, as this study was observational in nature. Participants received information regarding the study, and those who did not wish to participate were given the option to withdraw without any penalties.

Data Availability Statement: The data presented in this study are available upon reasonable request from the corresponding author. Due to privacy restrictions, data containing patient information are not publicly available.

Conflicts of Interest: The authors declare no conflicts of interest.

References

1. Gravallese, E.M.; Firestein, G.S. Rheumatoid arthritis—Common origins, divergent mechanisms. *N. Engl. J. Med.* **2023**, *388*, 529–542. [CrossRef] [PubMed]
2. Gough, A.K.; Lilley, J.; Eyre, S.; Holder, R.L.; Emery, P. Generalised bone loss in patients with early rheumatoid arthritis. *Lancet* **1994**, *344*, 23–27. [CrossRef]
3. Kroot, E.J.; Nieuwenhuizen, M.G.; de Waal Malefijt, M.C.; van Riel, P.L.; Pasker-de Jong, P.C.; Laan, R.F. Change in bone mineral density in patients with rheumatoid arthritis during the first decade of the disease. *Arthritis Rheum.* **2001**, *44*, 1254–1260. [CrossRef]
4. Laan, R.F.; Buijs, W.C.; Verbeek, A.L.; Draad, M.P.; Corstens, F.H.; van de Putte, L.B.; van Riel, P.L. Bone mineral density in patients with recent onset rheumatoid arthritis: Influence of disease activity and functional capacity. *Ann. Rheum. Dis.* **1993**, *52*, 21–26. [CrossRef]
5. Chan, E.; Pandith, V.; Towheed, T.E.; Brouillard, D.; Zee, B.; Anastassiades, T.P. Comparison of the combined cortical thickness of the second metacarpal with Sharp's method for scoring hand microradiographs in rheumatoid arthritis. *J. Rheumatol.* **1998**, *25*, 1290–1294. [PubMed]
6. Bayraktar, H.H.; Morgan, E.F.; Niebur, G.L.; Morris, G.E.; Wong, E.K.; Keaveny, T.M. Comparison of the elastic and yield properties of human femoral trabecular and cortical bone tissue. *J. Biomech.* **2004**, *37*, 27–35. [CrossRef] [PubMed]
7. Aguado, F.; Revilla, M.; Villa, L.F.; Rico, H. Cortical bone resorption in osteoporosis. *Calcif. Tissue Int.* **1997**, *60*, 323–326. [CrossRef] [PubMed]
8. Böttcher, J.; Pfeil, A.; Heinrich, B.; Lehmann, G.; Petrovitch, A.; Hansch, A.; Heyne, J.; Mentzel, H.; Malich, A.; Hein, G.; et al. Digital radiogrammetry as a new diagnostic tool for estimation of disease-related osteoporosis in rheumatoid arthritis compared with pQCT. *Rheumatol. Int.* **2005**, *25*, 457–464. [CrossRef]
9. Bottcher, J.; Pfeil, A. Diagnosis of periarticular osteoporosis in rheumatoid arthritis using digital X-ray radiogrammetry. *Arthritis Res. Ther.* **2008**, *10*, 103. [CrossRef]
10. Alenfeld, F.E.; Diessel, E.; Brezger, M.; Sieper, J.; Felsenberg, D.; Braun, J. Detailed analyses of periarticular osteoporosis in rheumatoid arthritis. *Osteoporos. Int.* **2000**, *11*, 400–407. [CrossRef] [PubMed]
11. Deodhar, A.A.; Brabyn, J.; Jones, P.W.; Davis, M.J.; Woolf, A.D. Longitudinal study of hand bone densitometry in rheumatoid arthritis. *Arthritis Rheum.* **1995**, *38*, 1204–1210. [CrossRef] [PubMed]
12. Sambrook, P.N. The skeleton in rheumatoid arthritis: Common mechanisms for bone erosion and osteoporosis. *J. Rheumatol.* **2000**, *27*, 2541–2542. [PubMed]
13. Dolan, A.L.; Moniz, C.; Abraha, H.; Pitt, P. Does active treatment of rheumatoid arthritis limit disease-associated bone loss. *Rheumatology* **2002**, *41*, 1047–1051. [CrossRef]
14. Wolfe, F.; Sharp, J.T. Radiographic outcome of recent-onset rheumatoid arthritis: A 19-year study of radiographic progression. *Arthritis Rheum.* **1998**, *41*, 1571–1582. [CrossRef] [PubMed]
15. Lems, W.F. Bisphosphonates and glucocorticoids: Effects on bone quality. *Arthritis Rheum.* **2007**, *56*, 3518–3522. [CrossRef] [PubMed]
16. Kong, Y.Y.; Feige, U.; Sarosi, I.; Bolon, B.; Tafuri, A.; Morony, S.; Capparelli, C.; Li, J.; Elliott, R.; McCabe, S.; et al. Activated T cells regulate bone loss and joint destruction in adjuvant arthritis through osteoprotegerin ligand. *Nature* **1999**, *402*, 304–309. [CrossRef] [PubMed]
17. Haugeberg, G.; Ørstavik, R.E.; Kvien, T.K. Effects of rheumatoid arthritis on bone. *Curr. Opin. Rheumatol.* **2003**, *15*, 469–475. [CrossRef]

18. Güler-Yüksel, M.; Allaart, C.F.; Goekoop-Ruiterman, Y.P.M.; de Vries-Bouwstra, J.K.; van Groenendael, J.H.L.M.; Mallée, C.; de Bois, M.H.W.; Breedveld, F.C.; Dijkmans, B.A.C.; Lems, W.F. Changes in hand and generalised bone mineral density in patients with recent-onset rheumatoid arthritis. *Ann. Rheum. Dis.* **2009**, *68*, 330–336. [CrossRef] [PubMed]
19. Kalla, A.A.; Meyers, O.L.; Chalton, D.; Heath, S.; Brown, G.M.M.; Smith, P.R.; Burger, M.C. Increased metacarpal bone mass following 18 months of slow-acting antirheumatic drugs for rheumatoid arthritis. *Br. J. Rheumatol.* **1991**, *30*, 91–100. [CrossRef]
20. Jensen, T.; Hansen, M.; Jensen, K.E.; Podenphant, J.; Hansen, T.M.; Hyldstrup, L. Comparison of dual X-ray absorptiometry (DXA), digital X-ray radiogrammetry (DXR), and conventional radiographs in the evaluation of osteoporosis and bone erosions in patients with rheumatoid arthritis. *Scand. J. Rheumatol.* **2005**, *34*, 27–33. [CrossRef]
21. Pfeil, A.; Haugeberg, G.; Renz, D.M.; Reinhardt, L.; Jung, C.; Franz, M.; Wolf, G.; Böttcher, J. Digital X-ray radiogrammetry and its sensitivity and specificity for the identification of rheumatoid arthritis-related cortical hand bone loss. *J. Bone Min. Metab.* **2017**, *35*, 192–198. [CrossRef]
22. Hoff, M.; Haugeberg, G.; Kvien, T.K. Hand bone loss as an outcome measure in established rheumatoid arthritis: 2-year observational study comparing cortical and total bone loss. *Arthritis Res. Ther.* **2007**, *9*, R81. [CrossRef] [PubMed]
23. Book, C.; Algulin, J.; Nilsson, J.A.; Saxne, T.; Jacobsson, L. Bone mineral density in the hand as a predictor for mortality in patients with rheumatoid arthritis. *Rheumatology* **2009**, *48*, 1088–1091. [CrossRef]
24. Wilczek, M.L.; Kälvesten, J.; Algulin, J.; Beiki, O.; Brismar, T.B. Digital X-ray radiogrammetry of hand or wrist radiographs can predict hip fracture risk—A study in 5,420 women and 2,837 men. *Eur. Radiol.* **2013**, *23*, 1383–1391. [CrossRef] [PubMed]
25. Haara, M.; Heliövaara, M.; Impivaara, O.; A Arokoski, J.P.; Manninen, P.; Knekt, P.; Kärkkäinen, A.; Reunanen, A.; Aromaa, A.; Kröger, H. Low metacarpal index predicts hip fracture: A prospective population study of 3,561 subjects with 15 years of follow-up. *Acta Orthop.* **2006**, *77*, 9–14. [CrossRef]
26. Towheed, T.E.; Brouillard, D.; Yendt, E.; Anastassiades, T. Osteoporosis in rheumatoid arthritis: Findings in the metacarpal, spine, and hip and a study of the determinants of both localized and generalized osteopenia. *J. Rheumatol.* **1995**, *22*, 440–443.
27. Arnett, F.C.; Edworthy, S.M.; Bloch, D.A.; Mcshane, D.J.; Fries, J.F.; Cooper, N.S.; Healey, L.A.; Kaplan, S.R.; Liang, M.H.; Luthra, H.S. The American Rheumatism Association 1987 revised criteria for the classification of rheumatoid arthritis. *Arthritis Rheum.* **1988**, *31*, 315–324. [CrossRef] [PubMed]
28. Hamilton, S. Unilateral rheumatoid arthritis in hemiplegia. *J. Can. Assoc. Radiol.* **1983**, *34*, 49–50. [PubMed]
29. Zangger, P.; Keystone, E.C.; Bogoch, E.R. Asymmetry of small joint involvement in rheumatoid arthritis: Prevalence and tendency towards symmetry over time. *Jt. Bone Spine.* **2005**, *72*, 241–247. [CrossRef] [PubMed]
30. Roldan, J.F.; Del Rincon, I.; Escalante, A. Loss of cortical bone from the metacarpal diaphysis in patients with rheumatoid arthritis: Independent effects of systemic inflammation and glucocorticoids. *J. Rheumatol.* **2006**, *33*, 508–516.
31. Aletaha, D.; Neogi, T.; Silman, A.J.; Funovits, J.; Felson, D.T.; Bingham, C.O.; Birnbaum, N.S.; Burmester, G.R.; Bykerk, V.P.; Cohen, M.D.; et al. 2010 rheumatoid arthritis classification criteria: An American College of Rheumatology/European League Against Rheumatism collaborative initiative. *Ann. Rheum. Dis.* **2010**, *69*, 1580–1588. [CrossRef]
32. Levin, A.; Stevens, P.E. Summary of KDIGO 2012 CKD Guideline: Behind the scenes, need for guidance, and a framework for moving forward. *Kidney Int.* **2014**, *85*, 49–61. [CrossRef] [PubMed]
33. Steinbrocker, O.; Traeger, C.H.; Batterman, R.C. Therapeutic criteria in rheumatoid arthritis. *J. Am. Med. Assoc.* **1949**, *140*, 659–662. [CrossRef]
34. Vehmas, T.; Solovieva, S.; Riihimaki, H.; Luoma, K.; Leino-Arjas, P. Hand workload and the metacarpal cortical index. a study of middle-aged teachers and dentists. *Osteoporos. Int.* **2005**, *16*, 672–680. [CrossRef]
35. Hagino, H. Revised osteoporosis diagnostic criteria and Japanese practice guideline on osteoporosis. *Clin. Calcium.* **2014**, *24*, 11–18. [PubMed]
36. Clarke, G.S.; Buckland-Wright, J.C.; Grahame, R. Symmetry of radiological features in the wrist and hands of patients with early to moderate rheumatoid arthritis: A quantitative microfocal radiographic study. *Br. J. Rheumatol.* **1994**, *33*, 249–254. [CrossRef]
37. Halla, J.T.; Fallahi, S.; Hardin, J.G. Small joint involvement: A systematic roentgenographic study in rheumatoid arthritis. *Ann. Rheum. Dis.* **1986**, *45*, 327–330. [CrossRef]
38. Koh, J.H.; Jung, S.M.; Lee, J.J.; Kang, K.Y.; Kwok, S.-K.; Park, S.-H.; Ju, J.H. Radiographic structural damage is worse in the dominant than the non-dominant hand in individuals with early rheumatoid arthritis. *PLoS ONE* **2015**, *10*, e0135409. [CrossRef] [PubMed]
39. Yaku, A.; Hashimoto, M.; Furu, M.; Ito, H.; Yamakawa, N.; Yamamoto, W.; Fujii, T.; Matsuda, F.; Mimori, T.; Terao, C. Relationship between handedness and joint involvement in rheumatoid arthritis. *Sci. Rep.* **2016**, *6*, 39180. [CrossRef]
40. Zakaria, D.; Robertson, J.; MacDermid, J.; Hartford, K.; Koval, J. Work-related cumulative trauma disorders of the upper extremity: Navigating the epidemiologic literature. *Am. J. Ind. Med.* **2002**, *42*, 258–269. [CrossRef] [PubMed]
41. Miyadera, H.; Tokunaga, K. Associations of human leukocyte antigens with autoimmune diseases: Challenges in identifying the mechanism. *J. Hum. Genet.* **2015**, *60*, 697–702. [CrossRef] [PubMed]
42. Zheng, H.F.; Tobias, J.H.; Duncan, E.; Evans, D.M.; Eriksson, J.; Paternoster, L.; Yerges-Armstrong, L.M.; Lehtimäki, T.; Bergström, U.; Kähönen, M.; et al. WNT16 influences bone mineral density, cortical bone thickness, bone strength, and osteoporotic fracture risk. *PLoS Genet.* **2012**, *8*, e1002745. [CrossRef] [PubMed]

43. Hoff, M.; Kvien, T.K.; Kälvesten, J.; Elden, A.; Haugeberg, G. Adalimumab therapy reduces hand bone loss in early rheumatoid arthritis: Explorative analyses from the PREMIER study. *Ann. Rheum. Dis.* **2009**, *68*, 1171–1176. [CrossRef]
44. Baker, J.F.; Long, J.; Mostoufi-Moab, S.; Denburg, M.; Jorgenson, E.; Sharma, P.; Zemel, B.S.; Taratuta, E.; Ibrahim, S.; Leonard, M.B. Muscle Deficits in Rheumatoid Arthritis Contribute to Inferior Cortical Bone Structure and Trabecular Bone Mineral Density. *J. Rheumatol.* **2017**, *44*, 1777–1785. [CrossRef]

Journal of
Clinical Medicine

MDPI

Article

Mortality and Predictive Factors for Death Following the Diagnosis of Interstitial Lung Disease in Patients with Rheumatoid Arthritis: A Retrospective, Long-Term Follow-Up Study

Shunsuke Mori [1,*], Fumikazu Sakai [2], Mizue Hasegawa [3], Kazuyoshi Nakamura [4] and Kazuaki Sugahara [4]

1 Department of Rheumatology, Clinical Research Center for Rheumatic Diseases, National Hospital Organization (NHO) Kumamoto Saishun Medical Center, Kohshi, Kumamoto 861-1196, Japan
2 Department of Radiology, Kanagawa Cardiovascular and Respiratory Center, Yokohama, Kanagawa 236-0051, Japan; fmksakai@yahoo.co.jp
3 Department of Respiratory Medicine, Tokyo Women's Medical University Yachiyo Medical Center, Yachiyo, Chiba 276-8524, Japan; hasemizue@yahoo.co.jp
4 Department of Respiratory Medicine, NHO Kumamoto Saishun Medical Center, Kohshi, Kumamoto 861-1196, Japan; nakamura.kazuyoshi.cy@mail.hosp.go.jp (K.N.); sugahara.kazuaki.ve@mail.hosp.go.jp (K.S.)
* Correspondence: mori.shunsuke.ra@mail.hosp.go.jp; Tel.: +81-96-242-1000

Abstract: Objective: The aim of this study was to determine mortality and predictive factors for death in patients with rheumatoid arthritis (RA) diagnosed with and without interstitial lung disease (ILD). **Methods:** We retrospectively performed a long-term follow-up study of patients diagnosed with RA at our medical center between April 2001 and June 2023. The diagnosis and classification of ILD were made based on pulmonary high-resolution computed tomography (HRCT), taken at RA diagnosis and during follow-up. **Results:** Among 781 patients with RA, 78 were diagnosed with ILD; all cases except one were subclinical. The most common HRCT pattern was definite usual interstitial pneumonia (UIP) followed by nonspecific interstitial pneumonia (NSIP)/UIP, probable UIP, NSIP, and early UIP. During follow-up (mean of 10.0 years), the crude incidence rate of death (95% confidence interval [CI]) was 7.1 (5.2–10.0) and 1.5 (1.0–1.9) per 100 person-years in RA patients with and without ILD. Poor control of RA activity was associated with increased incidence rates of death. The standardized mortality ratio (95% CI) compared with the general population was 1.32 (1.11–1.53) for all RA patients, 2.09 (1.45–2.73) for RA-ILD patients, and 1.16 (0.95–1.38) for non-ILD RA patients. Lung cancer and respiratory failure were the most common causes of death in RA-ILD patients. The Multivariable Fine-Gray regression analysis revealed that ILD (adjusted hazard ratio [HR] 2.97 [95% CI 1.95–4.53]), advanced age (1.08 per additional year [1.05–1.10]), and low body mass index (3.07 [2.10–4.49]) were strong predictive factors for mortality in RA patients. HRCT patterns did not affect the risk of death in RA-ILD patients. **Conclusions:** Regardless of HRCT pattern, RA-ILD contributes to the increased mortality risk in patients with RA.

Keywords: interstitial lung disease; rheumatoid arthritis; mortality; predictive factors for death; HRCT pattern

1. Introduction

Rheumatoid arthritis (RA) is a chronic immune-mediated rheumatic disease that primarily involves multiple synovial joints [1,2]; however, systemic inflammation associated with RA can cause extra-articular damage to various tissues and organs such as the lungs, heart, blood vessels, renal system, skin, nervous system, and eyes [3–5]. The incidence of extra-articular manifestations has been decreasing since 2000, but the mortality risk continues to be high in RA patients with extra-articular manifestations and comorbidities [6,7]. In particular, respiratory disease, malignancies, and cardiovascular disease lead to increased mortality in RA patients [8–11]. Although RA-related mortality has improved over time, there remains a persistent mortality gap between RA patients and the general population or non-RA controls [9,11–13].

The respiratory system is a common target of extra-articular manifestations. Although there is extensive heterogeneity among prevalence studies of lung involvement in RA, interstitial lung disease (ILD) has the greatest estimated prevalence, followed by airway disease, pleural effusion, and rheumatoid nodules [14–16]. Subclinical and clinical ILD are increasingly recognized throughout the entire RA disease course; interstitial lung abnormalities can be detected in up to 60% of RA patients by high-resolution computed tomography (HRCT), and symptomatic ILD likely occurs in 5% to 17% of patients [14,16,17]. Advanced age, male sex, smoking, and RA-related autoantibodies are recognized as patient-level risk factors for developing RA-ILD [18]. Despite advances in the management of RA, ILD may continue to be a major contributor to mortality in RA. Several population-based cohort studies have shown an increased mortality associated with RA-ILD compared with non-ILD RA [19–25]. Other comparison studies between RA patients and the general population or non-RA patients also suggest that ILD contributes to excess mortality in RA [11,26–29]. Delayed diagnosis, lack of biological or targeted drugs for RA-ILD, the existence of rapidly progressive fibrosis, and serious complications (such as lung cancer, pulmonary infection, respiratory failure, and pulmonary hypertension) cause poor outcomes associated with RA-ILD [6,15,30].

It is important to explore whether clinical characteristics and HRCT patterns could predict death outcomes for RA-ILD patients. Although a variety of HRCT patterns are seen in RA-ILD patients, the most common patterns may be usual interstitial pneumonia (UIP) and nonspecific interstitial pneumonia (NSIP) [14,16,31]. However, UIP and NSIP patterns on a HRCT scan often overlap, and indeterminate patterns for UIP can be observed [32–35], which may obscure the impact of HRCT patterns on mortality in RA-ILD patients in previous studies [36–38].

To evaluate mortality, cause of death, and predictive factors for death in RA patients with ILD, we retrospectively conducted a long-term follow-up study of patients diagnosed with RA at our rheumatology department between April 2001 and June 2023. The diagnosis and classification of ILD were made based on pulmonary HRCT, taken at RA diagnosis and during follow-up. Mortality estimates and causes of death were compared between RA patients with and without ILD. Using Fine-Gray competing risk regression analysis, we examined the effect of each baseline characteristic on death outcome over time. We also calculated standardized mortality ratios (SMRs) in our RA cohort with and without ILD compared with the general population in Japan. Additionally, we explored the impact of RA activity control on poor outcomes based on the 28-joint disease activity score using C-reactive protein (DAS28-CRP).

2. Materials and Methods

2.1. Patients

We used a real-world database including patients who received a diagnosis of RA at the rheumatology department of National Hospital Organization (NHO) Kumamoto Saishun Medical Center between April 2001 and June 2023. Participants in this study were required to meet the 2010 American College of Rheumatology (ACR)/European League Against Rheumatism (EULAR) criteria for diagnosis of RA [39]. Participants were also required to be 18 years of age or older. We excluded patients from this study if they had any of the following histories prior to RA diagnosis: (1) other collagen vascular diseases/autoimmune diseases; (2) exposure to asbestos or silica; or (3) thoracic radiation for cancer therapy.

2.2. Study Design

The diagnosis of RA-associated ILD (RA-ILD) was made based on pulmonary HRCT taken at RA diagnosis and during follow-up, irrespective of the presence or absence of clinical symptoms. We reviewed patient medical records and collected clinical data when the diagnosis of RA-ILD was made (baseline characteristics of patients), which included demographic characteristics; RA-related data (duration of joint signs and symptoms, DAS28-CRP, Steinbrocker stage, anticyclic citrullinated peptide antibodies [anti-CCP], and rheumatoid factor [RF]); smoking history; body mass index (BMI); and comorbidities such as type 2 diabetes, malignancy history, and cardiovascular disease (CVD) history. CVD included angina pectoris, cardiac infarction, and stroke. The entry year was also recorded. For RA patients without ILD, clinical data at the time of RA diagnosis were used as the baseline characteristics. For patients who were diagnosed with RA or RA-ILD before a commercially available enzyme-linked immunosorbent assay (ELISA) kit was available, we used sera that were collected at the time of each diagnosis and stored at −80 °C. Detailed methods for the measurement of anti-CCP are described in our previous study [40].

Follow-up started on the day of the HRCT-based diagnosis of ILD (for RA-ILD patients) or RA diagnosis (for RA patients without ILD) and ended with death, loss to follow-up, or the last follow-up visit before 31 December 2023, whichever occurred first. Patients who missed two or more scheduled clinical appointments were classified as lost to follow-up. We determined the cause of death according to each treating physician's judgment.

2.3. Pulmonary Function Tests and ILD Severity

For RA-ILD patients, we collected data of pulmonary function tests (PFTs) at the time of RA-ILD diagnosis. The forced vital capacity (FVC), forced expiratory volume in the first second (FEV_1), maximal mid-expiratory flow (MMF; also called forced expiratory flow from 25% to 75% of vital capacity [$FEF_{25–75}$]), and diffusing capacity of carbon monoxide (DL_{CO}) were measured using a rolling-seal type of spirometer. The results were expressed as a ratio of the measured to the predicted values (% predicted). The predicted values were calculated based on the age, sex, and height of the individual. An abnormal PFT was defined as a % predicted value < 80% for each PFT. The FEV_1/FVC ratio was also calculated; an abnormal FEV_1/FVC ratio was defined as <70%. Additionally, we collected data on exercise-induced oxygen desaturation, which was defined as a drop in percutaneous oxygen saturation (SpO_2) < 90% during a 6 min walk, at the time of diagnosis of RA-ILD. Disease severity staging at that time was determined based on the arterial partial pressure of oxygen (PaO_2) at rest and SpO_2 during the 6 min walk test according to the Japanese Respiratory Society Guidelines [41,42].

2.4. Classification of HRCT Pattern of ILD

Pulmonary HRCT images of ILD patients taken at RA diagnosis and during subsequent follow-ups were collected from our database and viewed in random order and independently by three observers (one board-certified radiologist [F. Sakai] and two board-certified pulmonologists [M. Hasegawa and K. Nakamura]) who were blinded to the patients' clinical status and PFT results. Final decisions were made by discussing whether there was disagreement among the three experts after the first assessment. We did not determine the inter-reader agreement in assessing the HRCT features by kappa statistics because all observers were very experienced at identifying abnormalities on pulmonary

HRCT, especially of parenchymal and airway lung diseases. HRCT abnormalities included the following findings: bronchiectasis or bronchiolectasis, bronchial wall thickening, centrilobular micro-nodules and a branching structure, cysts, ground-glass opacity (GGO), intralobular reticular opacity, airspace consolidation, honeycombing, traction bronchiectasis, architectural distortion, and emphysema. The distribution of HRCT abnormalities was evaluated according to six zones (upper, middle, and lower zones; involvement in at least 5% of any lung zone). We also examined whether these abnormalities had a predominantly subpleural or non-subpleural distribution.

Each patient with RA-ILD was classified as having one of the following four HRCT patterns: definite UIP, probable UIP, indeterminate for UIP, and alternative diagnosis according to the updated official American Thoracic Society (ATS)/European Respiratory Society (ERS)/Japanese Respiratory Society (JRS)/Latin American Thoracic Society (ALAT) clinical practice guideline for idiopathic pulmonary fibrosis (IPF) [43,44]. In this study, ILD patients with coexisting airway abnormalities such as bronchiolitis or bronchiectasis on HRCT scans were classified as RA-ILD, because a high prevalence of airway abnormalities has been observed in the RA population [32,45]. We further classified the "indeterminate for UIP" pattern into early UIP and NSIP/UIP based on the modified HRCT classification for RA-ILD that was reported by Yamakawa et al. [46]. In brief, honeycombing with a subpleural, basal-predominant distribution is a distinguishing feature of the definite UIP pattern. It can be seen with or without peripheral traction bronchiectasis/bronchiolectasis. Subpleural, basal-predominant reticulation with peripheral traction bronchiectasis/bronchiolectasis was considered the probable UIP pattern. The early UIP pattern was assigned when there were HRCT features consisting of subpleural, basal-predominant mild reticulation or GGO without traction bronchiectasis/bronchiolectasis. If central or diffuse distribution of GGO or reticulation as the component of NSIP and subpleural reticulation with traction bronchiectasis/bronchiolectasis, with or without honeycombing as the component of UIP, were both observed, the NSIP/UIP pattern was assigned. HRCT features showing lower lobe-predominant, central or diffuse GGO with limited or no reticulation and the absence of honeycombing were consistent with the NSIP pattern. In the present study, all patients who had an alternative diagnosis were finally diagnosed as NSIP.

2.5. DMARD Use and Control of RA Activity During Follow-Up

The exposure to disease-modifying antirheumatic drugs (DMARDs) during follow-up were examined using patient medical records. Based on a mean of DAS28-CRP values measured for 6 months prior to the end of follow-up, each patient was classified into a group with good control of RA activity (remission or low disease activity [DAS28-CRP < 2.7]) and a group with poor control of RA activity (moderate or high disease activity [DAS28-CRP ≥ 2.7]).

2.6. Statistical Analysis

The mean and standard deviation (SD) were used as descriptive statistics for data with continuous distribution, which included non-normally distributed data [47,48]. Number (percentage) was used for categorical data. We compared the baseline characteristics between the two patient groups using Fisher's exact probability test for categorial variables and the independent-measures t-test for continuous variables. There were no missing baseline measurements.

Crude incidence rates of death and 95% confidence intervals (CIs) were calculated by dividing the number of death cases by the number of corresponding follow-up person-years (PYs).

SMRs and 95% CIs in RA patients with and without ILD, in male and female patients separately, compared with the general population in Japan, were calculated as the ratio of the observed number of deaths in our cohort divided by the expected number of deaths in the reference population from 2001 to 2023. For the reference population, we used mortality data in the Japanese general population reported by Japanese Health and Wealth (http://www.stat.go.jp/english/index.html (accessed on 2 December 2024)). The expected number of deaths was calculated based on age- and sex-specific population mortality rates at each calendar year for patients at risk during follow-up.

We used the cumulative incidence function (CIF) to estimate the probability of death before a given time, because we considered the presence of competing risks (i.e., loss to follow-up). Gray's test was used to test the equality of CIF mortality estimates over time between RA patients with ILD and those without ILD [49]. For the same reason, Fine-Gray competing risk regression analysis was used to calculate the adjusted hazard ratios (HRs) with 95% CIs for death outcome over time. As predictor variables, we selected a set of baseline characteristics based on previous knowledge about the clinical relevance and importance of each variable, which included demographic data, RA-related data, RA-ILD diagnosis, smoking history, BMI, comorbidities, and entry year. For RA-ILD patients, HRCT patterns (definite UIP, probable UIP, indeterminate for UIP, and NSIP patterns) and HRCT abnormalities (honeycombing, traction bronchiectasis, and emphysema) were included as predictor variables. Predictor variables with p-values < 0.10 in univariable analyses were used in a multivariable Fine-Gray regression analysis. A forced entry procedure was selected in the multivariable analysis.

Two-sided p-values < 0.05 were considered to indicate statistical significance. For all statistical calculations, we used PASW Statistics version 27 (SPSS Japan Inc., Tokyo, Japan) and Easy R (Saitama Medical Center, Jichi Medical University, Saitama, Japan) [50].

3. Results

3.1. Baseline Characteristics of RA Patients with and Without ILD

A total of 781 patients were included in this study (Figure S1). Based on the HRCT findings taken at RA diagnosis and subsequent follow-up, 78 patients were diagnosed with RA-ILD (10.0%) and 703 were diagnosed without ILD. Clinical characteristics at baseline are shown in Table 1. No patients had missing data for baseline characteristics. RA-ILD patients had a mean age of 70.6 years, which was significantly higher than RA patients without ILD (62.4 years) (p < 0.001). Male patients were predominant in the RA-ILD group compared with the group without RA-ILD (55.1% vs. 22.6%, p < 0.001). The mean duration from the onset of joint symptoms was similar in patients with and without ILD (3.6 vs. 3.7 years). Approximately 90% of patients had high or moderate disease activity at baseline, and no significant difference in DAS28-CRP levels was observed between patient groups. Rates of anti-CCP-positive patients and RF-positive patients were significantly higher in RA-ILD patients than in RA patients without ILD (anti-CCP-positive, 96.2% vs. 86.6%, p = 0.011; RF-positive, 97.4% vs. 86.3%, p = 0.003). Smoking history was also significantly associated with the presence of RA-ILD (41.0% in RA-ILD patients vs. 10.0% in RA patients without ILD, p < 0.001). Additionally, RA-ILD patients more frequently had a history of CVD compared with RA patients without ILD (17.9% vs. 8.3%, p = 0.011).

Table 1. Baseline characteristics of RA patients with and without ILD.

	Overall (n = 781)	With RA-ILD (n = 78)	Without RA-ILD (n = 703)	p *
Age, years, mean (SD)	63.2 (12.8)	70.6 (8.1)	62.4 (13.0)	<0.001
≥18 and <45 years, number (%)	76 (9.7)	0	76 (10.8)	0.002
≥45 and <65 years, number (%)	285 (36.5)	17 (21.8)	268 (38.1)	0.004
≥65 years, number (%)	420 (53.8)	61 (78.2)	359 (51.1)	<0.001
Male, number (%)	202 (25.9)	43 (55.1)	159 (22.6)	<0.001
Duration of joint symptoms †, years, mean (SD)	3.7 (7.6)	3.6 (7.8)	3.7 (7.6)	0.99
DAS28-CRP, index, mean (SD)	4.3 (1.3)	4.2 (1.1)	4.3 (1.3)	0.25
High or moderate, number (%)	696 (89.1)	67 (85.9)	629 (89.5)	0.34
Steinbrocker stages III/IV, number (%)	265 (33.9)	31 (39.7)	234 (33.3)	0.26
Anti-CCP-positive, number (%)	684 (87.6)	75 (96.2)	609 (86.6)	0.011
RF-positive, number (%)	683 (87.5)	76 (97.4)	607 (86.3)	0.003
Smoking ≥ 30 pack-years ‡, number (%)	102 (13.1)	32 (41.0)	70 (10.0)	<0.001
BMI < 17, number (%)	80 (10.2)	11 (14.1)	69 (9.8)	0.24
Type 2 diabetes, number (%)	95 (12.2)	9 (11.5)	86 (12.2)	1.00
CKD stages ≥ 3, number (%)	27 (3.5)	4 (5.1)	23 (3.3)	0.34
Malignancy history, number (%)	42 (5.4)	7 (9.0)	35 (5.0)	0.18
CVD history, number (%)	72 (9.2)	14 (17.9)	58 (8.3)	0.011
Entry prior to 2011, number (%)	370 (47.4)	31 (39.7)	339 (48.2)	0.19

Data were obtained when patients were diagnosed with RA-ILD. For RA patients without ILD, data were obtained at the time of RA diagnosis. * Compared between RA patients with and without RA-ILD using Fisher's exact probability test for categorical variables and independent-measures t-test for continuous variables. † Defined as duration from onset of joint symptoms and signs, which referred to patient self-reports. ‡ Current smokers stopped smoking according to smoking cessation instructions following RA diagnosis. RA, rheumatoid arthritis; ILD, interstitial lung disease; RA-ILD, RA-associated ILD; DAS28-CRP, 28-joint disease activity score using C-reactive protein; anti-CCP, anti-cyclic citrullinated peptide antibodies; RF, rheumatoid factor; BMI, body mass index; CKD, chronic kidney disease; CVD cardiovascular disease; SD, standard deviation.

3.2. Baseline Features of RA-ILD

Characteristics of patients with ILD are shown in Table 2. Among 78 RA-ILD patients, 65 (83.3%) were diagnosed with ILD at the same time as their RA diagnosis. ILD preceded their RA diagnosis in three patients (3.8%). The most common HRCT pattern was definite UIP (37.2%) followed by NSIP/UIP (26.9%), probable UIP (17.9%), NSIP (11.5%), and early UIP (6.4%). Honeycombing was observed in all patients with definite UIP and in 10 patients with NSIP/UIP. Traction bronchiectasis was seen in all patients with probable UIP and in most patients with definite UIP or NSIP/UIP. Emphysema was observed in 46.2% of RA-ILD patients. Mean values of the % predicted for FVC and FEV_1 were within the normal range. The mean % predicted for DL_{CO}, an index of restrictive interstitial disease, was 83.2%. The FEV_1/FVC ratio, a sensitive index of overall airway obstruction, was 125.5%. It is worth noting that the mean % predicted for MMF, a specific index of small airway function, was 70.4%, indicating that obstructive changes in small airways are present in RA-ILD patients. Only one patient showed desaturation with exercise (SpO_2 < 90% during a 6 min walk) and disease severity stage III. This patient had clinical symptoms at the time of ILD diagnosis.

Table 2. Clinical, radiological, and functional features of RA-ILD at baseline.

	RA-ILD Patients (n = 78)
Age at RA diagnosis, years, mean (SD)	68.7 (9.8)
ILD onset, number (%)	
Before RA diagnosis	3 (3.8)
Simultaneous diagnosis	65 (83.3)
Within 10 years after RA diagnosis	6 (7.7)
More than 10 years after RA diagnosis	4 (5.1)
HRCT patterns, number (%)	
Definite UIP pattern	29 (37.2)
Probable UIP pattern	14 (17.9)
Indeterminate for UIP pattern	26 (33.3)
Early UIP	5 (6.4)
NSIP/UIP	21 (26.9)
NSIP	9 (11.5)
HRCT abnormalities, number (%)	
Honeycombing	39 (50)
Traction bronchiectasis	62 (79.5)
Emphysema	36 (46.2)
Pulmonary function test †, mean (SD)	
FVC, % predicted (n = 70)	95.3 (19.0)
FEV_1, % predicted (n = 70)	113.6 (12.6)
FEV_1/FVC ratio (n = 70)	125.5 (35.8)
MMF, % predicted (n = 70)	70.4 (30.0)
DL_{CO}, % predicted (n = 64)	83.2 (20.3)
SpO_2 < 90% during a 6 min walk, number (%)	1 (1.3)
Disease severity staging of ILD ‡, number (%)	
I	77 (98.7)
II	0
III	1 (1.3)
IV	0

Data were obtained when patients were diagnosed with RA-ILD. † Expressed as a ratio of the measured to the predicted values (% predicted), except the FEV_1/FVC ratio. ‡ Determined based on PaO_2 at rest and SpO_2 during the 6 min walk test according to the Japanese Respiratory Society Guidelines. RA, rheumatoid arthritis; ILD, interstitial lung disease; RA-ILD, RA-associated ILD; HRCT, high-resolution computed tomography; UIP, usual interstitial pneumonia; NSIP, non-specific interstitial pneumonia; SpO_2, oxygen saturation as measured using pulse oximeter; PaO_2, arterial partial pressure of oxygen; FVC, forced vital capacity; FEV_1, forced expiratory volume in one second; MMF, maximal mid-expiratory flow; DL_{CO}, diffusing capacity of carbon monoxide.

3.3. Mortality in RA Patients with and Without ILD

After the diagnosis of RA-ILD or RA was made, patients were followed for a mean of 10.0 years. As shown in Table 3, 128 patients (16.4%) were lost to follow-up. Death events occurred in 152 patients (19.5%; 41 RA-ILD patients [52.6%] and 111 RA patients without ILD [15.8%]). The crude incidence rate of death was significantly higher in RA-ILD patients than in RA patients without ILD (7.1 per 100 PYs [95% CI, 5.2–10.0] for RA-ILD patients and 1.5 per 100 PYs [95% CI, 1.0–1.9] for patients without RA-ILD). There were significant differences in the CIF-estimated cumulative incidence of death over time between patient groups ($p < 0.001$ with Gray's test). For example, the cumulative incidence (mortality rate) at 5 years was estimated to be 18.6% (95% CI, 10.5–28.6) for RA-ILD patients and 3.4% (95% CI, 2.2–5.0) for RA patients without ILD. The CIF plots for the probability of death events in RA-ILD patients grouped according to HRCT patterns are shown in Figure S1. There was no significant difference in CIF mortality estimates among these four patterns ($p = 0.57$ with Gray's test with post hoc Holm test).

Table 3. Mortality in RA patients with and without ILD.

	Total (n = 781)	With RA-ILD (n = 78)	Without RA-ILD (n = 703)
Follow-up [†], years, mean (SD)	10.0 (5.2)	7.4 (4.5)	10.2 (5.2)
Follow-up [†], years, median (IQR)	9.7 (5.9–13.9)	6.8 (3.8–10.7)	10.0 (6.1–14.1)
Lost to follow-up, number (%)	128 (16.4)	3 (3.8)	125 (17.8)
Death, number (%)	152 (19.5)	41 (52.6)	111 (15.8)
Crude incidence rate of death per 100 PYs (95% CI)	2.0 (1.7–2.0)	7.1 (5.2–10.0)	1.5 (1.0–1.9)
Cumulative incidence of death [‡] (%)			
1-year mortality rate (95% CI) [§]	0.8 (0.3–1.6)	2.6 (0.5–8.1)	0.7 (0.3–1.6)
5-year mortality rate (95% CI) [§]	4.7 (3.3–6.4)	18.6 (10.5–28.6)	3.4 (2.2–5.0)
10-year mortality rate (95% CI) [§]	14.9 (12.3–17.8)	52.5 (38.9–64.4)	11.4 (9.0–14.1)

[†] Follow-up began with the diagnosis of RA-ILD. For RA patients without ILD, follow-up began with the diagnosis of RA. [‡] Cumulative incidence (probability) of death during the follow-up period was estimated by the CIF. Gray's test was used to compare CIF mortality estimates over time between patients with and without RA-ILD ($p < 0.001$). [§] Cumulative incidence of death at 1, 5, and 10 years was expressed as the estimated 1-year, 5-year, and 10-year mortality rates (%). RA, rheumatoid arthritis; ILD, interstitial lung disease; RA-ILD, RA-associated ILD; PYs, person-years; CIF, cumulative incidence function; SD, standard deviation; IQR, interquartile range; 95% CI, 95% confidence interval.

The SMRs in our RA cohort compared with the general population in Japan were 1.32 (95% CI, 1.11–1.53) for overall RA patients, 2.09 (95% CI, 1.45–2.73) for RA-ILD patients, and 1.16 (95% CI, 0.95–1.38) for RA patients without ILD.

3.4. Cause of Death in RA Patients with and Without ILD

Among RA-ILD patients, 13 (31.7%) died due to malignancy, primarily lung cancer (Table 4). Twelve RA-ILD patients (29.3%) developed respiratory failure due to an acute exacerbation of ILD. Six patients (14.6%) died from serious infections. Among RA patients without ILD, malignancy was the most common cause of death (30.6%), followed by cardiovascular events (22.5%) and serious infection (13.5%). Death due to lung cancer and respiratory failure occurred more frequently in RA-ILD patients than in RA patients without ILD (lung cancer, 24.4% vs. 2.7%, $p < 0.001$; respiratory failure, 29.3% vs. 5.4%, $p < 0.001$). The rate of cardiovascular events as the cause of death was lower in RA-ILD patients than in RA patients without ILD (4.9% vs. 22.5%, $p = 0.015$). Overall malignancies or serious infection caused death at similar rates between RA patients with and without ILD.

Table 4. Cause of death in RA patients with and without ILD.

Cause of Death	With RA-ILD (n = 41)	Without RA-ILD (n = 111)	p *
Age at death, years (SD)	81.2 (8.1)	77.6 (9.9)	0.042
Malignancy, number (%)	13 (31.7)	34 (30.6)	1.00
Lung cancer, number (%)	10 (24.4)	3 (2.7)	<0.001
Respiratory failure, number (%)	12 (29.3)	6 (5.4)	<0.001
Serious infection, number (%)	6 (14.6)	15 (13.5)	1.00
Cardiovascular events, number (%)	2 (4.9)	25 (22.5)	0.015
Death of old age, number (%)	5 (12.2)	13 (11.7)	0.59
Aspiration pneumonia, number (%)	2 (4.9)	5 (4.5)	1.00
Others, number (%)	1 (2.4)	13 (11.7)	0.11

* Comparison between RA patients with and without ILD using Fisher's exact probability test for categorical variables and independent-measures t-test for continuous variables. RA, rheumatoid arthritis; ILD, interstitial lung disease; RA-ILD, RA-associated ILD; SD, standard deviation.

3.5. DMARD Use During Follow-Up and RA Control Within 6 Months Prior to the End of Follow-Up

As shown in Table S1, approximately 90% of RA patients without ILD received MTX as monotherapy or in combination therapy with other DMARDs during follow-up, whereas more than 40% of RA-ILD patients never received MTX, most likely because of concerns over ILD exacerbation. Instead of MTX treatment, RA-ILD patients were more often prescribed other csDMARDs. Additionally, IL-6 inhibitors and abatacept were prescribed more frequently for RA-ILD patients than for RA patients without ILD. The rates of the TNF inhibitor and JAK inhibitor use were similar between the two patient groups. Exposure duration to MTX was longer in RA patients without ILD than in RA-ILD patients. Exposure duration to other DMARDs did not differ significantly between RA-ILD patients and RA patients without ILD. Limited to RA-ILD patients, MTX users more often received other csDMARDs compared with non-MTX users. The rate of TNF inhibitor use was significantly higher among MTX users because TNF inhibitors are recommended to be used concomitantly with MTX (Table S2).

The status of RA control in each patient for 6 months before the end of follow-up was determined based on the mean DAS28-CRP value measured during this period and used to explore the influence of RA activity on mortality. The rate of poor control of RA activity was significantly higher in RA patients with ILD than in those without ILD (19.2% vs. 8.8%, $p = 0.008$), which may be explained by the restriction of DMARD use, especially MTX use, in RA-ILD patients. As shown in Table 5, the crude incidence rate of death events was significantly higher in the poor RA control group compared with the good RA control group (8.3 per 100 PYs [95% CI, 6.4–11.0] vs. 1.3 per 100 PYs [95% CI, 1.1–1.6]). These data suggested that the poor control of RA activity was associated with an increased risk of death in RA patients. There was no significant difference in incidence rates of death between patients with and without RA-ILD in the poor RA control group. In contrast, RA-ILD patients had a higher incidence rate of death than RA patients without ILD in the good RA control group. Thus, the increased mortality in RA-ILD patients was not explained simply by poor RA control due to the restriction of DMARD use.

Table 5. Mortality in RA patients with and without ILD, grouped by the status of RA activity control.

	Poor Control † (n = 77)			Good Control ‡ (n = 704)		
	Total (n = 77)	With RA-ILD (n = 15)	Without RA-ILD (n = 62)	Total (n = 704)	With RA-ILD (n = 63)	Without RA-ILD (n = 641)
Follow-up §, years, mean (SD)	8.9 (5.5)	7.3 (4.8)	9.3 (5.6)	10.1 (5.2)	7.5 (4.5)	10.3 (5.2)
Follow-up §, years, median (IQR)	8.1 (5.2–12.4)	6.7 (2.9–10.4)	8.2 (5.7–12.5)	9.8 (6.1–14.0)	6.9 (4.1–11.0)	10.1 (6.2–14.3)
Lost to follow-up, number (%)	9 (11.7)	0	9 (14.5)	119 (16.9)	3 (4.8)	116 (18.1)
Death, number (%)	57 (74.0)	13 (86.7)	44 (71.0)	95 (44.4)	28 (44.4)	67 (10.5)
Crude incidence rate of death per 100 PYs (95% CI)	8.3 (6.4–11.0)	11.9 (6.9–20.5)	7.7 (5.7–10.3)	1.3 (1.1–1.6)	5.9 (4.1–9.0)	1.0 (0.8–1.3)

† Defined as high or moderate disease activity using DAS28-CRP values in the 6 months before the end of follow-up. ‡ Defined as remission or low disease activity using DAS28-CRP values in the 6 months before the end of follow-up. § Follow-up began with the diagnosis of RA-ILD. For RA patients without ILD, follow-up began with the diagnosis of RA. RA, rheumatoid arthritis; ILD, interstitial lung disease; RA-ILD, RA-associated ILD; DAS28-CRP, 28-joint disease activity score using C-reactive protein; PYs, person-years; SD, standard deviation; IQR, interquartile range; 95% CI, 95% confidence interval.

3.6. Predictive Factors for Death in Overall RA Patients and RA-ILD Patients

The results from the univariable and multivariable Fine-Gray regression analyses for overall RA patients are shown in Table 6. Through multivariate modeling, age (adjusted HR 1.08 per additional year [95% CI, 1.05–1.10], $p < 0.001$), RA-ILD (adjusted HR 2.97 [95% CI, 1.95–4.53], $p < 0.001$), BMI < 17 (adjusted HR 3.07 [95% CI, 2.10–4.49], $p < 0.001$), anti-CCP-positive (adjusted HR 2.87 [95% CI, 1.25–6.56], $p = 0.013$), and male sex (adjusted HR 1.61 [95% CI, 1.02–2.53], $p = 0.042$) at baseline were identified as independent predictive factors for death.

Table 6. Predictive factors for death in overall RA patients.

Variables	Unadjusted HRs (95% CI)	p *	Adjusted HRs (95% CI)	p *
Age per additional year	1.09 (1.06–1.11)	<0.001	1.08 (1.05–1.10)	<0.001
Male vs. female	1.95 (1.41–2.71)	<0.001	1.61 (1.02–2.53)	0.042
Disease duration per additional year	1.02 (1.00–1.03)	0.026	0.99 (0.97–1.01)	0.46
DAS28-CRP per additional unit	0.98 (0.87–1.11)	0.75	–	–
Stages III/IV vs. I/II	1.31 (0.96–1.79)	0.090	0.98 (0.69–1.39)	0.91
Anti-CCP-positive vs. Anti-CCP-negative	3.00 (1.41–6.40)	0.005	2.87 (1.25–6.56)	0.013
RF-positive vs. RF-negative	2.19 (1.12–4.30)	0.022	1.07 (0.50–2.28)	0.87
RA-ILD, yes vs. no	5.84 (4.08–8.34)	<0.001	2.97 (1.95–4.53)	<0.001
Smoking > 30 PYs vs. no history	2.40 (1.64–3.51)	<0.001	1.31 (0.78–2.17)	0.31
BMI < 17, yes vs. no	2.89 (2.00–4.17)	<0.001	3.07 (2.10–4.49)	<0.001
Type 2 diabetes, yes vs. no	0.51 (0.27–0.97)	0.040	0.52 (0.27–1.01)	0.054
CKD stage ≥ 3, yes vs. no	1.98 (1.10–3.56)	0.020	1.52 (0.72–3.19)	0.27
Malignancy history, yes vs. no	1.34 (0.69–2.60)	0.38	–	–
CVD history, yes vs. no	1.57 (0.95–2.57)	0.080	1.14 (0.65–1.99)	0.65
Entry before 2011, yes vs. no	1.48 (1.04–2.10)	0.030	1.42 (0.98–2.07)	0.65

* Univariable and multivariable Fine-Gray competing risk regression analyses were conducted for overall RA patients. RA, rheumatoid arthritis; ILD, interstitial lung disease; RA-ILD-RA-associated ILD; anti-CCP, anti-cyclic citrullinated peptide antibodies; RF, rheumatoid factor; BMI, body mass index; CKD, chronic kidney disease; CVD, cardiovascular disease; PY, pack-years; HR, hazard ratio; 95% CI, 95% confidence interval.

The results for RA-ILD patients are shown in Table 7. Age (adjusted HR 1.08 per additional year [95% CI, 1.03–1.13], $p = 0.002$), BMI < 17 (adjusted HR 5.29 [95% CI, 2.28–12.27], $p < 0.001$), and CVD (adjusted HR 0.26, 95% CI, 0.08–0.85], $p = 0.030$) at baseline were independent predictive factors for mortality. Neither HRCT patterns nor HRCT abnormalities were identified as factors associated with death outcomes.

Table 7. Predictive factors for mortality in RA-ILD patients.

Variables	Unadjusted HR (95% CI)	p *	Adjusted HR (95% CI)	p *
Age per additional year	1.07 (1.03–1.12)	0.001	1.08 (1.03–1.13)	0.002
Male vs. female	1.47 (0.79–2.71)	0.22	–	–
Disease duration per additional year	0.99 (0.95–1.02)	0.43	–	–
DAS28-CRP per additional unit	1.04 (0.81–1.33)	0.77	–	–
Steinbrocker stages III/IV vs. I/II	0.80 (0.43–1.47)	0.47	–	–
Anti-CCP-positive vs. Anti-CCP-negative	0.70 (0.15–3.46)	0.87	–	–
RF-positive vs. RF-negative	0.27 (0.07–1.07)	0.060	0.40 (0.09–1.78)	0.23
HRCT patterns of ILD				
NSIP	1 (reference)	–	–	–
Early UIP	0.51 (0.14–1.87)	0.31	–	–
NSIP/UIP	0.51 (0.17–1.51)	0.22		
Probable UIP	0.42 (0.13–1.36)	0.15	–	–
Definite UIP	0.66 (0.29–1.53)	0.33	–	–
HRCT abnormalities				
Honeycomb, yes vs. no	1.43 (0.77–2.67)	0.26	–	–
Traction bronchiectasis, yes vs. no	0.80 (0.42–1.52)	0.49	–	–
Emphysema, yes vs. no	1.06 (0.58–1.94)	0.85	–	–
Smoking > 30 PYs vs. no history	1.54 (0.83–2.85)	0.17	–	–
BMI < 17.0, yes vs. no	4.59 (1.64–12.83)	0.004	5.29 (2.28–12.27)	<0.001
Type 2 diabetes, yes vs. no	0.17 (0.02–1.46)	0.11	–	–
CKD stage ≥ 3, yes vs. no	0.48 (0.05–4.43)	0.51	–	–
Malignancy history, yes vs. no	1.58 (0.84–2.96)	0.16	–	–
CVD history, yes vs. no	0.21 (0.07–0.68)	0.009	0.26 (0.08–0.85)	0.030
Entry before 2011, yes vs. no	1.34 (0.71–2.51)	0.36	–	–

* Univariable and multivariable Fine-Gray competing risk regression analyses were conducted for RA-ILD patients. RA, rheumatoid arthritis; ILD, interstitial lung disease; RA-ILD, RA-associated ILD; anti-CCP, anti-cyclic citrullinated peptide antibodies; RF, rheumatoid factor; HRCT, high-resolution computed tomography; UIP, unusual interstitial pneumonia; NSIP, non-specific interstitial pneumonia; BMI, body mass index; CKD, chronic kidney disease; CVD, cardiovascular disease; PY, pack-years; HR, hazard ratio; 95% CI, 95% confidence interval.

4. Discussion

In the present study, we showed that approximately 10% of RA patients developed ILD during the course of the disease. The most common HRCT pattern was definitive UIP followed by NSIP/UIP, probable UIP, NSIP, and early UIP. Lung cancer and respiratory failure were the most common causes of death in RA-ILD patients. During follow-up over a mean of 10.0 years, the crude incident rate of death was 5 times higher in RA-ILD patients than in RA patients without ILD, although all ILD cases except one were subclinical at the time of first diagnosis. The SMRs (95% CI) compared with the general population were 1.32 (1.11–1.53) for all RA patients, 2.09 (1.45–2.73) for RA-ILD patients, and 1.16 (0.95–1.38) for RA patients without ILD. Patients whose RA activity was poorly controlled had a significantly higher incidence rate of death compared with patients in the good RA control group. According to multivariable Fine-Gray regression analysis, ILD, advanced age, and low BMI were predictive factors for increased mortality in RA patients. HRCT patterns did not affect the risk of death in RA-ILD patients.

Using data from the French national claims database from 2013 to 2018, Juge et al. showed that RA-ILD patients had a 3.4-fold increase (95% CI, 3.1–3.9) in mortality rate compared with RA patients without ILD, especially in patients aged <75 years and in male patients [25]. Using the Medicare claims database from 2008 to 2017, Sparks et al. reported that RA-ILD had an HR of 1.66 (95% CI, 1.60–1.72) for total mortality compared with RA without ILD [21]. In a population-based cohort study in Denmark between 2004 and 2016, the HR ratio for death during follow-up > 5 to 10 years was 2.7 times higher (95% CI, 1.9–3.9) for RA-ILD compared with RA without ILD and it was higher in male patients [20]. Using data from the US Centers for Disease and Control Prevention, Gao et al. showed that the mortality rate ratio of RA-ILD to RA was 6.90 from 1999 to 2003 and 6.49 from 2014 to 2018, and they suggested that RA-ILD may contribute to the reduced life expectancy [22]. In the present study, we showed that the HRCT-based diagnosis of ILD, albeit subclinical, was a strong predictive factor for increased mortality in RA patients (adjusted HR 2.97 [95% CI, 1.95–4.53]). Thus, RA-ILD is associated with an increased mortality risk compared with RA without ILD.

In a national, matched-cohort study with the United States Veterans Health Administration database from 2000 to 2017 (RA vs. non-RA), Johnson et al. showed that ILD was the cause of death most strongly associated with RA (adjusted HR 3.39 [95% CI, 2.88–3.99]) [11]. In a retrospective cohort study using the Australian Rheumatology Association database from 1995 to 2020, Black et al. showed that ILD is an important cause of death in RA patients (cause-specific SMR 7.64 [95% CI, 3.98–14.69]) [29]. In a cohort study using the Korean National Statistical Office from 2001 to 2007, Kim et al. showed that death from ILD was significantly higher in RA patients (cause-specific SMR 18.18 [95% CI, 2.20–65.64]) [26]. In the present study, SMRs compared with the Japanese general population were 1.32 (95% CI, 1.11–1.53) for all RA patients and 2.09 (95% CI, 1.45–2.73) for RA-ILD patients. There was no significant difference in mortality rates in RA patients without ILD compared with the general population. These findings indicate that ILD contributes to excess death in RA patients compared with the general population or non-RA patients.

The effect of HRCT pattern on mortality in RA-ILD patients remains controversial. Some studies have shown that the UIP pattern is associated with an increased mortality risk in RA-ILD patients [51–59]. However, other studies have shown that the extent of lung involvement or severity of lung disease, rather than the baseline UIP pattern, independently predicts mortality [60–65]. Another study showed that survival in RA-ILD patients did not differ between the UIP and NSIP patterns [66]. Recently, Yamakawa et al. developed a modified HRCT classification for RA-ILD according to the latest guideline of IPF, in which the "indeterminate for UIP" pattern was further classified into early UIP and NSIP/UIP patterns [46]. Using the modified HRCT classification, Yamakawa et al. showed that their RA-ILD cohort included NSIP/UIP (27%), definite UIP (21%), probable UIP (20%), NSIP (14%), and early UIP (3%). In that study, the HRCT pattern was not a predictive factor for mortality in a multivariable Cox regression analysis [46]. In the present study, we followed the modified HRCT classification by Yamakawa et al. and found that in our RA cohort, the most common HRCT pattern was definite UIP (37.2%), followed by NSIP/UIP (26.9%), probable UIP (17.9%), NSIP (11.5%), and early UIP (6.4%). The HRCT pattern was not related to mortality risk in our RA-ILD patients. In both studies, most patients with the "indeterminate for UIP" pattern were classified as having the NSIP/UIP pattern. In other previous studies, the NSIP/UIP pattern might have been simply diagnosed as NSIP or UIP, which could have resulted in different conclusions regarding the effect of HRCT pattern on mortality risk in RA-ILD patients. In our statistical analyses, the presence of ILD was a strong predictive factor for death, and the NSIP pattern did not have a significantly better prognosis than the UIP, NSIP/UIP, or early UIP pattern, which suggests that, regardless of HRCT pattern, RA patients with ILD are at increased risk of death. Jacob et al. showed that the individual extents of fibrosis, reticulation, and honeycombing on HRCT scans could independently predict the development of progressive fibrosis and poor outcomes in RA-ILD patients [67]. In this respect, HRCT examinations for ILD at RA diagnosis and during follow-up can provide insight into the extents of these abnormalities.

There is some evidence of associations between RA disease activity and progression of ILD/death outcome in RA-ILD patients [68]. In a retrospective, single-center cohort study of RA-ILD patients in China, Chai et al. showed that high RA disease activity and an advanced extent of lung involvement were independent risk factors for the progression of radiologic fibrosis [63]. In a multicenter, prospective cohort study of US veterans with RA-ILD, Brooks et al. indicated that uncontrolled RA disease activity and the functional status of joints, as well as the severity of lung disease, were associated with increased mortality in this patient population [69]. In a retrospective, single-center cohort study of RA-ILD patients in China, Liu et al. showed that in addition to the UIP pattern, high RA disease activity and advanced fibrosis were independent risk factors for RA-ILD progression [58]. In a prospective study with data from the Korean Rheumatoid Arthritis-Interstitial Lung Disease cohort, Chang et al. found no association between the risk of deterioration of ILD/mortality and RA disease activity [64]. In the present study, the crude incidence rate of death events was significantly higher in the poor RA control group compared with the good RA control group. Thus, the poor control of RA activity was associated with the increased risk of death. The restriction of DMARD use in RA-ILD patients may have resulted in the higher rate of poor control of RA activity in this patient group compared with RA patients without ILD. Concerns about lung injury are greatest in patients receiving MTX, but a causal effect between MTX and fibrotic ILD has not been established [30,70]. The overall risk of worsening lung disease attributable to MTX is currently unclear. Recent studies do not support the idea that RA-ILD progression is increased in patients receiving MTX [71,72]. The 2021 ACR guidelines for treatment of RA include a conditional recommendation for MTX for the treatment of RA patients with clinically diagnosed mild and stable airway or parenchymal lung disease who have moderate to high disease activity [73]. The appropriate use of MTX considering RA disease activity would be important for the management of RA-associated ILD. The use of IL-6 inhibitors and abatacept may be considered in the treatment for RA-ILD patients because concomitant MTX use is not necessarily required for these DMARD therapies.

In the present study, all ILD cases, except one, were subclinical at baseline. Nevertheless, the mortality rate was 2.1 times higher in RA-ILD patients compared with the general population during long-term follow-up with a mean of 10 years. Among RA-ILD patients, the most common cause of death was respiratory failure due to acute exacerbation of ILD and lung cancer. Some RA patients with ILD are known to experience acute exacerbation, with sudden progression of fibrosis and short-term mortality. Unfortunately, it is difficult to predict which patients with RA-ILD are at a high risk of ILD progression. The regular monitoring of RA-ILD patients is important for the prompt identification of ILD progression and early intervention to preserve lung function [68,74]. Recently, we reported that the standardized incidence ratios of lung cancer in our RA cohort compared with the general population was 2.53 (95% CI, 1.29–3.77) for male patients. The presence of ILD was a strong predictive factor for lung cancer occurring in RA patients over time [75]. During follow-up, increased lung cancer-related mortality was observed in RA patients compared with non-RA patients (crude incidence rate: 0.29 per PY vs. 0.10 per PY). The presence of combined pulmonary fibrosis and emphysema was identified as an independent predictive factor for lung cancer-related mortality [76]. Non-surgical cancer treatment includes chemotherapy and radiation therapy, which are well known to exacerbate pulmonary fibrosis. Limited options for lung cancer treatment and treatment-associated complications may be associated with the increased lung cancer-related mortality observed in RA-ILD patients.

There are at least four potential limitations concerning the results of this study. First, this was a retrospective long-term observational study, in which there might be some difficulty in tracing subjects. However, the electronic medical records in the database of our medical center allowed us to obtain accurate clinical and HRCT data obtained at RA-ILD diagnosis as well as RA diagnosis, time from RA-ILD diagnosis (or RA diagnosis) to death, information about DMARD use during follow-up, and DAS28-CRP for the last 6 months. Second, we could not include the exposure history of individual DMARDs during follow-up as a predictor variable in the Fine-Gray regression analysis because it was a time-varying covariate. Instead, we classified each patient into good and poor RA activity control groups based on the mean DAS28-CRP value for the 6 months before the end of follow-up and found that the rate of poor control of RA activity was significantly higher in RA patients with ILD than in those without ILD. There was a negative effect of poor RA activity control on mortality in RA patients with and without ILD. However, the increased mortality observed in RA-ILD patients was not simply explained by poor RA control due to the restriction of DMARD use. Third, although lung biopsy is the gold standard for the classification of UIP patterns, we could not obtain lung biopsy samples from fibrosis lesions in RA-ILD patients. Histological confirmation of alternative diagnosis was not required in daily practice for RA-ILD patients because RA was definitively diagnosed as the cause of ILD in these cases. Additionally, there is the risk of biopsy-related complications. Considering the risk of lung biopsy and the benefit of establishing a definite diagnosis of UIP patterns, treating physicians did not perform lung biopsy in many cases. Finally, this study was conducted in our medical center located in the Kyushu area of Japan. Therefore, our findings might not be generalizable to other geographical areas.

5. Conclusions

Compared with the general population, the mortality rate was 2.1 times higher in patients with RA-ILD. The presence of ILD appeared to contribute to the excess death in RA patients, although all ILD cases except one were subclinical at the first diagnosis. RA-ILD patients had a mortality risk three times higher than that of RA patients without ILD. The HRCT pattern at baseline was not associated with mortality risk in patients with RA-ILD. Poor control of RA activity had a negative impact on prognosis in RA patients. Even if RA disease activity was well controlled, however, the presence of ILD was a strong predictive factor for mortality Although the generalizability of the current results must be established in future research, the present study has enhanced our understanding of the relationship between mortality risk and RA-ILD. We had expected that the early detection of ILD at RA diagnosis and during follow-up with HRCT examinations would improve patient outcomes by the timely initiation of treatment for ILD and careful therapeutic decisions for RA. However, subclinical ILD at baseline contributed to the increased risk for death in RA-ILD patients during long-term follow-up. In addition to HRCT screening for the early detection of ILD, regularly monitoring RA-ILD patients for the prompt identification of ILD progression and the development of comorbidities, such as lung cancer and acute exacerbation, is critical in improving patient outcome. A multidisciplinary approach is required for optimizing the management of each RA-ILD patient.

Supplementary Materials: The following supporting information can be downloaded at: https://www.mdpi.com/article/10.3390/jcm14041380/s1, Table S1. DMARD use during follow-up in overall RA patients. Table S2. DMARD use during follow-up in RA-ILD patients. Figure S1. Participant flow diagram. ACR, American College of Rheumatology; EULAR, European League Against Rheumatism; RA, rheumatoid arthritis; SLE, systemic lupus erythematosus; SSc, systemic sclerosis; ILD, interstitial lung disease; RA-ILD, RA-associated ILD; HRCT, high-resolution computed tomography. Figure S2. Probabilities of death events in RA-ILD patients over time grouped by HRCT patterns. Probability of death events during the follow-up period was estimated by the CIF. Gray's test with a post hoc Holm test was used for the comparisons of CIF plots over time among RA-ILD patients grouped according to HRCT patterns. There were no significant differences among HRCT patterns ($p = 0.57$). Numbers below the graph indicate RA-ILD patients remaining in the follow-up. RA, rheumatoid arthritis; ILD, interstitial lung disease; RA-ILD, RA-associated ILD; HRCT, high-resolution computed tomography; CIF, cumulative incidence function; UIP, usual interstitial pneumonia; NSIP, non-specific interstitial pneumonia.

Author Contributions: Conceptualization, S.M. and K.N.; Methodology, S.M. and K.N.; Validation, S.M., F.S., M.H., and K.N.; Formal Analysis, S.M.; Investigation, S.M., F.S., M.H., K.N., and K.S.; Resources, S.M., F.S., M.H., K.N., and K.S.; Data Curation, S.M.; Writing—Original Draft Preparation, S.M.; Writing—Review and Editing, S.M., F.S., M.H., K.N., and K.S.; Visualization, S.M.; Supervision, S.M. and K.N.; Project Administration, S.M.; Funding Acquisition, S.M. All authors have read and agreed to the published version of the manuscript.

Funding: This study was supported by internal research funds from the National Hospital Organization (NHO), Japan. The funder had no role in the study design; data collection, analysis, and interpretation; decision to publish; or manuscript preparation. No external funding was received for this study.

Institutional Review Board Statement: This study was conducted in accordance with the principles of the Declaration of Helsinki. The protocol of this study met the requirements of the Ethical Guidelines for Medical and Health Research Involving Human Subjects, Japan, and was approved by the Human Research Ethics Committee at the NHO Kumamoto Saishun Medical Center (No. 4-18; 16 January 2023).

Informed Consent Statement: Because the study involved a retrospective review of patient records and data were analyzed anonymously, our ethics committees waived the requirement for patient informed consent to participate.

Data Availability Statement: All data supporting the findings are available from the Human Research Ethics Committee of National Hospital Organization Kumamoto Saishun Medical Center for all interested researchers who meet the criteria for access to confidential data. Because these data include patients' personal information, the Committee does not recommend that such data be made unnecessarily public. Please contact Mr. Masahiro Hamaguchi, the Control Manager of the Committee, at 616-syol@mail.hosp.go.jp to request the data.

Conflicts of Interest: S. Mori received honoraria for lectures from AbbVie GK; Eli Lilly Japan K.K.; Pfizer Japan Inc.; Chugai Pharmaceutical Co., Ltd.; Eli Lilly Japan K.K.; Eisai Co., Ltd.; and Taisho

Pharma Co., Ltd. These companies had no role in the study design; data collection, analysis, and interpretation; decision to publish; or manuscript preparation. The other authors declare that they have no financial relationships that could create a potential conflict of interest or the appearance of a conflict of interest with regard to the work.

References

1. Smolen, J.S.; Aletaha, D.; McInnes, I.B. Rheumatoid arthritis. *Lancet* **2016**, *388*, 2023–2038. [CrossRef] [PubMed]
2. McInnes, I.B.; Schett, G. Pathogenetic insights from the treatment of rheumatoid arthritis. *Lancet* **2017**, *389*, 2328–2337. [CrossRef] [PubMed]
3. Figus, F.A.; Piga, M.; Azzolin, I.; McConnell, R.; Iagnocco, A. Rheumatoid arthritis: Extra-articular manifestations and comorbidities. *Autoimmun. Rev.* **2021**, *20*, 102776. [CrossRef] [PubMed]
4. Taylor, P.C.; Atzeni, F.; Balsa, A.; Gossec, L.; Muller-Ladner, U.; Pope, J. The Key Comorbidities in Patients with Rheumatoid Arthritis: A Narrative Review. *J. Clin. Med.* **2021**, *10*, 509. [CrossRef] [PubMed]
5. Wu, D.; Luo, Y.; Li, T.; Zhao, X.; Lv, T.; Fang, G.; Ou, P.; Li, H.; Luo, X.; Huang, A.; et al. Systemic complications of rheumatoid arthritis: Focus on pathogenesis and treatment. *Front. Immunol.* **2022**, *13*, 1051082. [CrossRef] [PubMed]
6. Myasoedova, E.; Matteson, E.L. Updates on interstitial lung disease and other selected extra-articular manifestations of rheumatoid arthritis. *Curr. Opin. Rheumatol.* **2024**, *36*, 203–208. [CrossRef] [PubMed]
7. Kimbrough, B.A.; Crowson, C.S.; Davis, J.M., 3rd; Matteson, E.L.; Myasoedova, E. Decline in Incidence of Extra-Articular Manifestations of Rheumatoid Arthritis: A Population-Based Cohort Study. *Arthritis Care Res.* **2024**, *76*, 454–462. [CrossRef] [PubMed]
8. Simard, J.F.; Ekberg, S.; Johansson, A.L.; Askling, J. What is the impact of chronic systemic inflammation such as rheumatoid arthritis on mortality following cancer? *Ann. Rheum. Dis.* **2016**, *75*, 862–866. [CrossRef]
9. Lacaille, D.; Avina-Zubieta, J.A.; Sayre, E.C.; Abrahamowicz, M. Improvement in 5-year mortality in incident rheumatoid arthritis compared with the general population-closing the mortality gap. *Ann. Rheum. Dis.* **2017**, *76*, 1057–1063. [CrossRef]
10. Widdifield, J.; Paterson, J.M.; Huang, A.; Bernatsky, S. Causes of death in rheumatoid arthritis: How do they compare to the general population? *Arthritis Care Res.* **2018**, *70*, 1748–1755. [CrossRef] [PubMed]
11. Johnson, T.M.; Yang, Y.; Roul, P.; Sauer, B.C.; Cannon, G.W.; Kunkel, G.; Michaud, K.; Baker, J.F.; Mikuls, T.R.; England, B.R. A narrowing mortality gap: Temporal trends of cause-specific mortality in a national matched cohort study in US veteranswith rheumatoid arthritis. *Arthritis Care Res.* **2023**, *75*, 1648–1658. [CrossRef] [PubMed]
12. Zhang, Y.; Lu, N.; Peloquin, C.; Dubreuil, M.; Neogi, T.; Avina-Zubieta, J.A.; Rai, S.K.; Choi, H.K. Improved survival in rheumatoid arthritis: A general population-based cohort study. *Ann. Rheum. Dis.* **2017**, *76*, 408–413. [CrossRef]
13. Holmqvist, M.; Ljung, L.; Askling, J. Mortality following new-onset Rheumatoid Arthritis: Has modern Rheumatology had an impact? *Ann. Rheum. Dis.* **2018**, *77*, 85–91. [CrossRef] [PubMed]
14. Wang, D.; Zhang, J.; Lau, J.; Wang, S.; Taneja, V.; Matteson, E.L.; Vassallo, R. Mechanisms of lung disease development in rheumatoid arthritis. *Nat. Rev. Rheumatol.* **2019**, *15*, 581–596. [CrossRef]
15. Farquhar, H.; Vassallo, R.; Edwards, A.L.; Matteson, E.L. Pulmonary Complications of Rheumatoid Arthritis. *Semin. Respir. Crit. Care Med.* **2019**, *40*, 194–207. [CrossRef]
16. Kadura, S.; Raghu, G. Rheumatoid arthritis-interstitial lung disease: Manifestations and current concepts in pathogenesis and management. *Eur. Respir. Rev.* **2021**, *30*, 210011. [CrossRef]
17. McDermott, G.C.; Doyle, T.J.; Sparks, J.A. Interstitial lung disease throughout the rheumatoid arthritis disease course. *Curr. Opin. Rheumatol.* **2021**, *33*, 284–291. [CrossRef]
18. Matteson, E.L.; Matucci-Cerinic, M.; Kreuter, M.; Burmester, G.R.; Dieude, P.; Emery, P.; Allanore, Y.; Pope, J.; Khanna, D. Patient-level factors predictive of interstitial lung disease in rheumatoid arthritis: A systematic review. *RMD Open* **2023**, *9*, e003059. [CrossRef]
19. Putman, R.K.; Hatabu, H.; Araki, T.; Gudmundsson, G.; Gao, W.; Nishino, M.; Okajima, Y.; Dupuis, J.; Latourelle, J.C.; Cho, M.H.; et al. Association Between Interstitial Lung Abnormalities and All-Cause Mortality. *JAMA* **2016**, *315*, 672–681. [CrossRef]
20. Hyldgaard, C.; Hilberg, O.; Pedersen, A.B.; Ulrichsen, S.P.; Lokke, A.; Bendstrup, E.; Ellingsen, T. A population-based cohort study of rheumatoid arthritis-associated interstitial lung disease: Comorbidity and mortality. *Ann. Rheum. Dis.* **2017**, *76*, 1700–1706. [CrossRef]
21. Sparks, J.A.; Jin, Y.; Cho, S.K.; Vine, S.; Desai, R.; Doyle, T.J.; Kim, S.C. Prevalence, incidence and cause-specific mortality of rheumatoid arthritis-associated interstitial lung disease among older rheumatoid arthritis patients. *Rheumatology* **2021**, *60*, 3689–3698. [CrossRef] [PubMed]
22. Gao, J.; Xin, L.; Guo, Q.; Xu, K.; Zhang, G.; Yang, Y.; Ma, D.; Zhang, L. Twenty-year changes in mortality rates and underlying causes of death in patients with rheumatoid arthritis-associated interstitial lung disease. *Scand. J. Rheumatol.* **2021**, *50*, 360–364. [CrossRef]

23. Jeganathan, N.; Nguyen, E.; Sathananthan, M. Rheumatoid Arthritis and Associated Interstitial Lung Disease: Mortality Rates and Trends. *Ann. Am. Thorac. Soc.* **2021**, *18*, 1970–1977. [CrossRef] [PubMed]
24. Fidler, L.; Widdifield, J.; Fisher, J.H.; Shapera, S.; Gershon, A.S. Rheumatoid arthritis associated interstitial lung disease: Trends in epidemiology and mortality in Ontario from 2000 to 2018. *Respir. Med.* **2023**, 107282. [CrossRef] [PubMed]
25. Juge, P.A.; Wemeau, L.; Ottaviani, S.; Desjeux, G.; Zhuo, J.; Vannier-Moreau, V.; Flipo, R.M.; Crestani, B.; Dieude, P. Increased mortality in patients with RA-associated interstitial lung disease: Data from a French administrative healthcare database. *RMD Open* **2023**, *9*, e003491. [CrossRef]
26. Kim, Y.J.; Shim, J.S.; Choi, C.B.; Bae, S.C. Mortality and incidence of malignancy in Korean patients with rheumatoid arthritis. *J. Rheumatol.* **2012**, *39*, 226–232. [CrossRef] [PubMed]
27. England, B.R.; Sayles, H.; Michaud, K.; Caplan, L.; Davis, L.A.; Cannon, G.W.; Sauer, B.C.; Solow, E.B.; Reimold, A.M.; Kerr, G.S.; et al. Cause-Specific Mortality in Male US Veterans with Rheumatoid Arthritis. *Arthritis Care Res.* **2016**, *68*, 36–45. [CrossRef] [PubMed]
28. Sparks, J.A.; Chang, S.C.; Liao, K.P.; Lu, B.; Fine, A.R.; Solomon, D.H.; Costenbader, K.H.; Karlson, E.W. Rheumatoid Arthritis and Mortality Among Women During 36 Years of Prospective Follow-Up: Results From the Nurses' Health Study. *Arthritis Care Res.* **2016**, *68*, 753–762. [CrossRef]
29. Black, R.J.; Lester, S.; Tieu, J.; Sinnathurai, P.; Barrett, C.; Buchbinder, R.; Lassere, M.; March, L.; Proudman, S.M.; Hill, C.L. Mortality estimates and excess mortality in rheumatoid arthritis. *Rheumatology* **2023**, *62*, 3576–3583. [CrossRef] [PubMed]
30. Koduri, G.; Solomon, J.J. Identification, Monitoring, and Management of Rheumatoid Arthritis-Associated Interstitial Lung Disease. *Arthritis Rheumatol.* **2023**, *75*, 2067–2077. [CrossRef]
31. Sullivan, D.I.; Ascherman, D.P. Rheumatoid Arthritis-Associated Interstitial Lung Disease (RA-ILD): Update on Prevalence, Risk Factors, Pathogenesis, and Therapy. *Curr. Rheumatol. Rep.* **2024**, *26*, 431–449. [CrossRef] [PubMed]
32. Tanaka, N.; Kim, J.S.; Newell, J.D.; Brown, K.K.; Cool, C.D.; Meehan, R.; Emoto, T.; Matsumoto, T.; Lynch, D.A. Rheumatoid arthritis-related lung diseases: CT findings. *Radiology* **2004**, *232*, 81–91. [CrossRef] [PubMed]
33. Lee, J.Y.; Yang, C.C.; Hsu, M.M. Histopathology of persistent papules and plaques in adult-onset Still's disease. *J. Am. Acad. Dermatol.* **2005**, *52*, 1003–1008. [CrossRef] [PubMed]
34. Kim, E.J.; Collard, H.R.; King, T.E., Jr. Rheumatoid arthritis-associated interstitial lung disease: The relevance of histopathologic and radiographic pattern. *Chest* **2009**, *136*, 1397–1405. [CrossRef]
35. Kim, E.J.; Elicker, B.M.; Maldonado, F.; Webb, W.R.; Ryu, J.H.; Van Uden, J.H.; Lee, J.S.; King, T.E., Jr.; Collard, H.R. Usual interstitial pneumonia in rheumatoid arthritis-associated interstitial lung disease. *Eur. Respir. J.* **2010**, *35*, 1322–1328. [CrossRef] [PubMed]
36. Singh, N.; Varghese, J.; England, B.R.; Solomon, J.J.; Michaud, K.; Mikuls, T.R.; Healy, H.S.; Kimpston, E.M.; Schweizer, M.L. Impact of the pattern of interstitial lung disease on mortality in rheumatoid arthritis: A systematic literature review and meta-analysis. *Semin. Arthritis Rheum.* **2019**, *49*, 358–365. [CrossRef] [PubMed]
37. Qiu, M.; Jiang, J.; Nian, X.; Wang, Y.; Yu, P.; Song, J.; Zou, S. Factors associated with mortality in rheumatoid arthritis-associated interstitial lung disease: A systematic review and meta-analysis. *Respir. Res.* **2021**, *22*, 264. [CrossRef] [PubMed]
38. Groseanu, L.; Nita, C. A Systematic Review of the Key Predictors of Progression and Mortality of Rheumatoid Arthritis-Associated Interstitial Lung Disease. *Diagnostics* **2024**, *14*, 1890. [CrossRef] [PubMed]
39. Aletaha, D.; Neogi, T.; Silman, A.J.; Funovits, J.; Felson, D.T.; Bingham, C.O., 3rd; Birnbaum, N.S.; Burmester, G.R.; Bykerk, V.P.; Cohen, M.D.; et al. 2010 Rheumatoid arthritis classification criteria: An American College of Rheumatology/European League Against Rheumatism collaborative initiative. *Arthritis Rheum.* **2010**, *62*, 2569–2581. [CrossRef]
40. Mori, S.; Naito, H.; Ohtani, S.; Yamanaka, T.; Sugimoto, M. Diagnostic utility of anti-cyclic citrullinated peptide antibodies for rheumatoid arthritis in patients with active lung tuberculosis. *Clin. Rheumatol.* **2009**, *28*, 277–283. [CrossRef] [PubMed]
41. Mori, S. Management of rheumatoid arthritis patients with interstitial lung disease: Safety of biological antirheumatic drugs and assessment of pulmonary fibrosis. *Clin. Med. Insights Circ. Respir. Pulm. Med.* **2015**, *9*, 41–49. [CrossRef]
42. Homma, S.; Sugino, K.; Sakamoto, S. Usefulness of a disease severity staging classification system for IPF in Japan: 20 years of experience from empirical evidence to randomized control trial enrollment. *Respir. Investig.* **2015**, *53*, 7–12. [CrossRef] [PubMed]
43. Raghu, G.; Remy-Jardin, M.; Myers, J.L.; Richeldi, L.; Ryerson, C.J.; Lederer, D.J.; Behr, J.; Cottin, V.; Danoff, S.K.; Morell, F.; et al. Diagnosis of idiopathic pulmonary fibrosis: An official ATS/ERS/JRS/ALAT clinical practice guideline. *Am. J. Respir. Crit. Care Med.* **2018**, *198*, e44–e68. [CrossRef] [PubMed]
44. Raghu, G.; Remy-Jardin, M.; Richeldi, L.; Thomson, C.C.; Inoue, Y.; Johkoh, T.; Kreuter, M.; Lynch, D.A.; Maher, T.M.; Martinez, F.J.; et al. Idiopathic pulmonary fibrosis (an update) and progressive pulmonary fibrosis in adults: An official ATS/ERS/JRS/ALAT clinical practice guideline. *Am. J. Respir. Crit. Care Med.* **2022**, *205*, e18–e47. [CrossRef]
45. Wilsher, M.; Voight, L.; Milne, D.; Teh, M.; Good, N.; Kolbe, J.; Williams, M.; Pui, K.; Merriman, T.; Sidhu, K.; et al. Prevalence of airway and parenchymal abnormalities in newly diagnosed rheumatoid arthritis. *Respir. Med.* **2012**, *106*, 1441–1446. [CrossRef]

46. Yamakawa, H.; Sato, S.; Tsumiyama, E.; Nishizawa, T.; Kawabe, R.; Oba, T.; Kamikawa, T.; Horikoshi, M.; Akasaka, K.; Amano, M.; et al. Predictive factors of mortality in rheumatoid arthritis-associated interstitial lung disease analysed by modified HRCT classification of idiopathic pulmonary fibrosis according to the 2018 ATS/ERS/JRS/ALAT criteria. *J. Thorac. Dis.* **2019**, *11*, 5247–5257. [CrossRef] [PubMed]
47. Lydersen, S. Statistical review: Frequently given comments. *Ann. Rheum. Dis.* **2015**, *74*, 323–325. [CrossRef] [PubMed]
48. Lydersen, S. Mean and standard deviation or median and quartiles? *Tidsskr. Nor. Laegeforen.* **2020**, *140*, pii 20-0032. [CrossRef]
49. Austin, P.C.; Lee, D.S.; Fine, J.P. Introduction to the analysis of survival Data in the presence of competing risks. *Circulation* **2016**, *133*, 601–609. [CrossRef] [PubMed]
50. Kanda, Y. Investigation of the freely available easy-to-use software 'EZR' for medical statistics. *Bone Marrow Transpl.* **2013**, *48*, 452–458. [CrossRef] [PubMed]
51. Kelly, C.A.; Saravanan, V.; Nisar, M.; Arthanari, S.; Woodhead, F.A.; Price-Forbes, A.N.; Dawson, J.; Sathi, N.; Ahmad, Y.; Koduri, G.; et al. Rheumatoid arthritis-related interstitial lung disease: Associations, prognostic factors and physiological and radiological characteristics—A large multicentre UK study. *Rheumatology* **2014**, *53*, 1676–1682. [CrossRef] [PubMed]
52. Solomon, J.J.; Chung, J.H.; Cosgrove, G.P.; Demoruelle, M.K.; Fernandez-Perez, E.R.; Fischer, A.; Frankel, S.K.; Hobbs, S.B.; Huie, T.J.; Ketzer, J.; et al. Predictors of mortality in rheumatoid arthritis-associated interstitial lung disease. *Eur. Respir. J.* **2016**, *47*, 588–596. [CrossRef] [PubMed]
53. Yunt, Z.X.; Chung, J.H.; Hobbs, S.; Fernandez-Perez, E.R.; Olson, A.L.; Huie, T.J.; Keith, R.C.; Janssen, W.J.; Goldstein, B.L.; Lynch, D.A.; et al. High resolution computed tomography pattern of usual interstitial pneumonia in rheumatoid arthritis-associated interstitial lung disease: Relationship to survival. *Respir. Med.* **2017**, *126*, 100–104. [CrossRef]
54. Putman, R.K.; Gudmundsson, G.; Axelsson, G.T.; Hida, T.; Honda, O.; Araki, T.; Yanagawa, M.; Nishino, M.; Miller, E.R.; Eiriksdottir, G.; et al. Imaging Patterns Are Associated with Interstitial Lung Abnormality Progression and Mortality. *Am. J. Respir. Crit. Care Med.* **2019**, *200*, 175–183. [CrossRef]
55. Kim, H.C.; Lee, J.S.; Lee, E.Y.; Ha, Y.J.; Chae, E.J.; Han, M.; Cross, G.; Barnett, J.; Joseph, J.; Song, J.W. Risk prediction model in rheumatoid arthritis-associated interstitial lung disease. *Respirology* **2020**, *25*, 1257–1264. [CrossRef] [PubMed]
56. Mena-Vazquez, N.; Rojas-Gimenez, M.; Romero-Barco, C.M.; Manrique-Arija, S.; Francisco, E.; Aguilar-Hurtado, M.C.; Anon-Onate, I.; Perez-Albaladejo, L.; Ortega-Castro, R.; Godoy-Navarrete, F.J.; et al. Predictors of Progression and Mortality in Patients with Prevalent Rheumatoid Arthritis and Interstitial Lung Disease: A Prospective Cohort Study. *J. Clin. Med.* **2021**, *10*, 874. [CrossRef] [PubMed]
57. Chen, N.; Diao, C.Y.; Gao, J.; Zhao, D.B. Risk factors for the progression of rheumatoid arthritis-related interstitial lung disease: Clinical features, biomarkers, and treatment options. *Semin. Arthritis Rheum.* **2022**, *55*, 152004. [CrossRef]
58. Liu, L.; Fang, C.; Sun, B.; Bao, R.; Zhang, H. Predictors of progression in rheumatoid arthritis-associated interstitial lung disease: A single-center retrospective study from China. *Int. J. Rheum. Dis.* **2022**, *25*, 795–802. [CrossRef]
59. Song, Y.J.; Kim, H.; Cho, S.K.; Kim, H.W.; Lim, C.; Nam, E.; Choi, C.B.; Kim, T.H.; Jun, J.B.; Bae, S.C.; et al. Risk factors of mortality in patients with rheumatoid arthritis-associated interstitial lung disease: A single-centre prospective cohort study. *Arthritis Res. Ther.* **2024**, *26*, 137. [CrossRef] [PubMed]
60. Rojas-Serrano, J.; Herrera-Bringas, D.; Perez-Roman, D.I.; Perez-Dorame, R.; Mateos-Toledo, H.; Mejia, M. Rheumatoid arthritis-related interstitial lung disease (RA-ILD): Methotrexate and the severity of lung disease are associated to prognosis. *Clin. Rheumatol.* **2017**, *36*, 1493–1500. [CrossRef] [PubMed]
61. Fu, Q.; Wang, L.; Li, L.; Li, Y.; Liu, R.; Zheng, Y. Risk factors for progression and prognosis of rheumatoid arthritis-associated interstitial lung disease: Single center study with a large sample of Chinese population. *Clin. Rheumatol.* **2019**, *38*, 1109–1116. [CrossRef]
62. Kawano-Dourado, L.; Doyle, T.J.; Bonfiglioli, K.; Sawamura, M.V.Y.; Nakagawa, R.H.; Arimura, F.E.; Lee, H.J.; Rangel, D.A.S.; Bueno, C.; Carvalho, C.R.R.; et al. Baseline Characteristics and Progression of a Spectrum of Interstitial Lung Abnormalities and Disease in Rheumatoid Arthritis. *Chest* **2020**, *158*, 1546–1554. [CrossRef]
63. Chai, D.; Sun, D.; Wang, Y.; Song, Y.; Wu, N.; Ye, Q. Progression of radiographic fibrosis in rheumatoid arthritis-associated interstitial lung disease. *Front. Med.* **2023**, *10*, 1265355. [CrossRef]
64. Chang, S.H.; Lee, J.S.; Ha, Y.J.; Kim, M.U.; Park, C.H.; Lee, J.S.; Kim, J.W.; Chung, S.W.; Pyo, J.Y.; Lee, S.W.; et al. Lung function trajectory of rheumatoid arthritis-associated interstitial lung disease. *Rheumatology* **2023**, *62*, 3014–3024. [CrossRef]
65. Farquhar, H.J.; Beckert, L.; Edwards, A.L.; Matteson, E.L.; Frampton, C.M.A.; Ganly, E.; Yetton, R.; Thiessen, R.; Haslett, J.; Bucknall, D.; et al. Rheumatoid interstitial lung disease in Canterbury, Aotearoa New Zealand—A retrospective cohort study. *Semin. Arthritis Rheum.* **2024**, *64*, 152359. [CrossRef]
66. Zamora-Legoff, J.A.; Krause, M.L.; Crowson, C.S.; Ryu, J.H.; Matteson, E.L. Patterns of interstitial lung disease and mortality in rheumatoid arthritis. *Rheumatology* **2017**, *56*, 344–350. [CrossRef] [PubMed]

67. Jacob, J.; Hirani, N.; van Moorsel, C.H.M.; Rajagopalan, S.; Murchison, J.T.; van Es, H.W.; Bartholmai, B.J.; van Beek, F.T.; Struik, M.H.L.; Stewart, G.A.; et al. Predicting outcomes in rheumatoid arthritis related interstitial lung disease. *Eur. Respir. J.* **2019**, *53*, 1800869. [CrossRef] [PubMed]
68. Matteson, E.L.; Bendstrup, E.; Strek, M.E.; Dieude, P. Clinical Course of Interstitial Lung Disease in Patients With Rheumatoid Arthritis. *ACR Open Rheumatol.* **2024**, *6*, 836–845. [CrossRef] [PubMed]
69. Brooks, R.; Baker, J.F.; Yang, Y.; Roul, P.; Kerr, G.S.; Reimold, A.M.; Kunkel, G.; Wysham, K.D.; Singh, N.; Lazaro, D.; et al. The impact of disease severity measures on survival in U.S. veterans with rheumatoid arthritis-associated interstitial lung disease. *Rheumatology* **2022**, *61*, 4667–4677. [CrossRef]
70. Dawson, J.K.; Quah, E.; Earnshaw, B.; Amoasii, C.; Mudawi, T.; Spencer, L.G. Does methotrexate cause progressive fibrotic interstitial lung disease? A systematic review. *Rheumatol. Int.* **2021**, *41*, 1055–1064. [CrossRef]
71. Kim, K.; Woo, A.; Park, Y.; Yong, S.H.; Lee, S.H.; Lee, S.H.; Leem, A.Y.; Kim, S.Y.; Chung, K.S.; Kim, E.Y.; et al. Protective effect of methotrexate on lung function and mortality in rheumatoid arthritis-related interstitial lung disease: A retrospective cohort study. *Ther. Adv. Respir. Dis.* **2022**, *16*, 17534666221135314. [CrossRef]
72. Kim, J.W.; Chung, S.W.; Pyo, J.Y.; Chang, S.H.; Kim, M.U.; Park, C.H.; Lee, J.S.; Lee, J.S.; Ha, Y.J.; Kang, E.H.; et al. Methotrexate, leflunomide and tacrolimus use and the progression of rheumatoid arthritis-associated interstitial lung disease. *Rheumatology* **2023**, *62*, 2377–2385. [CrossRef] [PubMed]
73. Fraenkel, L.; Bathon, J.M.; England, B.R.; St Clair, E.W.; Arayssi, T.; Carandang, K.; Deane, K.D.; Genovese, M.; Huston, K.K.; Kerr, G.; et al. 2021 American College of Rheumatology Guideline for the Treatment of Rheumatoid Arthritis. *Arthritis Rheumatol.* **2021**, *73*, 1108–1123. [CrossRef] [PubMed]
74. Luppi, F.; Sebastiani, M.; Salvarani, C.; Bendstrup, E.; Manfredi, A. Acute exacerbation of interstitial lung disease associated with rheumatic disease. *Nat. Rev. Rheumatol.* **2022**, *18*, 85–96. [CrossRef]
75. Mori, S.; Hasegawa, M.; Sakai, F.; Nakashima, K.; Nakamura, K. Incidence of and predictive factors for lung cancer in patients with rheumatoid arthritis: A retrospective long-term follow-up study. *Mod. Rheumatol.* **2024**, roae084. [CrossRef]
76. Mori, S.; Ueki, Y.; Hasegawa, M.; Nakamura, K.; Nakashima, K.; Hidaka, T.; Ishii, K.; Kobayashi, H.; Miyamura, T. Impact of combined pulmonary fibrosis and emphysema on lung cancer risk and mortality in rheumatoid arthritis: A multicenter retrospective cohort study. *PLoS ONE* **2024**, *19*, e0298573. [CrossRef] [PubMed]

Journal of
Clinical Medicine

MDPI

Article

Clinical Significance of Antinuclear Antibodies in Patients with Rheumatoid Arthritis: From SETOUCHI-RA Registry

Kazuhisa Nakano [1,*], Shunichi Fujita [1], Sumie Hiramatsu-Asano [1], Akiko Nagasu [1], Shoko Tsuji [1], Yuka Koide [1], Masatomo Yamada [1], Yo Mizuta [1], Masakatsu Ikeda [1], Hiroyasu Hirano [2] and Yoshitaka Morita [1]

1 Department of Rheumatology, Kawasaki Medical School, 577 Matsushima, Kurashiki 701-0192, Okayama, Japan; shunichi@med.kawasaki-m.ac.jp (S.F.); h061eb@med.kawasaki-m.ac.jp (S.H.-A.); nagasu.a@med.kawasaki-m.ac.jp (A.N.); shoko.0513@med.kawasaki-m.ac.jp (S.T.); koidey1223@med.kawasaki-m.ac.jp (Y.K.); yamada.masatomo@med.kawasaki-m.ac.jp (M.Y.); y-mizuta@med.kawasaki-m.ac.jp (Y.M.); mimi2411113@med.kawasaki-m.ac.jp (M.I.); morita@med.kawasaki-m.ac.jp (Y.M.)

2 Department of General Internal Medicine 1, Kawasaki Medical School, 577 Matsushima, Kurashiki 701-0192, Okayama, Japan; h-hirano@med.kawasaki-m.ac.jp

* Correspondence: nakanok@med.kawasaki-m.ac.jp

Abstract: Background/Objectives: Rheumatoid arthritis (RA) is a representative systemic autoimmune rheumatic disease (SARD) characterized by synovial inflammation. While antinuclear antibodies (ANAs) positivity in patients with RA varies widely, the relationship between ANA patterns and clinical features remains unclear. This study aimed to evaluate the clinical significance of ANA in patients with RA. **Methods:** This single-center RA registry study included 814 Japanese patients after excluding those with coexisting SARDs. ANA titers and staining patterns were assessed by indirect immunofluorescence assays on HEp-2 cells. Clinical and laboratory features were analyzed, and logistic regression was used to identify risk factors for pulmonary involvement. Hierarchical clustering and statistical analyses were performed to explore associations between ANA patterns and clinical features. **Results:** ANA positivity was observed in 41.5% of patients, with the speckled and homogeneous patterns being the most common. ANA-positive patients exhibited significantly higher rheumatoid factor (RF) and anti-cyclic citrullinated peptide antibody (ACPA) positivity rates and titers, along with elevated disease activity markers, including Evaluator's Global Assessment and Swollen Joint Count. Nucleolar pattern positivity was independently associated with pulmonary complications, predominantly interstitial lung disease, and higher rates of JAK inhibitor use. Discrete-speckled pattern-positive patients exhibited high ANA titers but lower RF and ACPA levels, reflecting a distinct subset of RA. **Conclusions:** ANA staining patterns and titers are clinically relevant in RA, with nucleolar and discrete-speckled patterns indicating distinct clinical and pathophysiological profiles. ANA should be interpreted alongside other serological markers and clinical parameters rather than as a standalone tool. Further studies are needed to refine its clinical applicability and integration into RA management.

Keywords: rheumatoid arthritis; antinuclear antibodies; pulmonary complications

1. Introduction

Rheumatoid arthritis (RA) is a representative systemic autoimmune rheumatic disease (SARD) primarily characterized by inflammation of the synovium [1]. If left untreated, RA can lead to joint destruction and irreversible organ damage. Although the etiology remains unknown, autoimmunity with the production of various autoantibodies plays a crucial role in RA-related inflammation. Rheumatoid factor (RF) and anti-cyclic citrullinated peptide antibody (ACPA), both well-recognized autoantibodies in RA, serve as key serological markers used in the diagnosis of RA and as indicators of poor prognosis [1,2].

Antinuclear antibodies (ANA) refer to a diverse group of autoantibodies targeting various nuclear and cytoplasmic components. The indirect immunofluorescence assay (IIFA) using HEp-2 cells has long been recognized as the gold standard for ANA detection. The observed fluorescence patterns reflect different cellular components, including nuclear, cytoplasmic, and mitotic structures. In recent years, the International Consensus on ANA Patterns (ICAP) initiative has established standardized nomenclature and definitions for ANA patterns [3]. ANA fluorescence patterns, along with antibody titers (or fluorescence intensity), are known as significant biomarkers for SARDs, such as systemic lupus erythematosus (SLE) and Sjögren's syndrome (SS) [4,5]. However, in patients with RA, ANA positivity rates have been reported to vary widely (14–77%) [6–9]. The relationship between ANA titers or staining patterns (e.g., homogeneous nuclear, speckled nuclear, and cytoplasmic speckled patterns) and clinical manifestations, disease course, or treatment selection in RA remains inconclusive.

To purely assess the clinical significance of ANA in patients with RA, it is essential to exclude patients with coexisting SARDs. The presence of SARDs may influence the frequency of ANA positivity and the clinical manifestations, thereby complicating the interpretation of the specific significance of ANA in RA.

This study aimed to evaluate the differences in clinical characteristics between ANA-positive and ANA-negative patients with RA, specifically excluding those with coexisting SARDs. Additionally, the impacts of ANA titers and staining patterns on disease activity, treatment selection, and prognosis were examined to comprehensively elucidate the clinical significance of ANA in RA.

2. Materials and Methods

2.1. Patients

All of the study participants were recruited from the prospective comprehensive single-center cohort (SurvEillance of Treatment Outcome of RA patients in Clinics and HospItals: SETOUCHI-RA registry) [10]. All patients are Japanese RA patients, and each has a diagnosis of RA based on the 1987 American College of Rheumatology (ACR) criteria [11] and/or 2010 ACR/European League Against Rheumatism (EULAR) classification criteria for RA [12].

2.2. Data Collection

Of the 917 patients with RA aged 18 years or older who visited the hospital between October 2022 and January 2023, 877 patients underwent disease activity assessment using the Clinical Disease Activity Index (CDAI) and serological assessment including ANA. Treatment histories and clinical data were collected with a data-collecting system and evaluated. The 814 patients were included in the analysis, excluding 63 patients with SARDs other than RA (Figure 1, Supplementary Table S1). This study was approved by the Ethics Committee of our hospital (Ethics Application No. 5564-04) and conducted in accordance with the Ethical Guidelines for Medical and Health Research Involving Human Subjects.

Malignancy was defined as the presence of a currently treated or monitored malignant tumor, as well as a history of previously treated malignancy. RA-lung disease was defined as the presence of pulmonary manifestations, including interstitial lung diseases (ILD), airway-related diseases, pulmonary vasculature involvement, and pleural involvement [13–15], with the majority of cases being ILD. These conditions were confirmed by a rheumatologist and/or pulmonologist based on clinical evaluation, imaging studies (e.g., chest computed tomography), and/or pulmonary function tests, as appropriate. Difficult-to-treat rheumatoid arthritis (D2T-RA) was defined according to the EULAR criteria [16] as patients who required two or more biologics or JAK inhibitors with different modes of action but still had a CDAI score of 10 or higher, or required glucocorticoids equivalent to 7.5 mg/day or more of prednisolone.

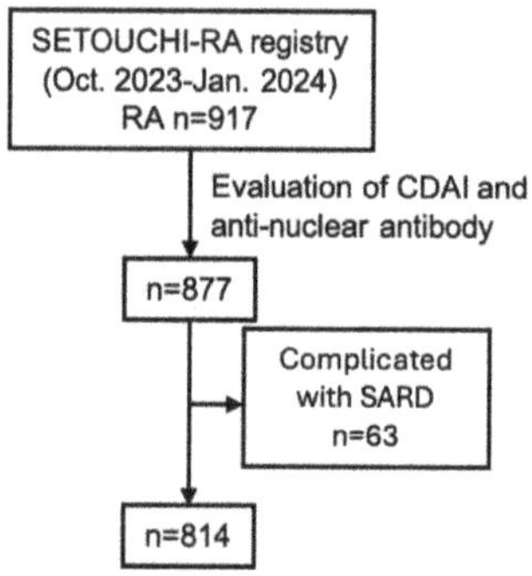

Figure 1. Process of patient selection.

ANA was determined by the fluorescent antibody method (SRL Co., Inc. Tokyo, Japan). Baseline ANA levels more than 1:40 were regarded as positive. ACPA was quantified by the ARCHITECT anti-CCP assay (Abbott Japan, Tokyo, Japan). IgM-rheumatoid factor (RF) was quantified by latex–turbidimetric immunoassay, using the N-Assay LA RF-K Nittobo (Nittobo Medical, Koriyama, Japan). The cutoff levels of the antibodies were set according to the manufacturers' instructions (ACPA < 4.5 U/mL, RF < 15 IU/mL).

2.3. Statistical Analysis

JMP version 17.0 (SAS Institute Japan Ltd., Tokyo, Japan) was used for statistical analyses. Descriptive summary statistics are provided in Table 1 and Supplementary Table S2 for all continuous variables with parametric or non-parametric data, analyzed using the chi-square test or Wilcoxon rank-sum test, as appropriate. Differences were considered statistically significant at a two-tailed $p < 0.05$ level. The clinical information and laboratory data items of patients with RA were subjected to hierarchical clustering using Ward's method and visualized as a heat map. A multivariable logistic regression analysis was then performed to investigate the factors associated with RA-associated lung disease in the univariable analysis ($p < 0.1$).

Table 1. Clinical and laboratory features in patients with rheumatoid arthritis stratified by anti-nuclear antibody status.

	Total	ANA-Negative	ANA-Positive	*p*-Value
Number	814	476 (41.5)	338 (58.5)	
Gender: Female (%)	613 (75.3)	346 (72.7)	267 (80.0)	0.048
Age, y	66 (56, 75)	66 (57, 74)	66 (55.8, 75)	0.83
Disease duration, M	131 (67, 200)	129 (69, 191)	137 (61, 203)	0.39
BMI, kg/m^2	22.5 (20.0, 25.0)	22.6 (19.9, 24.8)	22.5 (20.1, 25.4)	0.55
RA Family history (%)	164 (20.3)	92 (19.4)	72 (21.5)	0.48
Smoking history (%)	319 (39.2)	192 (40.5)	127 (37.6)	0.42
Positivity of RF (%)	594 (73.0)	321 (67.4)	273 (80.8)	<0.0001

Table 1. *Cont.*

	Total	ANA-Negative	ANA-Positive	p-Value
Positivity of ACPA (%)	629 (77.3)	352 (74.0)	277 (82.0)	0.007
Erosive X-ray (%)	416 (51.4)	238 (50.2)	178 (53.0)	0.31
Pain VAS	15 (2, 40)	10 (2, 30)	20 (2, 40)	0.21
Fatigue VAS	20 (10, 50)	20 (10, 50)	27.5 (10, 50)	0.41
PGA	20 (5, 40)	17 (3, 30)	20 (10, 40)	0.12
EGA	0 (0, 10)	0 (0, 10)	10 (0, 10)	0.04
TJ	0 (0, 0)	0 (0, 0)	0 (0, 0)	0.91
TJ28	0 (0, 0)	0 (0, 0)	0 (0, 0)	0.84
SJ	0 (0, 0)	0 (0, 0)	0 (0, 0.25)	0.09
SJ28	0 (0, 0)	0 (0, 0)	0 (0, 0)	0.03
CDAI	3 (1, 6)	2 (1, 6)	3 (1, 7)	0.17
HAQ	0 (0, 0.5)	0 (0, 0.5)	0 (0, 0.625)	0.81
EQ-5D	0.77 (0.65, 1)	0.77 (0.67, 1)	0.77 (0.65, 1)	0.68
D2T-RA (%)	24 (2.9)	14 (2.9)	10 (3.0)	1.00
		Complication		
Lung disease (%)	106 (13.0)	65 (13.7)	41 (12.1)	0.60
Malignancy (%)	137 (16.8)	80 (16.8)	57 (16.9)	1.00
Osteoarthritis (%)	180 (22.1)	107 (22.5)	73 (21.6)	0.80
Mental disorders (%)	34 (4.2)	17 (3.6)	17 (5.0)	0.37
		Laboratory data		
RF, IU/mL	42 (10, 135)	29.5 (0, 121)	54 (21, 163)	<0.0001
ACPA, U/mL	60.9 (6.7, 339)	47.5 (4.0, 255)	81.1 (10.8, 429.4)	0.0009
ESR, mm/h	14 (6, 29)	12 (5, 25)	18 (8, 33)	<0.0001
CRP, mg/dL	0.12 (0.05, 0.33)	0.11 (0.04, 0.32)	0.12 (0.06, 0.33)	0.33
WBC, /μL	5510 (4435, 6875)	5480 (4460, 6863)	5640 (4390, 6900)	0.98
Hb, g/dL	13.1 (12.2, 14)	13.1 (12.2, 14)	13.1 (12.1, 14)	0.28
Plt, $\times 10^3/\mu L$	232 (190, 278)	232 (190.8, 208.3)	230 (190, 273)	0.96
TP, g/dL	7.1 (6.9, 7.4)	7.1 (6.8, 7.4)	7.2 (6.9, 7.5)	<0.0001
Alb/Glob ratio	1.4 (1.2, 1.6)	1.4 (1.2, 1.6)	1.3 (1.2, 1.5)	<0.0001
IgG, mg/dL	1257 (1069, 1473)	1196 (1032, 1406)	1353 (1136, 1598)	<0.0001
IgA, mg/dL	256 (186, 341)	247 (174, 331)	266 (205, 354)	0.003
IgM, mg/dL	89 (64, 126)	82 (57, 113)	102 (75, 141)	<0.0001
		Previously Used DMARDs		
MTX (%)	717 (88.1)	423 (88.9)	294 (87.0)	0.44
bDMARDs (%)	478 (58.7)	267 (56.1)	211 (62.4)	0.07
TNFi (%)	391 (48.0)	212 (44.5)	179 (53.0)	0.02
IL-6Ri (%)	167 (20.5)	108 (22.7)	59 (17.5)	0.08
ABT (%)	94 (11.5)	49 (10.3)	45 (13.4)	0.22
JAKi (%)	125 (15.4)	74 (15.6)	51 (15.1)	0.92
Glucocorticoid (%)	524 (64.4)	312 (65.6)	212 (62.7)	0.41
		DMARDs in Current Use		
MTX (%)	498 (61.2)	295 (62.0)	203 (60.1)	0.61
TNFi (%)	169 (20.7)	83 (17.4)	86 (25.4)	0.01
IL-6Ri (%)	96 (11.8)	65 (13.7)	31 (9.2)	0.06
ABT (%)	56 (6.9)	31 (6.5)	25 (7.4)	0.67
JAKi (%)	103 (12.7)	60 (12.6)	43 (12.7)	1.00
Glucocorticoid (%)	148 (18.2)	93 (19.5)	55 (16.3)	0.27

Data are median (IQR, Interquartile range) except where noted. BMI = body mass index; RA = rheumatoid arthritis; RF = rheumatoid factor; ACPA = anti-citrullinated peptide antibody; VAS = visual analog scale; PGA = physician's global assessment; EGA = evaluator's global assessment; TJ = tender joint; SJ = Swollen joint; CDAI = clinical disease activity index; HAQ = Health Assessment Questionnaire; ESR = erythrocyte sedimentation rate; CRP = C-reactive protein; DAS = disease activity score; DMARDs = disease-modifying anti-rheumatic drugs; MTX = methotrexate; bDMARDs = biologic DMARDs; TNFi = TNF inhibitors; IL-6i = IL-6 inhibitor; ABT = abatacept; JAKi = JAK inhibitor.

RF and ACPA titers were classified into quintiles as follows: RF titer—Q0 (<15), Q1 (15–<33), Q2 (33–<78), Q3 (78–<190), Q4 (≥190); ACPA titer—Q0 (<5), Q1 (5–<34), Q2 (34–<120), Q3 (120–<480), Q4 (≥480).

3. Results

3.1. Clinical and Laboratory Features in ANA-Positive Patients with Rheumatoid Arthritis

Among the 814 patients with RA analyzed, 338 (41.5%) were ANA-positive, while 476 (58.5%) were ANA-negative. The clinical and laboratory features stratified by ANA positivity are summarized in Table 1. No significant differences were observed in age or disease duration. However, ANA-positive patients were more likely to be female and showed significantly higher positivity rates and titers of RF and ACPA. They also had elevated Evaluator's Global Assessment (EGA) and Swollen Joint Count (SJ-28). Additionally, ANA-positive patients exhibited higher levels of IgG, IgA, IgM, total protein, and erythrocyte sedimentation rate (ESR), while their albumin/globulin (A/G) ratio was lower. Regarding treatment history, ANA-positive patients were significantly more likely to have used tumor necrosis factor (TNF) inhibitors.

3.2. Association Between ANA Staining Patterns and Titers

The most frequent ANA staining patterns were the speckled pattern (313 patients) and the homogeneous pattern (269 patients), as shown in Table 2. Most homogeneous pattern-positive patients also tested positive for the speckled pattern (Supplementary Figure S1). ANA titers for the speckled and homogeneous patterns were predominantly low, with titers of 1:40 observed in 71% and 74% of patients, respectively, and 1:80 in 20% and 19%, respectively. Nucleolar pattern-positive patients showed titers up to 1:80, whereas approximately 60% of discrete-speckled pattern-positive patients exhibited high titers of 1:320 or greater (Table 2).

Table 2. The pattern and titer of immunofluorescence staining for antinuclear antibodies in patients with rheumatoid arthritis.

	ANA Positive Number	ANA-Titer, Number (%)					
		1:40	1:80	1:160	1:320	1:640	1:1280
Homogeneous	269	199 (74)	51 (19)	14 (5)	5 (2)	0 (0)	0 (0)
Speckled	313	223 (71)	63 (20)	16 (5)	9 (3)	2 (1)	0 (0)
Nucleolar	19	11 (58)	8 (42)	0 (0)	0 (0)	0 (0)	0 (0)
Discrete Speckled	16	1 (6)	2 (13)	2 (13)	6 (38)	3 (19)	2 (13)

ANA = anti-nuclear antibody.

3.3. Relationship Between ANA Titer, Staining Patterns, and Clinical Features

Hierarchical clustering was performed to examine the relationship between ANA titer, staining patterns, and clinical and laboratory features (Figure 2). The heatmap suggests that patient groups with moderate disease activity (MDA) or high disease activity (HDA), including those with D2T-RA, were not consistently associated with ANA positivity. Patients with speckled or homogeneous patterns exhibited a wide range of clinical variables with no clear trends, likely due to the high prevalence of these patterns.

In contrast, nucleolar pattern-positive patients tended to have older age at RA onset, a higher proportion of patients with low disease activity (LDA), and a notable association with pulmonary complications. On the other hand, discrete-speckled pattern-positive patients had higher ANA titers but lower RF and ACPA titers, and their RA disease activity was controlled at CDAI-LDA or below.

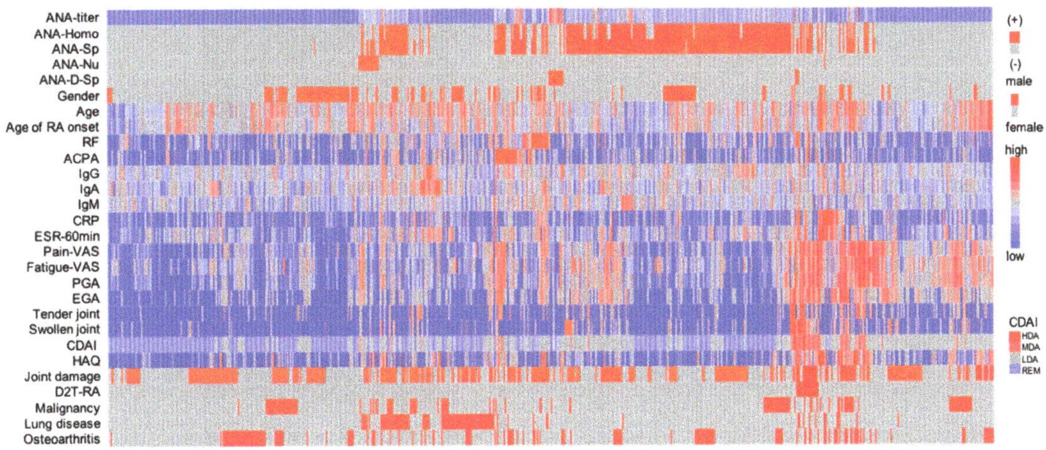

Figure 2. Hierarchical clustering heatmap of clinical and laboratory features in rheumatoid arthritis.

When assessing the clinical significance of ANA patterns in ANA-positive patients (Supplementary Table S2), speckled pattern positivity was significantly associated with higher RF positivity and titers, as well as higher ACPA titers. These features were not observed in homogeneous pattern-positive patients. Nucleolar pattern positivity was associated with older age, a higher prevalence of pulmonary complications, and a greater likelihood of JAK inhibitor use. Conversely, discrete speckled pattern positivity was significantly associated with lower RF positivity.

3.4. RF and ACPA in Speckled and/or Homogeneous ANA Patterns

Speckled pattern positivity was associated with significantly higher RF positivity and RF and ACPA titers. To further evaluate the relationship, RF and ACPA titers were assessed in ANA-positive patients with speckled and/or homogeneous patterns using both actual values and quartiles (Figure 3). RF and ACPA titers were significantly higher in ANA-positive patients at 1:40 compared to ANA-negative patients (Figure 3a,c). Additionally, in ANA titers of 1:40 or greater, the proportion of RF-negative and ACPA-negative patients decreased by approximately half, while the population in Q3 and Q4 increased (Figure 3b,d).

3.5. Risk Factors for Pulmonary Involvement in RA

Pulmonary complications are a critical aspect of RA management. Logistic regression analysis was performed to identify risk factors for pulmonary involvement in RA, including ANA staining patterns. Five variables with $p < 0.1$ in univariate analysis—gender, age, RF titer, ACPA titer, and ANA nucleolar pattern positivity—were included in multivariate analysis (Table 3). The independent risk factors identified were age (odds ratio 1.04, 95% confidence interval (CI) 1.02–1.06) and ANA nucleolar pattern positivity (odds ratio 3.71, 95% CI 1.30–9.82). Among ANA-positive patients, nucleolar pattern positivity was associated with lung involvement, whereas speckled and homogeneous patterns showed no significant correlation with specific extra-articular manifestations.

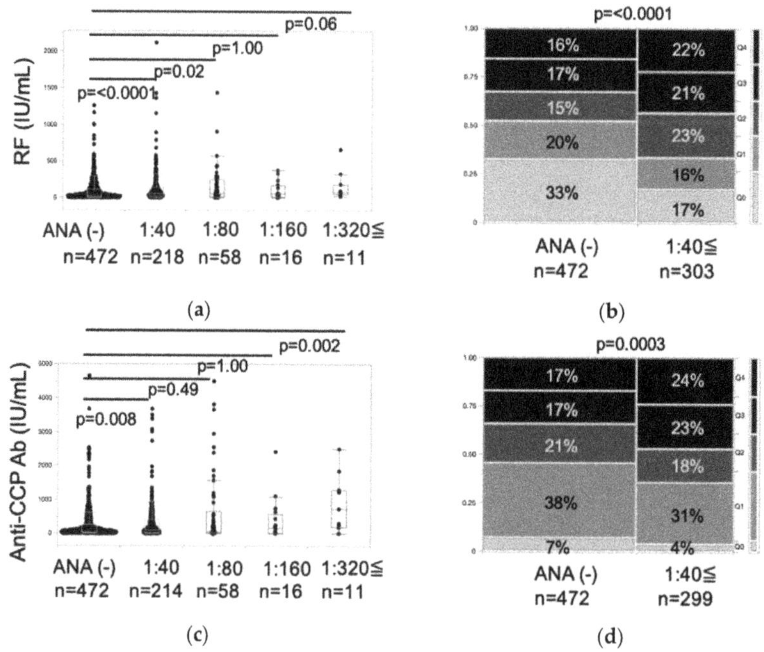

Figure 3. Association between ANA positivity (speckled and/or homogeneous pattern) and RF/ACPA titer in rheumatoid arthritis. For panels (**a**,**c**), non-parametric comparisons with the ANA-negative group were conducted using Dunn's test. For panels (**b**,**d**), statistical significance was assessed using the exact test for the Cochran–Armitage trend test. In panels B and D, RF and ACPA titers were classified into quintiles as follows: RF titer—Q0 (<15), Q1 (15–<33), Q2 (33–<78), Q3 (78–<190), Q4 (≥190); ACPA titer—Q0 (<5), Q1 (5–<34), Q2 (34–<120), Q3 (120–<480), Q4 (≥480).

Table 3. Clinical risk factors for lung involvement in rheumatoid arthritis.

	Univariable				Multivariable			
	Odds Ratio	95% CI		*p*-Value	Odds Ratio	95% CI		*p*-Value
		Lower	Upper			Lower	Upper	
Gender; male	1.61	1.027	2.485	0.038	1.32	0.822	2.094	0.245
Age	1.04	1.024	1.061	<0.0001	1.04	1.018	1.057	<0.0001
BMI	0.96	0.912	1.016	0.171				
RA family history	0.68	0.377	1.171	0.172				
Smoking history	1.27	0.839	1.917	0.256				
Drug allergy	1.17	0.668	1.963	0.569				
RF titer	1.00	1.001	1.002	0.001	1.00	1.000	1.002	0.056
ACPA titer	1.00	1.000	1.001	0.003	1.00	1.000	1.001	0.059
ANA-Speckled	0.84	0.543	1.279	0.419				
ANA-Homogeneous	0.77	0.487	1.203	0.260				
ANA-Nucleolar	4.10	1.495	10.447	0.008	3.71	1.303	9.817	0.016
ANA-D-Sp	0.44	0.024	2.206	0.373				

CI = confidence interval; BMI = body mass index; RA = rheumatoid arthritis; RF = rheumatoid factor; ACPA = anti-citrullinated peptide antibody; ANA = anti-nuclear antibody; D-Sp = discrete speckled.

4. Discussion

In this study, we comprehensively evaluated the clinical characteristics of ANA-positive and ANA-negative patients with RA using registry data, and identified several key findings.

First, ANA-positive patients exhibited higher positivity rates and titers of RF and ACPA, suggesting an association with heightened autoimmune activity. Speckled and homogeneous pattern-positive patients demonstrated higher RF and ACPA titers, indicating the potential involvement of these staining patterns in RA pathogenesis. Furthermore, nucleolar pattern positivity was identified as an independent risk factor for pulmonary complications in patients with RA. This finding highlights the potential utility of the nucleolar pattern as a novel marker for assessing pulmonary risk, in addition to conventional RF and ACPA [13–15,17,18].

The reported ANA positivity rates in RA range from 14% to 77%, with major differences likely arising from population characteristics (e.g., ethnicity, disease duration) and concomitant treatments, rather than detection methods, as all studies utilized HEp-2 cell-based IIF ANA testing. Although the ICAP has contributed to standardizing ANA interpretation, variability between institutions and among individual observers may still affect results. In our study, the ANA positivity rate was 42%. In contrast, Paknikar et al. reported a 25% ANA positivity rate among patients with RA within 90 days of diagnosis [8], and Liu et al. found a 77% positivity rate in patients with RA compared to other arthritis patients and healthy controls, matched by age and sex [9]. Ethnic and genetic factors significantly influence ANA prevalence and patterns in RA. Studies suggest that ANA positivity is more common in certain populations, such as Asian cohorts, potentially due to genetic predispositions (e.g., HLA associations) [19]. Additionally, ANA positivity is generally more frequent in females and older individuals, reflecting broader autoimmune susceptibility trends. The prevalence of certain autoimmune diseases, including SLE and SS, is also higher in non-white populations, which may contribute to variations in ANA profiles [19]. Additionally, Ishikawa et al. demonstrated that ANA positivity is more likely with TNF inhibitor use [20], emphasizing the need to consider factors such as ethnicity, disease severity, and treatment effects.

TNF inhibitors are known to induce ANA positivity in a subset of RA patients. Previous studies have suggested that this may be mediated through the cross-regulation of TNF-α and interferon (IFN)-α pathways. TNF-α suppresses IFN-α production by inhibiting the differentiation and activation of plasmacytoid dendritic cells [21]. Thus, TNF blockade may lead to sustained IFN-α secretion, which could contribute to ANA induction and, in some cases, lupus-like manifestations [21]. However, it remains unclear whether TNF inhibitor-induced ANA positivity has direct clinical relevance in RA management. Further studies are needed to determine the impact of this mechanism on treatment effectiveness and disease progression.

The interpretation of ANA staining patterns in patients with RA also warrants further discussion. Liu et al. reported that homogeneous patterns were the most common, followed by speckled patterns in 60% of cases [9]. However, in our study, most homogeneous pattern-positive patients were also positive for the speckled pattern. These differences in staining pattern detection may be attributed to variability in interpretation, despite the standardization efforts led by ICAP [3], and could depend on institutional practices or technician expertise [4,5].

Generally, high-titer ANA positivity with homogeneous patterns is strongly associated with SLE, whereas speckled patterns are linked to a variety of autoimmune diseases, including SS and SLE [4,5,22,23]. In our study, patients with RA with other SARDs were excluded, which likely explains the predominance of discrete speckled patterns at high titers ($\geq$1:320). Discrete speckled pattern positivity is almost synonymous with anti-centromere antibody positivity, a disease-specific marker for systemic sclerosis (SSc) [24], and is also a risk factor for primary SS [25]. However, many SSc cases may be limited cutaneous types, making the identification of typical SSc findings challenging [24].

In ANA-positive patients with RA, female predominance, higher RF/ACPA levels, and elevated γ-globulin percentages have been reported [6,9]. In our study, we confirmed these findings, along with higher levels of swollen joint counts and EGA. Although ANA-positive patients with RA without SARD symptoms exhibit normal IL-1β and IL-6 levels compared to healthy individuals, they have significantly higher type I IFN signature gene expression in peripheral blood [26]. This suggests enhanced autoimmune responses mediated by type I IFN signaling [27], which may contribute to the prevalence of homogeneous and speckled patterns in ANA-positive patients. The biological mechanisms underlying ANA positivity in RA are not yet fully elucidated. However, recent studies suggest that type I IFN signaling plays a critical role in the autoimmune process, contributing to both ANA production and disease pathogenesis, particularly in genetically susceptible individuals [27]. Future research should focus on clarifying the interplay between ANA and RA-specific immune pathways to establish its role in disease progression and treatment response.

For the evaluation of connective-tissue disease-associated ILD, markers such as RF, ACPA, anti-Scl-70 and anti-melanoma differentiation-associated gene 5 (MDA5), anti-tRNA synthetase antibodies are considered useful [28]. Nucleolar pattern positivity is strongly associated with SSc and related autoantibodies, such as anti-U3 RNP, anti-Th/To, anti-NOR 90, and anti-PM/Scl antibodies [29]. Furthermore, while nucleolar ANA positivity was associated with pulmonary complications, we found no strong correlation between other ANA patterns and extra-articular organ involvement. This highlights the need for further studies to delineate the clinical implications of different ANA staining patterns in RA. Among patients with RA with ILD, nucleolar pattern positivity may suggest the presence of an SSc spectrum disease, which could influence therapeutic decisions. Recent studies have demonstrated the utility of JAK inhibitors in RA with ILD [30–32]. Patients with nucleolar pattern positivity had a significantly higher rate of JAK inhibitor use, possibly reflecting a higher prevalence of pulmonary complications in this subgroup. In contrast, ANA-positive patients with speckled or homogeneous patterns were more likely to receive TNF inhibitors, possibly due to their higher RF and ACPA titers. However, our study does not assess treatment effectiveness, and further prospective studies are needed to confirm these associations. Nonetheless, whether JAK inhibitors are optimal in the context of SSc spectrum diseases warrants further investigation.

Discrete speckled pattern-positive patients exhibited high ANA titers but low RF/ACPA levels, suggesting a distinct pathophysiological subset among patients with RA. Clinical differences between ANA-positive patients with speckled or homogeneous patterns and those with discrete speckled or nucleolar patterns underscore the potential utility of ANA staining patterns in clinical practice and therapeutic decision-making.

This study has several limitations. First, ANA detection was performed using the IIF method, which is subject to variability in staining pattern interpretation due to institutional practices or technician experience. Future studies should incorporate specific ANA subtypes, such as anti-SSA, anti-dsDNA, and antiphospholipid antibodies, using highly specific assays such as immunoblot, ELISA, or Crithidia luciliae indirect immunofluorescence test (CLIFT). This would provide a more detailed immunological profile and further clarify the clinical implications of ANA positivity in RA patients. As a single-center study, generalizability may be limited, and multi-center studies are needed to validate our findings. Furthermore, due to the cross-sectional design, we could not assess the longitudinal impact of ANA positivity on disease progression and treatment response. Additionally, the effects of treatment on ANA results cannot be fully excluded, especially considering reports that TNF inhibitors can induce ANA positivity. Future prospective studies should address these gaps to refine the clinical significance of ANA in RA. Furthermore, while this study excluded patients with multiple coexisting SARDs, secondary SS is relatively common in RA and can be challenging to diagnose accurately [33]. We focused on the primary disease states of SARD and did not treat secondary SS as an independent condition. In our RA registry, if other SARDs were diagnosed based on their respective classification or diagnostic criteria, they were counted as SARDs coexisting with RA. However, we did not comprehensively evaluate detailed autoimmune features. Additionally, when diagnosing RA based on the 2010 ACR/EULAR classification criteria [12], the presence of a confirmed SARD diagnosis can make it unclear whether the case truly represents RA. To ensure that we analyzed a population that could be diagnosed as "pure RA", we excluded patients with other diagnosed SARDs from this study. Understanding the changes in ANA and other immune profiles caused by secondary autoimmune conditions remains an important area for future research.

To clarify the clinical significance of ANA in RA, multicenter prospective studies with larger cohorts, including treatment-naïve patients, are necessary. As this study is cross-sectional, it cannot determine whether ANA positivity actively contributes to disease progression or is simply a marker of immune activation. Longitudinal studies are required to evaluate its predictive value in disease progression and treatment response. Future research should also explore the biological mechanisms linking ANA positivity to disease activity and treatment response.

5. Conclusions

In this study, we demonstrated that ANA-positive RA patients exhibit distinct clinical and serological characteristics, with specific ANA staining patterns correlating with disease activity and pulmonary complications. While our findings suggest that ANA positivity may serve as a potential biomarker for patient stratification, its clinical applicability remains uncertain. Further studies incorporating specific autoantibody subtypes and longitudinal analyses are needed to refine its role in RA management. ANA testing should be interpreted in the context of other serological markers and clinical features, rather than as a standalone diagnostic or prognostic tool. Future research should explore the prognostic implications of ANA in RA and assess its role in guiding therapeutic decision-making, with the goal of integrating ANA testing into personalized RA management strategies.

Supplementary Materials: The following supporting information can be downloaded at: https://www.mdpi.com/article/10.3390/jcm14051553/s1, Table S1: Complicated systemic autoimmune arthritic diseases; Figure S1: Venn diagram of positive speckled and homogeneous patterns; Table S2: Clinical and laboratory features given by anti-nuclear antibody staining patterns in ANA-positive patients with rheumatoid arthritis.

Author Contributions: K.N. was involved in the conception and design of this study and the interpretation of results, and prepared the first draft of the paper. S.F. and Y.M. (Yoshitaka Morita) contributed to the discussion of the final draft and revised it critically for intellectual content. All authors were involved in the recruitment of patients. All authors have read and agreed to the published version of the manuscript.

Funding: This research received no external funding.

Institutional Review Board Statement: The study was conducted in accordance with the Declaration of Helsinki, and approved by the Ethics Committee of our hospital (Ethics Application No. 5564-04, approved on 15 February 2022).

Informed Consent Statement: Written informed consent for the use of clinical data was obtained from all subjects in accordance with the Helsinki declaration.

Data Availability Statement: All data generated or analyzed during the study are included in this published article.

Acknowledgments: The authors would like to thank Asami Kusumoto and Misako Tanno (Department of Rheumatology, Kawasaki Medical School) for their assistance in data collection and data cleaning.

Conflicts of Interest: The authors declare no conflicts of interest.

References

1. Gravallese, E.M.; Firestein, G.S. Rheumatoid Arthritis—Common Origins, Divergent Mechanisms. *N. Engl. J. Med.* **2023**, *388*, 529–542. [CrossRef] [PubMed]
2. Smolen, J.S.; Landewé, R.B.M.; Bergstra, S.A.; Kerschbaumer, A.; Sepriano, A.; Aletaha, D.; Caporali, R.; Edwards, C.J.; Hyrich, K.L.; Pope, J.E.; et al. EULAR recommendations for the management of rheumatoid arthritis with synthetic and biological disease-modifying antirheumatic drugs: 2022 update. *Ann. Rheum. Dis.* **2022**, *82*, 3–18. [CrossRef] [PubMed]
3. Damoiseaux, J.; Andrade, L.E.C.; Carballo, O.G.; Conrad, K.; Francescantonio, P.L.C.; Fritzler, M.J.; de la Torre, I.G.; Herold, M.; Klotz, W.; Cruvinel, W.d.M.; et al. Clinical relevance of HEp-2 indirect immunofluorescent patterns: The International Consensus on ANA patterns (ICAP) perspective. *Ann. Rheum. Dis.* **2019**, *78*, 879–889. [CrossRef] [PubMed]
4. Tan, E.M.; Kunkel, H.G. Specificity of speckled ANA patterns for autoimmune diseases including SS and SLE. *Arthritis Rheumatol.* **1969**, *12*, 419–425.
5. Satoh, M.; Vázquez-Del Mercado, M.; Chan, E.K.L. Clinical interpretation of antinuclear antibody tests in systemic rheumatic diseases. *Mod. Rheumatol.* **2009**, *19*, 219–228. [CrossRef]
6. Caspi, D.; Elkayam, O.; Eisinger, M.; Vardinon, N.; Yaron, M.; Burke, M. Clinical significance of low titer anti-nuclear antibodies in early rheumatoid arthritis: Implications on the presentation and long-term course of the disease. *Rheumatol. Int.* **2001**, *20*, 43–47. [CrossRef]
7. Wei, Q.; Jiang, Y.; Xie, J.; Lv, Q.; Xie, Y.; Tu, L.; Xiao, M.; Wu, Z.; Gu, J. Analysis of antinuclear antibody titers and patterns by using HEp-2 and primate liver tissue substrate indirect immunofluorescence assay in patients with systemic autoimmune rheumatic diseases. *J. Clin. Lab. Anal.* **2020**, *34*, e23362. [CrossRef]
8. Paknikar, S.S.; Crowson, C.S.; Davis, J.M.; Thanarajasingam, U. Exploring the Role of Antinuclear Antibody Positivity in the Diagnosis, Treatment, and Health Outcomes of Patients With Rheumatoid Arthritis. *ACR Open Rheumatol.* **2021**, *3*, 422–426. [CrossRef]
9. Liu, F.; Wang, X.Q.; Zou, J.W.; Li, M.; Pan, C.C.; Si, Y.Q. Association between serum antinuclear antibody and rheumatoid arthritis. *Front. Immunol.* **2024**, *15*, 1123456. [CrossRef]
10. Fujita, S.; Nakano, K.; Nagasu, A.; Hiramatsu-Asano, S.; Akagi, T.; Morita, Y. Prognosis and prognostic factors of lung cancer complications in patients with rheumatoid arthritis. *Int. J. Rheum. Dis.* **2024**, *27*, e15069. [CrossRef]
11. Arnett, F.C.; Edworthy, S.M.; Bloch, D.A.; McShane, D.J.; Fries, J.F.; Cooper, N.S.; Healey, L.A.; Kaplan, S.R.; Liang, M.H.; Luthra, H.S.; et al. The American Rheumatism Association 1987 revised criteria for the classification of rheumatoid arthritis. *Arthritis Rheum.* **1988**, *31*, 315–324. [CrossRef] [PubMed]
12. Aletaha, D.; Neogi, T.; Silman, A.J.; Funovits, J.; Felson, D.T.; Bingham, C.O., 3rd; Birnbaum, N.S.; Burmester, G.R.; Bykerk, V.P.; Cohen, M.D.; et al. 2010 Rheumatoid arthritis classification criteria: An American College of Rheumatology/European League Against Rheumatism collaborative initiative. *Arthritis Rheum.* **2010**, *62*, 2569–2581. [CrossRef] [PubMed]
13. Wang, D.; Zhang, J.; Lau, J.; Wang, S.; Taneja, V.; Matteson, E.L.; Vassallo, R. Mechanisms of lung disease development in rheumatoid arthritis. *Nat. Rev. Rheumatol.* **2019**, *15*, 581–596. [CrossRef]
14. Shaw, M.; Collins, B.F.; Ho, L.A.; Raghu, G. Rheumatoid arthritis-associated lung disease. *Eur. Respir. Rev.* **2015**, *24*, 1–16. [CrossRef] [PubMed]
15. Kadura, S.; Raghu, G. Rheumatoid arthritis-interstitial lung disease: Manifestations and current concepts in pathogenesis and management. *Eur. Respir. Rev.* **2021**, *30*, 210011. [CrossRef] [PubMed]
16. Nagy, G.; Roodenrijs, N.M.T.; Welsing, P.M.; Kedves, M.; Hamar, A.; van der Goes, M.C.; Kent, A.; Bakkers, M.; Blaas, E.; Senolt, L.; et al. EULAR definition of difficult-to-treat rheumatoid arthritis. *Ann. Rheum. Dis.* **2021**, *80*, 31–35. [CrossRef]
17. Azam, A.T.; Odeyinka, O.; Alhashimi, R.; Thoota, S.; Ashok, T.; Palyam, V.; Sange, I. Rheumatoid Arthritis and Associated Lung Diseases: A Comprehensive Review. *Cureus* **2022**, *14*, e31211. [CrossRef]
18. Joshua, V.; Hensvold, A.H.; Reynisdottir, G.; Hansson, M.; Cornillet, M.; Nogueira, L.; Serre, G.; Nyren, S.; Karimi, R.; Eklund, A.; et al. Association between number and type of different ACPA fine specificities with lung abnormalities in early, untreated rheumatoid arthritis. *RMD Open* **2020**, *6*, e001278. [CrossRef]
19. Satoh, M.; Chan, E.K.L.; Ho, L.A.; Rose, K.M.; Parks, C.G.; Cohn, R.D.; Jusko, T.A.; Walker, N.J.; Germolec, D.R.; Whitt, I.Z.; et al. Prevalence and sociodemographic correlates of antinuclear antibodies in the United States. *Arthritis Rheum.* **2012**, *64*, 2319–2327. [CrossRef]

20. Ishikawa, Y.; Hashimoto, M.; Ito, H.; Tanaka, M.; Yukawa, N.; Fujii, T.; Yamamoto, W.; Mimori, T.; Terao, C. Anti-nuclear antibody development is associated with poor treatment response to biological disease-modifying anti-rheumatic drugs in patients with rheumatoid arthritis. *Semin. Arthritis Rheum.* **2019**, *49*, 204–210. [CrossRef]
21. Palucka, A.K.; Blanck, J.P.; Bennett, L.; Pascual, V.; Banchereau, J. Cross-regulation of TNF and IFN-α in autoimmune diseases. *Proc. Natl. Acad. Sci. USA* **2005**, *102*, 3372–3377. [CrossRef] [PubMed]
22. Mariz, H.A.; Sato, E.I.; Barbosa, S.H.; Rodrigues, S.H.; Dellavance, A.; Andrade, L.E.C. Pattern on the antinuclear antibody–HEp-2 test is a critical parameter for discriminating antinuclear antibody–positive healthy individuals and patients with autoimmune rheumatic diseases. *Arthritis Rheumatol.* **2011**, *63*, 191–200. [CrossRef] [PubMed]
23. Al-Mughales, J.A. Anti-Nuclear Antibodies Patterns in Patients With Systemic Lupus Erythematosus and Their Correlation With Other Diagnostic Immunological Parameters. *Front. Immunol.* **2022**, *13*, 879456. [CrossRef] [PubMed]
24. Fritzler, M.J.; Rattner, J.B.; Luft, L.M.; Edworthy, S.M.; Casiano, C.A.; Peebles, C.; Mahler, M. Historical perspectives on the discovery and elucidation of autoantibodies to centromere proteins (CENP) and the emerging importance of antibodies to CENP-F. *Autoimmun. Rev.* **2011**, *10*, 194–200. [CrossRef]
25. Liu, Y.; Guo, L.; Lin, W.; Ning, X.; Liu, M.; Cao, J.; Su, Y.; Zheng, X.; Li, S.; Li, F.; et al. Anticentromere antibody positive patients with primary Sjögren's syndrome have distinctive clinical and immunological characteristics. *Clin. Exp. Rheumatol.* **2023**, *41*, 2371–2378. [CrossRef]
26. Hafiz, W.; Nori, R.; Bregasi, A.; Noamani, B.; Bonilla, D.; Lisnevskaia, L.; Silverman, E.; Bookman, A.A.M.; Johnson, S.R.; Landolt-Marticorena, C.; et al. Fatigue severity in anti-nuclear antibody-positive individuals does not correlate with pro-inflammatory cytokine levels or predict imminent progression to symptomatic disease. *Arthritis Res. Ther.* **2019**, *21*, 223. [CrossRef]
27. Lin, C.M.A.; Isaacs, J.D.; Cooles, F.A.H. Role of IFN-α in Rheumatoid Arthritis. *Curr. Rheumatol. Rep.* **2024**, *26*, 37–52. [CrossRef]
28. Kuwana, M.; Bando, M.; Kawahito, Y.; Sato, S.; Suda, T.; Kondoh, Y. Identification and management of connective tissue disease-associated interstitial lung disease: Evidence-based Japanese consensus statements. *Expert Rev. Respir. Med.* **2023**, *17*, 71–80. [CrossRef]
29. Cavazzana, I.; Vojinovic, T.; Airo', P.; Fredi, M.; Ceribelli, A.; Pedretti, E.; Lazzaroni, M.G.; Garrafa, E.; Franceschini, F. Systemic Sclerosis-Specific Antibodies: Novel and Classical Biomarkers. *Clin. Rev. Allergy Immunol.* **2023**, *64*, 412–430. [CrossRef]
30. Tardella, M.; Carlo, M.D.; Carotti, M.; Ceccarelli, L.; Giovagnoni, A.; Salaffi, F. A retrospective study of the efficacy of JAK inhibitors or abatacept on rheumatoid arthritis-interstitial lung disease. *Inflammopharmacology* **2022**, *30*, 705–712. [CrossRef]
31. Tsujii, A.; Isoda, K.; Yoshimura, M.; Nakabayashi, A.; Kim, D.-S.; Tamada, T.; Yamamoto, K.; Ohshima, S. Janus kinase inhibitors vs. abatacept about safety and efficacy for patients with rheumatoid arthritis-associated interstitial lung disease: A retrospective nested case-control study. *BMC Rheumatol.* **2024**, *8*, 4. [CrossRef] [PubMed]
32. Narváez, J.; Aguilar-Coll, M.; Roig-Kim, M.; Maymó-Paituvi, P.; Palacios-Olid, J.; Nolla, J.M.; LLop, D. Janus kinase inhibitors in rheumatoid arthritis-associated interstitial lung disease: A systematic review and meta-analysis. *Autoimmun. Rev.* **2024**, *23*, 103636. [CrossRef] [PubMed]
33. Alani, H.; Henty, J.; Thompson, N.; Jury, E.; Ciurtin, C. Systematic review and meta-analysis of the epidemiology of polyautoimmunity in Sjögren's syndrome (secondary Sjögren's syndrome) focusing on autoimmune rheumatic diseases. *Scand. J. Rheumatol.* **2017**, *47*, 141–154. [CrossRef] [PubMed]

Journal of
Clinical Medicine

MDPI

Article

Structural and Functional Outcomes in Rheumatoid Arthritis After 10-Year Therapy with Disease-Modifying Antirheumatic Drugs Under Tight Control: Evidence from Real-World Cohort Data

Shunsuke Mori [1,*], Akitomo Okada [2], Toshimasa Shimizu [3,4], Ayuko Takatani [3,5] and Tomohiro Koga [3]

1 Department of Rheumatology, Clinical Research Center for Rheumatic Diseases, National Hospital Organization Kumamoto Saishun Medical Center, Kohshi 861-1196, Japan
2 Department of Rheumatology, National Hospital Organization Nagasaki Medical Center, Omura 856-8562, Japan; akitomoo@hotmail.com
3 Department of Immunology and Rheumatology, Nagasaki University Graduate School of Biomedical Sciences, Nagasaki 852-8523, Japan; toshimasashimizu2000@yahoo.co.jp (T.S.); ayuko.takatani@nagasaki-u.ac.jp (A.T.); tkoga@nagasaki-u.ac.jp (T.K.)
4 Clinical Research Center, Nagasaki University Hospital, Nagasaki 852-8501, Japan
5 Department of Public Health, Nagasaki University Graduate School of Biomedical Sciences, Nagasaki 852-8523, Japan
* Correspondence: mori.shunsuke.ra@mail.hosp.go.jp; Tel.: +81-96-242-1000

Abstract: Objectives: To examine long-term outcomes and predictors of structural and functional remission in rheumatoid arthritis (RA) after 10-year disease-modifying antirheumatic drug (DMARD) therapy under tight control. **Methods**: We used real-world cohort data from RA patients who completed 10-year DMARD therapy toward remission or low disease activity based on every-3-month measurements between April 2001 and July 2024. Baseline characteristics, disease control during follow-up, and outcomes after 10 years were examined. **Results**: Among 204 patients, 76% received biological and/or non-biological targeted DMARDs. Clinical remission, structural remission defined as an increase in modified total Sharp score (mTSS) $\leq$ 5 per 10 years, and functional remission defined as health assessment questionnaire-disability index (HAQ-DI) $\leq$ 0.5 were achieved by 68.1%, 73.0%, and 81.4% of patients, respectively. The mean increase (Δ) in mTSS was 5.4 for 10 years (Δerosion score, 1.2; Δjoint space narrowing [JSN] score, 4.2), and 28.9% of patients had no structural progression (51% for erosion score and 34.8% for JSN score). Mean HAQ-DI was 0.26. During a 10-year follow-up, 8.8% of patients experienced high or moderate disease activity lasting for $\geq$12 months and they had a low structural remission rate (11.1%) and functional remission rate (16.6%). According to multivariable logistic regression analysis, baseline mTSS and JNS score (but not erosion score) were strong predictors for structural and functional remission after 10 years. **Conclusions**: Structural damage progression and functional loss are limited during 10-year tightly controlled DMARD therapy. Compared with bone erosion, JSN appears to be of much higher relevance to structural and functional outcomes.

Keywords: rheumatoid arthritis; structural remission; functional remission; joint space narrowing; tight control; predictive factors; long-term outcomes

1. Introduction

Rheumatoid arthritis (RA) is a chronic autoimmune disease characterized by synovial membrane inflammation, which causes progressive joint damage [1,2]. Joint damage is closely related to physical function in RA patients and health-related quality of life, especially as disease duration increases [3–5]. Systematic reviews of the literature between 1986 and 2001 showed that structural damage, which comprises bone erosion and cartilage degradation, starts early in the disease course and constantly progresses over the first 20 years [3,4]. However, management of RA has been revolutionized over the past decades. The availability of conventional, biological, and non-biological targeted disease-modifying antirheumatic drugs (DMARDs) has dramatically improved long-term outcomes. Early and aggressive intervention of DMARDs with increased treatment choice can induce the prompt suppression of inflammatory disease activity and a significant reduction in joint damage in RA patients [6–8].

Tight control of RA is a treatment strategy tailored to individual patients with the aim of achieving a predefined level of disease activity within a certain period of time. This treatment strategy is attained by careful and regular monitoring of disease activity as well as early therapeutic adjustments or switches of DMARD therapies that fail to control disease activity [9,10]. The development and widespread adoption of validated composite measures, which include joint assessment, have allowed disease activity to be quantified reliably [11,12]. Previous clinical trials have indicated that the tight-control strategy can not only adequately control clinical disease activity, but also substantially reduce radiographic progression compared with conventional approaches to the management of RA [13–16]. In these clinical trials, the treatment goal was clinical remission or low disease activity; measurements of disease activity were performed every 1 to 3 months and, until the desired treatment goal was reached, DMARD therapies were adjusted at least every 3 months [13–16]. The treat-to-target strategy, which was first developed in 2010 as the guideline principle for the treatment of RA, recommends that treatment be directed to reach and maintain remission or at least low disease activity, and be adjusted toward such a goal at least every 3 months based on the tight-control strategy [17,18]. A recent systematic review and meta-analysis of the literature between 1990 and 2023 indicated that the treat-to-target strategy has significant advantages in increasing clinical response and remission rates and improving health-related quality of life in RA patients [19]. However, there is limited information regarding long-term protective effects of the treat-to-target strategy under tight control on structural damage progression and functional loss, as well as predictive factors for structural and functional remission in real-world settings, especially after various biological and non-biological targeted DMARDs have become available in RA treatment.

Our objectives were to examine long-term outcomes and predictors for structural and functional remission in RA patients after 10-year DMARD therapy under tight control toward remission or at least low disease activity in daily practice. For this study, we conducted a retrospective, long-term follow-up study using real-world cohort data from RA patients who had completed 10-year tight-control DMARD therapy based on every-3-month measurements between April 2001 and July 2024. We examined the contribution of bone erosion and cartilage degradation to structural damage progression and functional loss at 10 years. Additionally, structural and functional outcomes were compared between patients with experience of high or moderate disease activity lasting $\geq$12 months and those with good disease control during 10-year DMARD therapy.

2. Materials and Methods

2.1. Patients

We used a real-world database of RA patients who visited the rheumatology division of the National Hospital Organization (NHO) Kumamoto Saishun Medical Center as of April 2001. From this database, we identified patients who started DMARD therapy between April 2001 and July 2014 and had been followed for ≥10 years by July 2024. All participants in this study were required to fulfill the 2010 American College of Rheumatology (ACR)/European Alliance of Associations for Rheumatology (EULAR, formerly the European League Against Rheumatism) criteria for diagnosis of RA [20] and were required to be 18 years of age or older. Patient enrollment flow diagram is shown in Figure 1. We excluded patients if they had any of the following characteristics at their first visit: (1) Steinbrocker radiological stage IV (because of the difficulty in precise scoring of joint damage); (2) previous use of biological DMARD (bDMARD) or targeted synthetic DMARD (tsDMARD); and (3) lack of baseline x-rays of hands and/or feet. We also excluded patients who had failed to receive 10-year DMARD therapy under tight control of clinical disease activity due to the following reasons: (1) discontinuation of DMARD therapy (adverse events or patient's preference) or (2) drop-out of tight control of clinical disease activity. We did not exclude patients who discontinued DMARD therapy temporarily for certain reasons (e.g., liver enzyme elevations, infection, surgical interventions) and then restarted within 1 month.

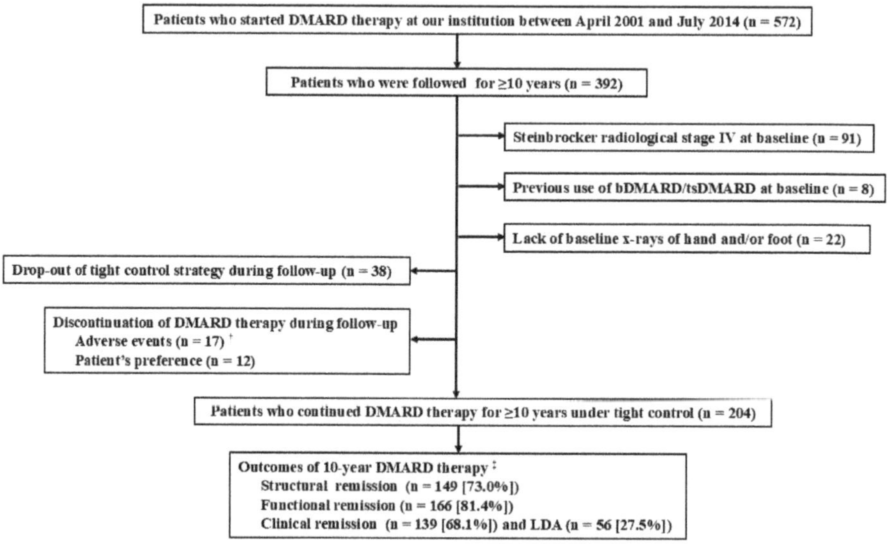

Figure 1. Patient enrollment flow diagram † Included infection (n = 4), fracture (n = 4), malignancy (n = 3), Fabry disease (n = 1), dementia (n = 1), de novo hepatitis B virus infection (n = 1), cardiac infarction (n = 1), chronic pulmonary embolism (n = 1), and lymphopenia (n = 1). We did not exclude patients who discontinued DMARD therapy temporarily and restarted within 1 month. ‡ Defined as ΔmTSS ≤ 5.0 for structural remission, HAQ-DI ≤ 0.5 for functional remission, CDAI ≤ 2.8 for clinical remission, and CDAI > 2.8 and ≤10 for LDA. CDAI clinical disease activity index; DMARD, disease-modifying antirheumatic drug; bDMARD, biological DMARD; tsDMARD, targeted synthetic DMARD; HAQ-DI, health assessment questionnaire-disability index; LDA, low disease activity; mTSS, van der Heijde-modified total Sharp score; RA, rheumatoid arthritis.

Tight control was defined as a treatment strategy in which (1) assessment of clinical disease activity should be performed at each scheduled visit (every 1–3 months) or at any time if patients had aggravation of their clinical signs or symptoms; and (2) DMARD therapy should be modified or changed if patients cannot achieve remission or at least low disease activity within 3 months or if patients suffer from a disease flare [9,10]. A disease flare was defined as a worsening of the disease activity index (a return to moderate or high activity) at any time during follow-up.

2.2. Data Collection at Baseline

We reviewed our patient records and collected clinical data at the time of their first visits (baseline characteristics), which included demographic characteristics (age and sex), RA-related factors (28-joint disease activity score based on erythrocyte sedimentation rate [DAS28-ESR], duration of joint signs and/or symptoms (disease duration), anti-cyclic citrullinated peptide antibodies [anti-CCP], and rheumatoid factor [RF]), smoking history, and body mass index (BMI). Sera that had been collected at the first visit and stored at −80 °C were used for the detection of anti-CCP and RF. Detailed methods for the measurement have been described in our previous study [21]. The previous use of conventional synthetic DMARDs (csDMARDs) and year of the patient's first visit at our institution were also recorded. The availability of DMARDs differed between 2001 and 2014. To explore the possibility that this difference in DMARD availability during the early stage of a patient's treatment might affect structural and functional outcomes after 10 years, we included the year of each patient's first visit in the baseline characteristics.

2.3. Monitoring Clinical Disease Activity During Follow-Up

For monitoring disease activity, we used DAS28-ESR between 2001 and 2005. Since 2006, the clinical disease activity index (CDAI) has been used to follow patients [11,22]. For CDAI, cut-off values for disease activity states were defined as follows: >22 for high disease activity; >10 and ≤22 for moderate disease activity; >2.8 and ≤10 for low disease activity; and ≤2.8 for remission [11]. For DAS28-ESR, the following definition was used: >5.1 for high disease activity; ≥3.2 and ≤5.1 for moderate disease activity; ≥2.6 and <3.2 for low disease activity; and <2.6 for remission [23]. For all patients, the disease activity state after 10-year DMARD therapy was determined based on CDAI values.

Based on the clinical disease activity during the 10-year follow-up, each RA patient was classified into a poor control group (patients with experience of high or moderate disease activity lasting for ≥12 months), a moderate control group (patients with experience of high or moderate disease activity lasting for 3–12 months), and a good control group (patients without experience of high or moderate disease activity lasting for ≥3 months).

2.4. Assessment of Joint Destruction

To assess structural damage, we use radiographic imaging of each patient's hands and feet taken both at baseline and after 10 years of DMARD therapy. Each radiograph was assessed independently by two rheumatologists who were well trained and competent to score radiographs using the van der Heijde-modified total Sharp score (mTSS) [24,25]. The readers were blinded to the patient's clinical status and treatment. To evaluate structural damage progression, a change in mTSS from baseline to 10 years later (ΔmTSS) was calculated for each patient. The mTSS is the sum of the erosion score (range 0–280) and the joint space narrowing (JSN) score (range 0–168). In addition to mTSS, we also reported erosion score and JSN score separately because these scores can provide complementary information on different aspects of structural damage [26,27]. The inter-observer agreement between the two readers was determined using the intraclass correlation coefficient (ICC). A two-way mixed-effects model with consistency definition and single rater type (ICC (3,1)) was applied [28]. The ICC (3,1) for ΔmTSS, erosion score, and JNS score were 0.907, 0.953, and 0.963, respectively, which indicated excellent agreement in radiographic scoring.

2.5. Outcomes of Interest

The outcomes of interest were structural changes defined as the ΔmTSS, functional impairment expressed by the health assessment questionnaire-disability index (HAQ-DI), and improvement of clinical disease activity after 10 years of DMARD therapy under tight control. Structural and functional remission were defined as ΔmTSS ≤ 5.0 per 10 years and HAQ-DI ≤ 0.5 at 10 years, respectively. Clinical remission was defined as CDAI ≤ 2.8 at 10 years.

2.6. Statistical Analysis

Mean and standard deviation (SD) were used as descriptive statistics for data with a continuous distribution, which included non-normally distributed data [29]. Number (percentage) was used for categorical data. We compared baseline characteristics and DMARD use between two patient groups using the independent-measures *t*-test for continuous variables and Fisher's exact probability test for categorical variables. Comparisons of outcomes between three patient groups were performed using a one-way analysis of variance (ANOVA) with post hoc Tukey's honestly significant difference (HSD) test for continuous variables and using Fisher's exact probability test with the post hoc Holm test for categorical variables. There were no missing measurements at baseline, clinical disease activity state and DMARD use during follow-up, or outcomes after 10 years.

Logistic regression analysis was performed to evaluate the association between structural or functional remission after 10-year DMARD therapy as a dependent variable and a set of baseline characteristics as independent variables that were considered to be clinically relevant based on previous knowledge, which included age, sex, RA-related factors, smoking history, BMI, previous use of csDMARDs, and year of the first visit. Additionally, mTSS (erosion score/JSN score) at baseline was introduced into this analysis as an independent variable. Univariable logistic regression analysis was performed first for each independent variable. Thereafter, all variables with p-values < 0.10 in the univariable models were introduced into multivariable logistic regression analysis. The mTSS and erosion score/JSN score were included separately in multivariable regression analysis (Model 1 for mTSS and Model 2 for erosion score/JSN score), because erosion score and JSN score are compositions of mTSS. A forced entry procedure was used in the multivariable model. The strength of association between structural or functional remission and the independent variables was estimated using odds ratios (ORs) and 95% confidence intervals (95% CIs). Receiver operating characteristic (ROC) curves and the corresponding area under the curve (AUC) values were calculated to provide an index of validity for the multivariable logistic regression model.

For all tests, p-values < 0.05 were considered to indicate statistical significance. All calculations were performed using PASW Statistics version 27 (SPSS Japan Inc., Tokyo, Japan) and Easy R (Saitama Medical Center, Jichi Medical University, Saitama, Japan) [30].

3. Results

3.1. Baseline Characteristics of RA Patients Grouped by Achievement of Structural and Functional Remission After 10-Year DMARD Therapy

As shown in Figure 1, we identified 204 patients with RA (50 males and 154 females) who completed 10-year DMARD therapy under tight control. Baseline characteristics are shown in Table 1. The mean age at baseline was 57.5 years, and the mean disease duration was 1.8 years. More than 80% of patients did not have previous use of any type of DMARDs at baseline. The mean DAS28-ESR was 4.8. The mean mTSS at baseline was 8.4 (erosion score, 3.2; JSN score, 5.2) and 30.9% had normal joint space without bone erosion at baseline (mTSS = 0).

Table 1. Baseline characteristics of RA patients grouped by achievement of structural and functional remission after 10-year tight-control DMARD therapy.

Baseline Characteristics	Total	Structural Remission ¶		p *	Functional Remission ¶		p *
	(n = 204)	Yes	No		Yes	No	
		(n = 149)	(n = 55)		(n = 166)	(n = 38)	
Age, years, mean (SD)	57.5 (10.4)	57.9 (10.8)	56.4 (9.3)	0.34	56.7 (9.9)	61.3 (11.7)	0.013
>65 years, number (%)	48 (23.5)	38 (25.5)	10 (18.2)	0.35	32 (19.0)	16 (44.4)	0.005
Male, number (%)	50 (24.5)	43 (28.9)	7 (12.7)	0.018	46 (27.4)	4 (11.1)	0.035
Anti-CCP positive, number (%)	179 (87.7)	127 (85.2)	52 (94.5)	0.092	144 (86.7)	35 (92.1)	0.58
RF positive, number (%)	162 (79.4)	114 (76.5)	48 (87.3)	0.12	131 (78.9)	31 (81.6)	0.83
DAS28-ESR, mean (SD)	4.8 (1.2)	4.7 (1.2)	5.1 (1.1)	0.030	4.7 (1.1)	5.4 (1.2)	<0.001
High (>5.1) number (%)	86 (42.2)	58 (38.9)	28 (50.9)	0.15	63 (38.0)	23 (60.5)	0.017
Disease duration †, years, mean (SD)	1.8 (3.5)	1.4 (2.9)	2.8 (4.7)	0.020	1.7 (3.5)	2.4 (3.5)	0.23
≤6 months, number (%)	126 (61.8)	94 (63.1)	32 (58.2)	0.52	106 (63.9)	20 (52.6)	0.20
Year of the first visit ‡, number (%)							
2001–2008	75 (36.8)	58 (38.9)	17 (30.9)	0.33	62 (37.3)	13 (34.2)	0.85
2009–2011	77 (37.7)	55 (36.9)	22 (40.0)	0.75	63 (38.0)	14 (36.8)	1.00
2012–2014	52 (25.5)	36 (24.2)	16 (29.1)	0.47	41 (24.7)	11 (28.9)	0.68
Previous csDMARD use, number (%)							
No use	173 (84.8)	129 (86.6)	44 (80)	0.27	141 (84.9)	32 (84.2)	1.00
Smoking history > 30 PYs, number (%)	31 (15.2)	27 (18.1)	4 (7.3)	0.077	28 (16.9)	3 (7.9)	0.21
BMI > 25, number (%)	32 (15.7)	19 (12.8)	13 (23.6)	0.081	24 (14.5)	8 (21.1)	0.13
mTSS (range 0–448) §, mean (SD)	8.4 (13.7)	5.8 (10.7)	15.5 (18.0)	<0.001	6.6 (11.6)	16.5 (18.7)	<0.001
0, number (%)	63 (30.9)	57 (38.3)	6 (10.9)	<0.001	60 (36.1)	3 (7.9)	<0.001
>0 and ≤5, number (%)	66 (32.4)	50 (33.6)	16 (29.1)	0.62	53 (31.9)	13 (34.2)	0.85
>5 and ≤25, number (%)	55 (27.0)	33 (22.1)	22 (40)	0.013	41 (24.5)	14 (36.8)	0.16
>25, number (%)	20 (9.8)	9 (6.0)	11 (20)	0.006	12 (7.2)	8 (21.1)	0.016
Erosion score, mean (SD)	3.2 (6.0)	2.4 (4.6)	5.5 (8.3)	<0.001	2.6 (4.6)	6.1 (9.6)	<0.001
No erosion, number (%)	94 (46.1)	75 (50.3)	19 (34.5)	0.057	85 (51.2)	9 (23.7)	0.002
>0 and ≤3, number (%)	63 (30.9)	46 (30.9)	17 (30.9)	1.00	46 (27.7)	17 (44.7)	0.051
>3 and ≤10, number (%)	26 (12.7)	19 (12.8)	7 (12.7)	1.00	22 (13.3)	4 (10.5)	0.79
>10, number (%)	21 (10.3)	9 (6.0)	12 (21.8)	0.003	13 (7.8)	8 (21.1)	0.033
Only erosion, number (%)	33 (16.2)	20 (13.4)	13 (23.6)	0.089	28 (16.9)	5 (13.2)	0.79
JSN score, mean (SD)	5.2 (8.7)	3.5 (6.6)	10.0 (11.5)	<0.001	4.0 (7.7)	10.4 (10.9)	<0.001
Normal joint space, number (%)	97 (47.5)	83 (55.7)	14 (25.5)	<0.001	89 (53.6)	8 (21.1)	<0.001
>0 and ≤3, number (%)	33 (16.2)	26 (17.4)	7 (12.7)	0.52	28 (16.9)	5 (13.2)	0.81
>3 and ≤10, number (%)	35 (17.2)	23 (15.4)	12 (21.8)	0.30	27 (16.3)	8 (21.1)	0.48
>10, number (%)	39 (19.1)	17 (11.4)	22 (40)	<0.001	22 (13.3)	17 (44.7)	<0.001
Only JSN, number (%)	36 (17.6)	28 (18.8)	8 (14.5)	0.54	30 (18.1)	6 (15.8)	0.61

* Compared between patients who achieved remission and those who failed in achieving remission, using Fisher's exact probability test for categorical variables and independent-measures t-test for continuous variables. † Defined as the time length from onset of joint symptoms and/or signs to the first visit at our institution. ‡ Available DMARDs: 2001–2008, TNF inhibitors; 2009–2011, plus IL-6 inhibitors and abatacept; 2012–2014, plus JAK inhibitors. § Determined as the sum of the erosion score (range 0–280) and the JSN score (range 0–168). ¶ Defined as ΔmTSS ≤ 5.0 per 10 years for structural remission and HAQ-DI ≤ 0.5 at 10 years for functional remission. anti-CCP, anti-cyclic citrullinated peptide antibodies; BMI, body mass index; csDMARDs, conventional synthetic DMARDs; DAS28-ESR, 28-joint disease activity score using erythrocyte sedimentation rate; DMARD, disease-modifying antirheumatic drug; HAQ-DI, health assessment questionnaire-disability index; IL-6, interleukin-6; JAK, Janus kinase; JSN, joint space narrowing; mTSS, van der Heijde-modified total Sharp score; PYs, pack-years; RA, rheumatoid arthritis; RF, rheumatoid factor; SD, standard deviation; TNF, tumor necrosis factor.

After 10-year DMARD therapy under tight control, 195 patients (95.6%) achieved clinical remission (68.1% for CDAI ≤ 2.8) or low disease activity (27.5% for CDAI > 2.8 and ≤10). In total, 149 patients (73.0%) in structural remission and 166 patients (81.4%) were in functional remission (Figure 1). As shown in Table 1, mean mTSS, erosion score, and JNS score at baseline were significantly lower in the structure remission and functional remission groups than in the non-remission groups (structural remission: 5.8 versus 15.5 for mTSS, 2.4 versus 5.5 for erosion score, 3.5 versus 10.0 for JSN score, $p < 0.001$; functional remission: 6.6 versus 16.5 for mTSS, 2.6 versus 6.1 for erosion score, 4.0 versus 10.4, for JSN score, $p < 0.001$). Regarding demographic characteristics, patients in the functional remission group were significantly younger compared with those in the non-remission group (56.7 versus 61.3 years, $p = 0.013$). Rates of male patients were higher in the structural remission and functional remission groups than in the non-remission groups (structural remission: 28.9% versus 12.7%, $p = 0.018$; functional remission: 27.4% versus 11.1%, $p = 0.035$).

Regarding RA-related characteristics, the mean DAS28-ESR values were lower in the structural remission and functional remission groups compared with the non-remission groups (structural remission: 4.7 versus 5.1, $p = 0.030$; functional remission: 4.7 versus 5.4, $p < 0.001$). Disease duration was significantly shorter in the structural remission group than in the non-remission group (1.4 years versus 2.8 years, $p = 0.020$).

3.2. *Clinical, Functional, and Structural Outcomes in RA Patients Grouped by Disease Activity Control During 10-Year DMARD Therapy*

Detailed clinical, functional, and structural outcomes after 10 years are shown in Table 2. Mean CDAI and HAQ-DI were 2.8 and 0.26, respectively. Mean mTSS was 13.8 (erosion score, 4.4; JSN score, 9.4). Mean increase in mTSS (ΔmTSS) for 10 years was 5.4 (Δerosion score, 1.2; ΔJSN score, 4.2). Median ΔmTSS was 2.0. Under tight control, 28.9% of patients had no structural changes for 10 years, 51.0% had no progression of bone erosion, and 34.8% had no changes in JSN (Table 2 and Figure 2). The contribution of JSN changes to joint damage progression was much higher compared with progression of erosive changes.

Table 2. Outcomes in RA patients grouped by experience of high or moderate disease activity during 10-year tight-control DMARD therapy.

Outcomes at 10 Years	Total	Good Control †	Moderate Control †	Poor Control †	p *
	(n = 204)	(n = 134)	(n = 52)	(n = 18)	
Clinical disease activity at 10 years					
CDAI, mean (SD)	2.8 (3.1)	1.9 (2.1)	3.5 (3.5)	7.6 (3.6)	<0.001
Remission (<2.8), number (%)	139 (68.1)	109 (81.3)	28 (53.8)	2 (11.1)	<0.001
Low (>2.8 and ≤10), number (%)	56 (27.5)	23 (17.2)	20 (38.5)	13 (72.2)	<0.001
Physical function at 10 years					
HAQ-DI, mean (SD)	0.26 (0.49)	0.12 (0.34)	0.35 (0.45)	1.05 (0.69)	<0.001
HAQ-DI ≤ 0.5 (remission), number (%)	166 (81.4)	126 (94.0)	37 (71.2)	3 (16.6)	<0.001
Structural changes for 10 years					
mTSS at 10 years, mean (SD)	13.8 (17.8)	7.8 (12.0)	22.5 (20.6)	34.1 (20.9)	<0.001
ΔmTSS, mean (SD)	5.4 (9.0)	1.7 (2.2)	8.6 (9.3)	22.9 (14.6)	<0.001
ΔmTSS, median (IQR)	2.0 (0, 6)	1.0 (0, 3.0)	5.3 (2.5, 13)	20.3 (9.9, 36.4)	<0.001
ΔmTSS ≤ 5 (remission), number (%)	149 (73.0)	121 (90.3)	26 (50.0)	2 (11.1)	<0.001
ΔmTSS = 0 (no progression), number (%)	59 (28.9)	55 (41.0)	4 (7.7)	0	<0.001
ΔmTSS ≥ 25, number (%)	10 (4.9)	0	2 (3.8)	8 (44.4)	<0.001
Changes in bone erosion for 10 years					
Erosion score at 10 years, mean (SD)	4.4 (6.9)	2.8 (4.9)	7.5 (9.8)	7.5 (6.0)	<0.001
Δerosion score, mean (SD)	1.2 (2.4)	0.4 (1.0)	2.0 (2.9)	4.8 (3.7)	<0.001
Δerosion score ≤ 3, number (%)	180 (88.2)	131 (97.8)	41 (78.8)	8 (44.4)	<0.001
Δerosion score = 0, number (%)	104 (51.0)	85 (63.4)	17 (32.7)	2 (11.1)	<0.001
Changes in joint space for 10 years					
JSN score at 10 years, mean (SD)	9.4 (12.4)	4.9 (7.8)	15.0 (13.0)	26.5 (17.1)	<0.001
ΔJSN score, mean (SD)	4.2 (7.3)	1.3 (1.9)	6.8 (7.2)	18.1 (12.5)	<0.001
ΔJSN score ≤ 3, number (%)	143 (70.1)	105 (91.3)	34 (51.5)	4 (17.4)	<0.001
ΔJSN score = 0, number (%)	71 (34.8)	58 (50.4)	13 (19.7)	0	<0.001

* Differences among the patient groups were assessed using one-way analysis of variance (ANOVA) with Tukey's HSD post hoc test for continuous variables and Fisher's exact probability test with the post hoc Holm test for categorical variables. † Defined as the experience of high or moderate disease activity continuing for ≥12 months (poor control), the experience of high or moderate disease activity continuing for 3–12 months (moderate control), and no experience of high or moderate disease activity continuing for ≥3 months (good control) during 10-year DMARD therapy. ANOVA, analysis of variance; CDAI, clinical disease activity index; DMARD, disease-modifying antirheumatic drug; HAQ-DI, health assessment questionnaire-disability index; HSD, honestly significant difference; IQR, interquartile range; JSN, joint space narrowing; mTSS, van der Heijde-modified total Sharp score; RA, rheumatoid arthritis; SD, standard deviation; Δ, a change from baseline to 10 years later.

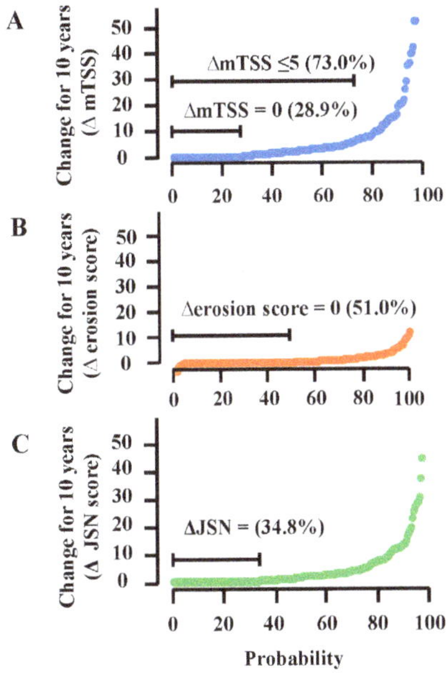

Figure 2. Cumulative probability plots of changes in mTSS (**A**), erosion score (**B**), and JSN score (**C**) for 10 years of DMARD therapy under tight control. JSN score, joint space narrowing score; mTSS, van der Heijde-modified total Sharp score.

We classified RA patients into three categories; that is, good, moderate, and poor control groups, based on the experience of high or moderate disease activity for 10 years (Table 2). In total, 134 patients (65.7%) had no experience of high or moderate disease activity lasting for ≥3 months (good control group). In contrast, 18 patients (8.8%) experienced high or moderate disease activity lasting for ≥12 months (poor control group), and 52 patients (25.5%) had high or moderate disease activity lasting for 3–12 months (moderate control group). Ten years later, the means of CDAI, HAQ-DI, mTSS, and ΔmTSS, as well as the rates of patients with clinical, functional, and structural remission, were significantly different among the three patient groups. In the good control group, more than 90% of patients were in structural remission and functional remission at 10 years. In contrast, the rates of structural remission and functional remission in the poor control group were 11.1% and 16.6%, respectively. Progression of bone erosion and JSN was significantly slower in the good control group compared with the poor and moderate control groups, but their contributions to structural changes were similar among the three control groups.

3.3. DMARD Use for 10 Years in RA Patients Under Tight Control

All patients, except those with contraindication for methotrexate (MTX), started DMARD therapy with MTX monotherapy. As shown in Table 3, 96.6% of patients used MTX. MTX exposure was significantly longer in the structural remission and functional remission groups than in the non-remission groups (structural remission: 109.1 versus 92.0 months; functional remission: 107.4 versus 89.7 months, $p < 0.001$). In total, 155 patients (76%) received bDMARD and/or tsDMARD. The rate of bDMARD/tsDMARD use for 10 years was significantly lower in the functional remission group compared with the non-remission group (71.7% versus 94.7%, $p = 0.001$). A similar trend was observed in a comparison between the structural remission group and the non-remission group (72.5% versus 85.5%, $p = 0.065$). The number of bDMARD/tsDMARD classes used per patient for 10 years was significantly smaller in the structural remission and functional remission groups compared with the non-remission groups (structural remission: 1.2 versus 1.9, $p < 0.001$; functional remission: 1.2 versus 2.3, $p < 0.001$). The number of failures per patient was significantly smaller in the structural remission and functional remission groups than in the non-remission groups (structural remission: 0.5 versus 1.2, $p < 0.001$; functional remission: 0.5 versus 1.5, $p < 0.001$). Thus, RA patients in the non-remission groups received more classes of bDMARD/tsDMARD and experienced more failures during 10-year DMARD therapy compared with those in the remission groups.

Table 3. DMARD use in RA patients grouped by structural and functional outcomes after 10-year tight-control therapy.

	Total	Structural Remission ††		p *	Functional Remission ††		p *
	(n = 204)	Yes	No		Yes	No	
		(n = 149)	(n = 55)		(n = 166)	(n = 38)	
MTX use, number (%)	197 (96.6)	142 (95.3)	55 (100)	0.19	161 (97.0)	36 (94.7)	0.62
Use as monotherapy, number (%)	49 (24.0)	41 (27.5)	8 (14.5)	0.065	47 (28.3)	2 (5.3)	0.001
Exposure, months, mean (SD) †	104.3 (28.0)	109.1 (22.7)	92.0 (35.9)	<0.001	107.4 (24.9)	89.7 (37.0)	<0.001
b/tsDMARD use ‡, number (%)	155 (76.0)	108 (72.5)	47 (85.5)	0.065	119 (71.7)	36 (94.7)	0.001
Use of 1 class, number (%)	79 (38.7)	61 (40.9)	18 (32.7)	0.33	69 (41.6)	10 (26.3)	0.10
Use of 2 classes, number (%)	40 (19.6)	29 (19.5)	11 (20.0)	1.00	30 (18.1)	10 (26.3)	0.26
Use of ≥3 classes, number (%)	36 (17.6)	18 (12.1)	18 (32.7)	0.001	20 (12.0)	16 (42.1)	<0.001
Number of classes used per patient, mean (SD)	1.4 (1.1)	1.2 (1.0)	1.9 (1.3)	<0.001	1.2 (1.0)	2.3 (1.3)	<0.001
Exposure, months, mean (SD) §	79.6 (36.1)	76.9 (37.7)	85.8 (31.4)	0.16	77.4 (36.8)	86.8 (32.9)	0.17
Time to the first use, months, mean (SD) §	23.3 (28.6)	23.7 (29.9)	22.3 (25.4)	0.79	24.0 (29.2)	21.0 (26.4)	0.58
b/tsDMARD failure per patient, number, mean (SD) §¶	0.7 (1.1)	0.5 (1.0)	1.2 (1.3)	<0.001	0.5 (0.9)	1.5 (1.4)	<0.001
No failure, number (%)	95 (61.3)	75 (69.4)	20 (42.6)	0.002	84 (70.6)	11 (30.6)	<0.001
Failure of 1 class, number (%)	26 (16.8)	15 (13.9)	11 (23.4)	0.16	17 (14.3)	9 (25.0)	0.14
Failure of 2 classes, number (%)	19 (12.3)	14 (13.0)	5 (10.6)	0.79	13 (10.9)	6 (16.7)	0.39
Failure of ≥3 classes, number (%)	15 (9.7)	4 (3.7)	11 (23.4)	<0.001	5 (4.2)	10 (27.8)	<0.001

* Compared between patients who achieved remission by 10-year DMARD therapy under tight control and those who failed in achieving remission, using Fisher's exact probability test for categorical variables and independent-measures t-test for continuous variables. † Determined for 197 patients who received MTX during 10-year DMARD therapy. ‡ Including four classes of b/tsDMARDs (TNF inhibitors used for 133 patients [55.4%], IL-6 inhibitors for 70 patients [34.3%], abatacept for 34 patients [16.7%)], and JAK inhibitors for 62 patients [30.4%]). § Determined for 155 patients who received one or more b/tsDMARDs during 10-year DMARD therapy (108 with structural remission and 47 without it; 119 with functional remission and 36 without it). ¶ Defined as failure to achieve remission or low disease activity within 3 months or occurrence of disease flare. †† Defined as ΔmTSS for 10 years ≤ 5.0 for structural remission and HAQ-DI after 10 years ≤ 0.5 for functional remission. DMARD, disease-modifying antirheumatic drug; b/tsDMARD, biological DMARD and targeted synthetic DMARD; HAQ-DI, health assessment questionnaire-disability index; IL-6, interleukin-6; JAK, Janus kinase; mTSS, van der Heijde-modified total Sharp score; MTX, methotrexate; RA, rheumatoid arthritis; SD, standard deviation; TNF, tumor necrosis factor.

3.4. Predictors of Structural Remission After 10-Year DMARD Therapy Under Tight Control

Univariable logistic regression analyses revealed that male sex, DAS28-ESR, disease duration, mTSS, erosion score, and JSN score at baseline were significantly associated with structural remission after 10 years (Table 4). Baseline mTSS and other baseline characteristics with $p < 0.10$ in the univariable analyses were introduced into the multivariable analysis as independent variables (Model 1), which showed that baseline mTSS was the only variable to predict structural remission after 10 years. Adjusted ORs (95% CIs) for baseline mTSS were 0.15 (0.05–0.46) for >5 and ≤25 ($p < 0.001$) and 0.12 (0.03–0.48) for >25 ($p = 0.003$) versus 0 (normal joint space without erosion at baseline). When baseline erosion score and JSN score, instead of mTSS, were introduced into the multivariable analysis as independent variables (Model 2), the JSN score and the first visit year were identified as variables for predicting structural remission after 10 years. Adjusted ORs (95% CIs) for JSN score were 0.29 (0.10–0.83) for >3 and ≤10 ($p = 0.021$) and 0.14 (0.04–0.47) for >10 ($p = 0.002$) versus 0 (normal joint space). Adjusted OR (95% CI) for the year of the first visit was 2.45 (1.04–5.77) for 2009–2011 versus 2001–2008 ($p = 0.040$).

Table 4. Predictors of structural remission after 10-year DMARD therapy under tight control.

Variables at Baseline	Univariable Analysis		Multivariable Analysis (Model 1)		Multivariable Analysis (Model 2)	
	Unadjusted OR (95% CI)	p *	Adjusted OR (95% CI)	p *	Adjusted OR (95% CI)	p *
Age per additional year	1.02 (0.99–1.05)	0.34	–	–	–	–
Age > 65 years, yes vs. no	1.54 (0.71–3.35)	0.28	–	–	–	–
Male vs. female	2.78 (1.17–6.63)	0.020	3.57 (0.97–13.16)	0.056	3.13 (0.83–11.77)	0.091
Anti-CCP, positive vs. negative	0.33 (0.10–1.16)	0.080	0.35 (0.09–1.43)	0.14	0.30 (0.07–1.29)	0.11
RF, positive vs. negative	0.48 (0.20–1.14)	0.097	–	–	–	–
RF > 200 U/mL, yes or no	0.49 (0.23–1.02)	0.060	0.44 (0.18–1.09)	0.076	0.43 (0.17–1.08)	0.073
DAS28-ESR per additional unit	0.74 (0.57–10.97)	0.030	0.74 (0.53–1.02)	0.066	0.74 (0.53–1.04)	0.083
High (>5.1), yes vs. no	0.62 (0.33–1.15)	0.13	–	–	–	–
Disease duration per additional day	1.00 (1.00–1.00)	0.030	1.00 (1.00–1.00)	0.71	1.00 (1.00–1.00)	0.98
≤6 months, yes vs. no	0.92 (0.49–1.75)	0.81	–	–	–	–
Year of the first visit						
2001–2008	1 (reference)	–	–	–	–	–
2009–2011	1.99 (0.97–4.06)	0.060	2.18 (0.95–5.00)	0.066	2.45 (1.04–5.77)	0.040
2012–2014	2.10 (0.93–4.74)	0.080	1.64 (0.63–4.24)	0.31	1.94 (0.73–5.17)	0.18
Previous csDMARD use, yes vs. no	0.62 (0.28–1.40)	0.25	–	–	–	–
Smoking history > 30 PYs, yes vs. no	2.82 (0.94–8.48)	0.060	2.57 (0.51–12.92)	0.25	2.58 (0.49–13.50)	0.26
BMI > 25, yes vs. no	0.47 (0.22–1.04)	0.060	0.56 (0.22–1.47)	0.24	0.49 (0.18–1.32)	0.16
mTSS						
0 (no erosion/normal joint space)	1 (reference)	–	1 (reference)	–	–	–
>0 and ≤5	0.33 (0.12–0.91)	0.030	0.38 (0.13–1.10)	0.074	–	–
>5 and ≤25	0.16 (0.06–0.43)	<0.001	0.15 (0.05–0.46)	<0.001	–	–
>25	0.09 (0.03–0.29)	<0.001	0.12 (0.03–0.48)	0.003	–	–
Erosion score						
0 (no erosion)	1 (reference)	–	–	–	1 (reference)	–
>0 and ≤3	0.69 (0.32–1.45)	0.32	–	–	1.16 (0.48–2.82)	0.75
>3 and ≤10	0.69 (0.25–1.87)	0.46	–	–	2.18 (0.57–8.37)	0.26
>10	0.19 (0.07–0.52)	0.001	–	–	0.76 (0.19–3.09)	0.70
JSN score						
0 (normal joint space)	1 (reference)	–	–	–	1 (reference)	–
>0 and ≤3	0.63 (0.23–1.72)	0.36	–	–	0.73 (0.23–2.24)	0.58
>3 and ≤10	0.32 (0.13–0.79)	0.014	–	–	0.29 (0.10–0.83)	0.021
>10	0.13 (0.06–0.31)	<0.001	–	–	0.14 (0.04–0.47)	0.002

* Univariable and multivariable logistic regression analyses were conducted to evaluate baseline characteristics associated with structural remission after 10 years of DMARD therapy under tight control. Structural remission was defined as ΔmTSS for 10 years ≤ 5.0. All variables with p-values < 0.10 in the univariable models were introduced into multivariable analysis as independent factors using a forced entry procedure. As independent factors, mTSS was introduced into Model 1, and erosion score and JSN score were introduced into Model 2. The multivariable model yielded an AUC-ROC of 0.80 (0.73–0.86, $p < 0.001$) for Models 1 and 0.80 (0.74–0.87, $p < 0.001$) for Model 2. anti-CCP, anti-cyclic citrullinated peptide antibodies; AUC, area under the curve; BMI, body mass index; csDMARDs, conventional synthetic DMARDs; DAS28-ESR, disease activity score 28 joints-erythrocyte sedimentation rate; DMARD, disease-modifying antirheumatic drug; JNS, joint space narrowing; mTSS, van der Heijde-modified total Sharp score; OR, odds ratio; PYs, pack-years; RA, rheumatoid arthritis; RF, rheumatoid factor; ROC, receiver operating characteristic; 95% CI, 95% confidence interval.

3.5. Predictors of Functional Remission After 10-Year DMARD Therapy Under Tight Control

In univariable logistic regression analyses, we identified advanced age, male sex, DAS28-ESR, mTSS, erosion score, and JSN score at baseline as variables significantly associated with functional remission after 10 years (Table 5). When baseline mTSS and other baseline characteristics with $p < 0.10$ in the univariable analyses were introduced into the multivariable analysis as independent variables (Model 1), mTSS, advanced age, male sex, and DAS28-ESR were identified as predictor variables of functional remission at 10 years. Adjusted ORs (95% CIs) for baseline mTSS were 0.17 (0.04–0.70) for >0 and ≤5 ($p = 0.014$), 0.10 (0.02–0.43) for >5 and ≤10 ($p = 0.002$), and 0.07 (0.01–0.34) for >10 ($p = 0.001$) versus 0 (norm joint space without erosion at baseline). Adjusted ORs (95% CIs) for age > 65 years, male sex, and DAS28-ESR per additional unit were 0.29 (0.12–0.70) ($p = 0.006$), 6.66 (1.91–23.15) ($p = 0.003$), and 0.55 (0.38–0.80) ($p = 0.002$), respectively. When we introduced baseline erosion score and JSN score, instead of mTSS, into multivariable analysis as independent variables (Model 2), JSN score, advanced age, male sex, and DAS28-

ESR were detected as variables to predict functional remission after 10 years. Adjusted ORs (95% CIs) for baseline JSN score were 0.17 (0.05–0.58) for >3 and ≤10 ($p = 0.005$) and 0.09 (0.02–0.38) for >10 ($p < 0.001$) versus 0 (normal joint space). Adjusted ORs (95% CIs) for age > 65 years, male sex, and for DAS28-ESR per additional unit was 0.27 (0.10–0.69) ($p = 0.006$), 6.15 (1.66–22.74) ($p = 0.006$), and 0.57 (0.39–0.85) ($p = 0.006$), respectively.

Table 5. Predictors of functional remission after 10-year DMARD therapy under tight control.

Variables at Baseline	Univariable Analysis		Multivariable Analysis (Model 1)		Multivariable Analysis (Model 2)	
	Unadjusted OR (95% CIs)	p *	Adjusted OR (95% CI)	p *	Adjusted OR (95% CI)	p *
Age per additional year	0.96 (0.92–0.99)	0.015	–	–	–	–
Age > 65 years, yes vs. no	0.33 (0.16–0.70)	0.004	0.29 (0.12–0.70)	0.006	0.27 (0.10–0.69)	0.006
Male vs. female	3.26 (1.10–9.70)	0.034	6.66 (1.91–23.15)	0.003	6.15 (1.66–22.74)	0.006
Anti-CCP, positive vs. negative	0.56 (0.16–1.98)	0.37	–	–	–	–
RF, positive vs. negative	0.85 (0.34–2.08)	0.71	–	–	–	–
RF > 200 U/mL, yes or no	1.27 (0.49–3.31)	0.62	–	–	–	–
DAS28-ESR per additional unit	0.58 (0.42–0.80)	<0.001	0.55 (0.38–0.80)	0.002	0.57 (0.39–0.85)	0.006
High (>5.1), yes vs. no	0.40 (0.19–0.82)	0.013	–	–	–	–
Disease duration per additional day	1.00 (1.00–1.00)	0.24	–	–	–	–
≤6 months, yes vs. no	1.59 (0.78–3.24)	0.20	–	–	–	–
Year of the first visit						
2001–2008	1 (reference)	–	–	–	–	–
2009–2011	1.59 (0.70–3.60)	0.27	–	–	–	–
2012–2014	1.40 (0.57–3.44)	0.46	–	–	–	–
Previous csDMARD use, yes vs. no	0.95 (0.36–2.50)	0.91	–	–	–	–
Smoking history > 30 PYs, yes vs. no	2.37 (0.68–8.24)	0.18	–	–	–	–
BMI > 25, yes vs. no	0.63 (0.26–1.55)	0.32	–	–	–	–
mTSS						
0 (no erosion/normal joint space)	1 (reference)	–	1 (reference)	–	–	–
>0 and ≤5	0.20 (0.055–0.75)	0.017	0.17 (0.04–0.70)	0.014	–	–
>5 and ≤10	0.15 (0.04–0.54)	0.004	0.10 (0.02–0.43)	0.002	–	–
>10	0.08 (0.02–0.32)	<0.001	0.07 (0.01–0.34)	0.001	–	–
Erosion score						
0 (no erosion)	1 (reference)	–	–		1 (reference)	–
>0 and ≤3	0.29 (0.12–0.69)	0.006	–		0.46 (0.17–1.25)	0.13
>3 and ≤10	0.58 (0.16–2.07)	0.40	–		2.00 (0.38–10.54)	0.42
>10	0.17 (0.06–0.53)	0.002	–		0.84 (0.17–4.19)	0.83
JSN score						
0 (normal joint space)	1 (reference)	–	–		1 (reference)	–
>0 and ≤3	0.50 (0.15–1.66)	0.26	–		0.52 (0.14–1.94)	0.33
>3 and ≤10	0.30 (0.10–0.89)	0.029	–		0.17 (0.05–0.58)	0.005
>10	0.12 (0.04–0.30)	<0.001	–		0.09 (0.02–0.38)	<0.001

* Univariable and multivariable logistic regression analyses were conducted to evaluate baseline characteristics associated with functional remission after 10 years of DMARD therapy under tight control. Functional remission was defined as HAQ-DI after 10 years ≤ 0.5. All variables with p-values < 0.10 in the univariable models were introduced into multivariable analysis as independent factors using a forced entry procedure. As independent factors, mTSS was introduced into Model 1, and erosion score and JSN score were introduced into Model 2. The multivariable model yielded an AUC-ROC of 0.80 (0.73–0.88, $p < 0.001$) for Model 1 and 0.83 (0.75–0.90, $p < 0.001$) for Model 2. anti-CCP, anti-cyclic citrullinated peptide antibodies; AUC, area under the curve; BMI, body mass index; csDMARDs, conventional synthetic DMARDs; DAS28-ESR, 28-joint disease activity score using erythrocyte sedimentation rate; DMARD, disease-modifying antirheumatic drug; HAQ-DI, health assessment questionnaire-disability index; JSN, joint space narrowing; mTSS, van der Heijde-modified total Sharp score; OR, odds ratio; PYs, pack-years; RA, rheumatoid arthritis; RF, rheumatoid factor; ROC, receiver operating characteristic; 95% CI, 95% confidence interval.

3.6. Sensitivity Analysis

Considering the influence of disease control for the 10-year follow-up on structural and functional outcomes, we performed univariable and multivariable logistic regression analyses for RA patients who experienced high or moderate disease activity lasting for ≥3 months (the poor and moderate control groups) (Tables S1 and S2). In multivariable logistic regression models, baseline mTSS (Model 1) and JSN score (Model 2) were identified as the strong predictors of structural and functional remission after 10 years.

4. Discussion

In the present study, 76% of RA patients were treated with bDMARDs and/or tsDMARDs. Clinical, structural, and functional remission were achieved in 68.1%, 73.0%, and 81.4%, respectively, of RA patients who completed 10-year DMARD therapy under tight control. Mean ΔmTSS per 10 years was 5.4 (Δerosion score, 1.2; ΔJNS score, 4.2), and 28.9% of patients had no structural progression for 10 years (51% without erosive progression and 34.8% without JNS progression). Mean HAQ-DI was 0.26. During 10-year DMARD therapy, 65.7% of patients showed good control of disease activity, but 8.8% experienced high or moderate disease activity lasting for ≥12 months. The disease control significantly affected structural and functional outcomes after 10 years. For all patients, baseline mTSS and JSN score (but not erosion score) were the strong predictors for structural and functional remission after 10 years. Even for patients who failed at good disease control during follow-up, baseline mTSS and JSN were identified as factors predicting structural and functional remission.

Radiographic progression and functional loss in the present study were limited compared with previous 10-year follow-up studies without tight control. A prospective cohort study for RA patients recruiting from 1993 to 1994 reported that the mean mTSS of hands and feet increased to 35.4 at 10 years from 5.8 at baseline (average annual progression rate, 2.96/year) [31]. Longitudinal follow-up studies for RA patients starting in 1992 (EURIDISS cohort) showed that the mean mTSS of hands (scale 0–280) worsened to 36.0 at 10 years from 6.8 at baseline (mean yearly progression rate, 2.8). Mean HAQ-DI at 10 years was 0.92 [32–34]. In a 10-year follow-up study of Japanese RA patients recruiting in 1995, the mean mTSS worsened from 5 to 35 after 10 years [35]. Most patients in those studies were treated with MTX and other csDMARDs without tight control during follow-up. In a systematic review and meta-analysis using data from longitudinal observational cohorts (follow-up range, 5–20 years), Carpenter et al. showed that the annual progression rate of structural joint damage in studies recruiting between 1990 and 2011 was significantly lower compared with that in studies recruiting between 1965 and 1989 because of critical changes in treatment practices [36].

Previous clinical trials have shown that the treat-to-target strategy with MTX monotherapy or combination with infliximab or adalimumab induced long-term protective effects on structural damage progression and functional loss in RA patients. The BeSt study compared four different treatment strategies, namely arms 1 and 2 starting with MTX monotherapy (switching to or adding other DMARD) and arms 3 and 4 starting with MTX combination therapy (prednisolone or infliximab) in patients with early RA. Those patients were recruited between 2000 and 2002 and received tightly controlled targeted treatment to achieve low disease activity [14]. For all strategies, subsequent treatment adjustments were done based on DAS44 measurements every 3 months [37]. Over 10 years, 82% had low disease activity (DAS44 ≤ 2.4) and 53% were in remission (DAS44 < 1.6). Mean estimated ΔmTSS during follow-up was 10.9, 8.4, 8.1, and 6.1 (median 2.0, 2.5, 3.0, and 1.5) for arms 1–4, respectively. Mean HAQ-DI after 10 years was 0.69, 0.72, 0.64, and 0.58 in arms 1–4, respectively. All treat-to-target strategies were equally effective in preventing functional disability and radiographic progression after 10 years [37,38]. The IMPROVED study determined 5-year outcomes of early remission induction therapy with MTX plus prednisolone followed by targeted treatment aiming at drug-free remission (DAS44 < 1.6) with a combination of MTX and other csDMARD (arm 1) and a combination of MT and adalimumab (arm 2) in early RA patients who were included between 2007 and 2010. Tight control was done based on DAS44 measures every 4 months [39,40]. After 5 years, 48% were in remission. Mean ΔmTSS was 2.0 (median 0.5) and 1.7 (median 0.29) in arms 1 and

2, respectively. Mean HAQ-DI was 0.83 and 0.82 in arms 1 and 2, respectively. There were no significant differences between the randomization arms [41].

In the 8-year open-label extension of PREMIER trials, patients with early RA who had completed an initial double-blinded clinical trial with adalimumab plus MTX (arm 1), adalimumab alone, (arm 2), and MTX alone (arm 3) for 2 years were then followed by adalimumab with and without MTX during the open-label extension for 8 years. For 10-year completers, patients in the arm 1 achieved remission more readily compared with arms 2 and 3 (75.6% in arm 1, 61.7% in arm 2, and 56.2% in arm 3). Patients initially randomized to arm 1 displayed better structural and functional outcomes after 10 years, particularly in the prevention of radiographic progression; mean ΔmTSS was 4.0, 8.8, and 11.0 for arms 1–3, respectively. Mean HAQ-DI was 0.4, 0.7, and 0.6 in arms 1–3, respectively. Initial intensive therapy in patients with early RA had long-term benefits, which persisted up to 10 years [42]. Similar results were obtained in the 9-year open-label extension of the DE019 study (a 1-year randomized controlled trial for adalimumab in patients with long-standing RA) [43].

In the present analysis of real-world cohort data, similar levels of annual mean ΔmTSS rate and mean HAQ-DI were observed to the above-mentioned results from the BeSt, IMPROVED, and PREMIER studies. Radiographic progression was well suppressed, and good functional ability was preserved after 10-year DMARD therapy under tight control. The majority of our patients started RA treatment with MTX monotherapy, and if the treatment target was not achieved within 3 months, MTX monotherapy was switched to bDMARD or tsDMARD therapy with or without MTX. For 10 years, 76% of patients received bDMARDs and/or tsDMARDs with and without MTX. Thus, tightly controlled DMARD therapy from the start of RA treatment can lead to favorable long-term structural and functional outcomes in RA patients after 10 years in the real-world setting.

In the present study, structural and functional outcomes were worse in RA patients who experienced high or moderate disease activity lasting for ≥12 months during 10-year DMARD therapy compared with those who maintained good disease activity control. In the ESPOIR cohort study recruiting between 2002 and 2005, 10-year radiographic and functional outcomes were better in patients in sustained remission compared with those in sustained low disease activity and those in sustained moderate or high disease activity [44]. In a post hoc analysis of 10-year results from the BeSt study, more RA patients who had initially received MTX combination therapy achieved early and continuous low disease activity than those who had started with MTX monotherapy. Regardless of initial therapy, however, RA patients with continuous low disease activity had similar long-term clinical and radiological outcomes [45]. In another post hoc analysis of 10-year BeSt results, disease flares were associated with long-term joint damage progression and functional deterioration with a dose–response relationship with the number of flares [46]. These results indicated that good control of clinical disease activity during a 10-year follow-up is important in achieving structural and functional remission. In the present study, RA patients in the non-remission groups received more classes of bDMARD/tsDMARD and experienced more failures during 10-year DMARD therapy compared with those in the structural remission and functional remission groups. The rate of users of ≥3 bDMARD/tsDMARD classes was significantly higher in the non-remission groups than in the remission groups. The users of ≥3 classes had 2 or more switches of a current bDMARD/tsDMARD to another one mainly because of the need for treatment adjustments to control clinical disease activity. In other words, these patients might experience high or moderate disease activity for a longer time than users of 1 or 2 bDMARD/tsDMARD classes. The data suggest that sustained remission or at least low disease activity during follow-up is important in achieving structural and functional remission after 10 years. In the present study, we assessed clinical disease activity every 1 to 3 months and, if at least low disease activity was not achieved within 3 months, DMARD therapy was modified or changed. However, more frequent monitoring and earlier switching or adjustments of DMARD therapy may be required for patients with high or moderate disease activity.

We showed that baseline mTSS was a strong predictor of structural remission at the end of a 10-year DMARD therapy under tight control. Ten-year cohort studies in Europe also showed that baseline radiographic damage in RA patients was predictive of long-term radiographic joint damage, although most patients in those studies were treated with csDMARDs [31,47]. In the post hoc analysis of patients with early RA in the ASPIRE study, the progression of bone erosions and JSN was compared between MTX monotherapy and infliximab plus MTX combination therapy. Among patients with development or progression of joint damage after 54 weeks, bone erosion occurred more often than JNS in both treatment groups, suggesting that progression of bone erosion and JSN are potentially independent events. In addition, there was a tendency for joints with existing erosions or JSN at baseline to have progression of the same type of damage, rather than development of new damage [48]. Long-term effects of bone erosion and JSN on joint damage progression were reported in the long-term extension of BeSt, IMPROVED, and DE019 trials, in which the JSN component (cartilage damage) appeared to drive the radiological progression compared with bone erosions regardless of initial treatment [43,49]. In the present study, baseline JSN score, but not erosion score, was significantly associated with future structural outcomes, and JNS was the predominant type of joint damage after 10 years of DMARD therapy. Cartilage destruction seems to be of much higher relevance to joint damage progression than bone destruction.

Physical dysfunction has been reported as a consequence of ongoing inflammatory activity and structural joint damage through the course of RA; in early RA, it is most associated with the extent of disease activity, and in late RA, with structural damage [50,51]. Physical dysfunction is partly reversible, which is mediated by disease activity. Reversibility of physical disability decreases with the duration of RA, and in the absence of disease activity, structural damage contributes to irreversible physical dysfunction [52]. A relationship between structural damage and impaired physical function was also shown in the EURIDISS 10-year follow-up studies. Structural damage and disease activity are independent contributors to impaired physical function early and late in the RA process. [32,34]. Using data from several clinical trials for TNF inhibitors in RA patients, Aletaha et al. showed that cartilage damage was more clearly associated with irreversible physical disability at the time of remission than bone damage [53]. We found that baseline JSN score (but not erosion score) was strongly associated with not only structural damage but also physical dysfunction after 10-year DAMRD therapy. In addition to JSN score, baseline DAS28-ESR was also a strong predictor for physical function after 10 years. High DAS28-ESR had a trend to contribute to poor structural outcomes, but this association was not statistically significant in the present study.

In previous 10-year follow-up studies, high levels of disease activity (especially exemplified by acute phase reactants and swollen joint counts) and the presence of autoantibodies at baseline have been reported as prognostic factors associated with progression of joint damage in RA [31,33,47], but these baseline characteristics were not identified as the predictors for poor structural outcomes in the present study. Using 5-year results from the IMPROVED study, van der Pol et al. showed that, in patients with these poor prognostic factors, there was a non-significant increase in the risk of joint damage progression as the number of these factors increased [54].

There are some limitations to this study. First, this was a long-term retrospective observational study, which may confer inherent limitations. However, the medical records in our database allowed us to obtain accurate clinical data at baseline, information about DMARD use and control status of clinical disease activity during follow-up, and structural and functional outcomes after 10 years. Second, the aim of this study was to evaluate long-term outcomes and identify baseline characteristics predicting structural and functional remission in RA patients who completed 10-year DMARD therapy under tight control. Therefore, we excluded patients who dropped out of tightly controlled DMARD therapy during the 10-year follow-up. However, we showed that, even in patients who completed 10-year tight-control therapy, approximately 8.8% experienced high or moderate disease activity lasting for ≥12 months, and these poorly controlled patients had significantly lower structural and functional remission rates compared with patients who maintained good disease activity control. Third, various types of bDMARDs and tsDMARDs were used with and without MTX during 10-year tight-control therapy. We could not examine the effects of each DMARD therapy on long-term outcomes because of the small number of patients in individual treatment groups and the various exposure times.

5. Conclusions

Tightly controlled DMARD therapy toward remission or at least low disease activity can contribute to the suppression of structural damage and physical dysfunction after 10 years in the real-world setting. Baseline mTSS was a strong predictor for structural and functional remission. JSN seems to be more clearly associated with joint damage progression and functional loss than bone erosion. Patients with the experience of high or moderate disease activity lasting for ≥12 months during follow-up are at increased risk of poor structural and functional outcomes. Even for patients who failed at good disease control during follow-up, baseline JSN is a strong factor predicting structural and functional remission. To obtain favorable long-term structural and functional outcomes, particular attention should be given to the prevention of cartilage damage progression during DMARD therapy under tight control in daily practice.

Supplementary Materials: The following supporting information can be downloaded at: https://www.mdpi.com/article/10.3390/jcm14196832/s1, Table S1. Predictors of structural remission after 10-year DMARD therapy in RA patients who had poor or moderate control of clinical disease activity; Table S2. Predictors of functional remission after 10-year DMARD therapy in RA patients who had poor or moderate control of clinical disease activity.

Author Contributions: Conceptualization, S.M. and T.K.; Methodology, S.M. and T.K.; Validation, S.M., A.O., T.S., A.T., and T.K.; Formal Analysis, S.M.; Investigation, S.M., A.O., T.S., A.T., and T.K.; Resources, S.M.; Data Curation, S.M.; Writing—original Draft Preparation, S.M.; Writing—Review and Edition, S.M., A.O., T.S., A.T., and T.K.; Visualization, S.M.; Supervision, S.M. and T.K.; Project Administration, S.M.; Funding Acquisition, S.M. All authors have read and agreed to the published version of the manuscript.

Funding: This study was supported by internal research funds from the National Hospital Organization (NHO), Japan. The funder had no role in the study design, data collection, analysis, and interpretation, decision to publish, or manuscript preparation. No external funding was received for this study.

Institutional Review Board Statement: This study was conducted in accordance with the principles of the Declaration of Helsinki. The protocol of this study also meets the requirements of the Ethical Guidelines for Medical and Health Research Involving Human Subjects, Japan and was approved by the Human Research Ethics Committee at NHO Kumamoto Saishun Medical Center (No. 6-1 approved on 16 May 2024).

Informed Consent Statement: Because the study involved a retrospective review of patient records and data were analyzed anonymously, our ethics committees waived the requirement for patient informed consent to participate.

Data Availability Statement: All data supporting the findings are available from the Human Research Ethics Committee of the NHO Kumamoto Saishun Medical Center for all interested researchers who meet the criteria for access to confidential data. Because these data include patients' personal information, the Committee does not recommend that such data be made public unnecessarily. Please contact Masahiro Hamaguchi, the Control Manager of the Committee, at 616-syol@mail.hosp.go.jp to request the data.

Conflicts of Interest: We have read the journal's policy and the authors of this manuscript have the following competing interests: S. Mori received honoraria for lectures from AbbVie GK, Chugai Pharmaceutical Co. Ltd., Eisai, Astellas Pharma Inc., and Taisho Pharma Co., Ltd. T. Koga received speaker's fees from AbbVie GK, Eli Lilly Japan K.K., Eisai, Gilead Sciences, Inc., and GSK. These companies had no role in the study design, data collection, analysis, and interpretation, decision to publish, or manuscript preparation. The other authors had no financial relationships that could create a potential conflict of interest or the appearance of a conflict of interest with regard to the work.

References

1. McInnes, I.B.; Schett, G. Pathogenetic insights from the treatment of rheumatoid arthritis. *Lancet* **2017**, *389*, 2328–2337. [CrossRef] [PubMed]
2. Smolen, J.S.; Aletaha, D.; Barton, A.; Burmester, G.R.; Emery, P.; Firestein, G.S.; Kavanaugh, A.; McInnes, I.B.; Solomon, D.H.; Strand, V.; et al. Rheumatoid arthritis. *Nat. Rev. Dis. Primers* **2018**, *4*, 18001. [CrossRef] [PubMed]
3. Scott, D.L.; Pugner, K.; Kaarela, K.; Doyle, D.V.; Woolf, A.; Holmes, J.; Hieke, K. The links between joint damage and disability in rheumatoid arthritis. *Rheumatology* **2000**, *39*, 122–132. [CrossRef]
4. Scott, D.L.; Smith, C.; Kingsley, G. Joint damage and disability in rheumatoid arthritis: An updated systematic review. *Clin. Exp. Rheumatol.* **2003**, *21*, S20–S27.
5. Bombardier, C.; Barbieri, M.; Parthan, A.; Zack, D.J.; Walker, V.; Macarios, D.; Smolen, J.S. The relationship between joint damage and functional disability in rheumatoid arthritis: A systematic review. *Ann. Rheum. Dis.* **2012**, *71*, 836–844. [CrossRef]
6. Fraenkel, L.; Bathon, J.M.; England, B.R.; St Clair, E.W.; Arayssi, T.; Carandang, K.; Deane, K.D.; Genovese, M.; Huston, K.K.; Kerr, G.; et al. 2021 American College of Rheumatology Guideline for the Treatment of Rheumatoid Arthritis. *Arthritis Rheumatol.* **2021**, *73*, 1108–1123. [CrossRef] [PubMed]
7. Smolen, J.S.; Landewe, R.B.M.; Bergstra, S.A.; Kerschbaumer, A.; Sepriano, A.; Aletaha, D.; Caporali, R.; Edwards, C.J.; Hyrich, K.L.; Pope, J.E.; et al. EULAR recommendations for the management of rheumatoid arthritis with synthetic and biological disease-modifying antirheumatic drugs: 2022 update. *Ann. Rheum. Dis.* **2023**, *82*, 3–18. [CrossRef]
8. Brown, P.; Pratt, A.G.; Hyrich, K.L. Therapeutic advances in rheumatoid arthritis. *BMJ* **2024**, *384*, e070856. [CrossRef]
9. Bakker, M.F.; Jacobs, J.W.; Verstappen, S.M.; Bijlsma, J.W. Tight control in the treatment of rheumatoid arthritis: Efficacy and feasibility. *Ann. Rheum. Dis.* **2007**, *66* (Suppl. 3), iii56–iii60. [CrossRef]
10. Mease, P.J. Improving the routine management of rheumatoid arthritis: The value of tight control. *J. Rheumatol.* **2010**, *37*, 1570–1578. [CrossRef]
11. Aletaha, D.; Smolen, J. The Simplified Disease Activity Index (SDAI) and the Clinical Disease Activity Index (CDAI): A review of their usefulness and validity in rheumatoid arthritis. *Clin. Exp. Rheumatol.* **2005**, *23*, S100–S108.
12. Aletaha, D.; Ward, M.M.; Machold, K.P.; Nell, V.P.; Stamm, T.; Smolen, J.S. Remission and active disease in rheumatoid arthritis: Defining criteria for disease activity states. *Arthritis Rheum.* **2005**, *52*, 2625–2636. [CrossRef]
13. Grigor, C.; Capell, H.; Stirling, A.; McMahon, A.D.; Lock, P.; Vallance, R.; Kincaid, W.; Porter, D. Effect of a treatment strategy of tight control for rheumatoid arthritis (the TICORA study): A single-blind randomised controlled trial. *Lancet* **2004**, *364*, 263–269. [CrossRef]
14. Goekoop-Ruiterman, Y.P.; de Vries-Bouwstra, J.K.; Allaart, C.F.; van Zeben, D.; Kerstens, P.J.; Hazes, J.M.; Zwinderman, A.H.; Ronday, H.K.; Han, K.H.; Westedt, M.L.; et al. Clinical and radiographic outcomes of four different treatment strategies in patients with early rheumatoid arthritis (the BeSt study): A randomized, controlled trial. *Arthritis Rheum.* **2005**, *52*, 3381–3390. [CrossRef]
15. Makinen, H.; Kautiainen, H.; Hannonen, P.; Mottonen, T.; Leirisalo-Repo, M.; Laasonen, L.; Korpela, M.; Blafield, H.; Hakola, M.; Sokka, T. Sustained remission and reduced radiographic progression with combination disease modifying antirheumatic drugs in early rheumatoid arthritis. *J. Rheumatol.* **2007**, *34*, 316–321.

16. Verstappen, S.M.; Jacobs, J.W.; van der Veen, M.J.; Heurkens, A.H.; Schenk, Y.; ter Borg, E.J.; Blaauw, A.A.; Bijlsma, J.W.; Utrecht Rheumatoid Arthritis Cohort study, g. Intensive treatment with methotrexate in early rheumatoid arthritis: Aiming for remission. Computer Assisted Management in Early Rheumatoid Arthritis (CAMERA, an open-label strategy trial). *Ann. Rheum. Dis.* **2007**, *66*, 1443–1449. [CrossRef] [PubMed]
17. Smolen, J.S.; Aletaha, D.; Bijlsma, J.W.; Breedveld, F.C.; Boumpas, D.; Burmester, G.; Combe, B.; Cutolo, M.; de Wit, M.; Dougados, M.; et al. Treating rheumatoid arthritis to target: Recommendations of an international task force. *Ann. Rheum. Dis.* **2010**, *69*, 631–637. [CrossRef]
18. Schoels, M.; Knevel, R.; Aletaha, D.; Bijlsma, J.W.J.; Breedveld, F.C.; Boumpas, D.T.; Burmester, G.; Combe, B.; Cutolo, M.; Dougados, M.; et al. Evidence for treating rheumatoid arthritis to target: Results of a systematic literature search. *Ann. Rheum. Dis.* **2010**, *69*, 638–643. [CrossRef] [PubMed]
19. Hao, Y.; Oon, S.; Nikpour, M. Efficacy and safety of treat-to-target strategy studies in rheumatic diseases: A systematic review and meta-analysis. *Semin. Arthritis Rheum.* **2024**, *67*, 152465. [CrossRef] [PubMed]
20. Aletaha, D.; Neogi, T.; Silman, A.J.; Funovits, J.; Felson, D.T.; Bingham, C.O., III; Birnbaum, N.S.; Burmester, G.R.; Bykerk, V.P.; Cohen, M.D.; et al. 2010 Rheumatoid arthritis classification criteria: An American College of Rheumatology/European League Against Rheumatism collaborative initiative. *Arthritis Rheum.* **2010**, *62*, 2569–2581. [CrossRef]
21. Mori, S.; Naito, H.; Ohtani, S.; Yamanaka, T.; Sugimoto, M. Diagnostic utility of anti-cyclic citrullinated peptide antibodies for rheumatoid arthritis in patients with active lung tuberculosis. *Clin. Rheumatol.* **2009**, *28*, 277–283. [CrossRef]
22. Aletaha, D.; Nell, V.P.; Stamm, T.; Uffmann, M.; Pflugbeil, S.; Machold, K.; Smolen, J.S. Acute phase reactants add little to composite disease activity indices for rheumatoid arthritis: Validation of a clinical activity score. *Arthritis Res. Ther.* **2005**, *7*, R796–R806. [CrossRef] [PubMed]
23. Inoue, E.; Yamanaka, H.; Hara, M.; Tomatsu, T.; Kamatani, N. Comparison of Disease Activity Score (DAS)28-erythrocyte sedimentation rate and DAS28-C-reactive protein threshold values. *Ann. Rheum. Dis.* **2007**, *66*, 407–409. [CrossRef]
24. van der Heijde, D.M.; van Riel, P.L.; Nuver-Zwart, I.H.; Gribnau, F.W.; vad de Putte, L.B. Effects of hydroxychloroquine and sulphasalazine on progression of joint damage in rheumatoid arthritis. *Lancet* **1989**, *1*, 1036–1038. [CrossRef]
25. van der Heijde, D. How to read radiographs according to the Sharp/van der Heijde method. *J. Rheumatol.* **2000**, *27*, 261–263.
26. van der Heijde, D. Erosions versus joint space narrowing in rheumatoid arthritis: What do we know? *Ann. Rheum. Dis.* **2011**, *70* (Suppl. 1), I116–I118. [CrossRef]
27. Lillegraven, S.; van der Heijde, D.; Uhlig, T.; Kvien, T.K.; Haavardsholm, E.A. What is the clinical relevance of erosions and joint space narrowing in RA? *Nat. Rev. Rheumatol.* **2012**, *8*, 117–120. [CrossRef]
28. Koo, T.K.; Li, M.Y. A Guideline of Selecting and Reporting Intraclass Correlation Coefficients for Reliability Research. *J. Chiropr. Med.* **2016**, *15*, 155–163. [CrossRef] [PubMed]
29. Lydersen, S. Statistical review: Frequently given comments. *Ann. Rheum. Dis.* **2015**, *74*, 323–325. [CrossRef] [PubMed]
30. Kanda, Y. Investigation of the freely available easy-to-use software 'EZR' for medical statistics. *Bone Marrow Transpl.* **2013**, *48*, 452–458. [CrossRef]
31. Courvoisier, N.; Dougados, M.; Cantagrel, A.; Goupille, P.; Meyer, O.; Sibilia, J.; Daures, J.P.; Combe, B. Prognostic factors of 10-year radiographic outcome in early rheumatoid arthritis: A prospective study. *Arthritis Res. Ther.* **2008**, *10*, R106. [CrossRef]
32. Odegard, S.; Landewe, R.; van der Heijde, D.; Kvien, T.K.; Mowinckel, P.; Uhlig, T. Association of early radiographic damage with impaired physical function in rheumatoid arthritis: A ten-year, longitudinal observational study in 238 patients. *Arthritis Rheum.* **2006**, *54*, 68–75. [CrossRef]
33. Syversen, S.W.; Gaarder, P.I.; Goll, G.L.; Odegard, S.; Haavardsholm, E.A.; Mowinckel, P.; van der Heijde, D.; Landewe, R.; Kvien, T.K. High anti-cyclic citrullinated peptide levels and an algorithm of four variables predict radiographic progression in patients with rheumatoid arthritis: Results from a 10-year longitudinal study. *Ann. Rheum. Dis.* **2008**, *67*, 212–217. [CrossRef]
34. Navarro-Compan, V.; Landewe, R.; Provan, S.A.; Odegard, S.; Uhlig, T.; Kvien, T.K.; Keszei, A.P.; Ramiro, S.; van der Heijde, D. Relationship between types of radiographic damage and disability in patients with rheumatoid arthritis in the EURIDISS cohort: A longitudinal study. *Rheumatology* **2015**, *54*, 83–90. [CrossRef]
35. Tanaka, N.; Sakahashi, H.; Ishii, S.; Sato, E.; Hirose, K.; Ishima, T. Synovial membrane enhancement and bone erosion by magnetic resonance imaging for prediction of radiologic progression in patients with early rheumatoid arthritis. *Rheumatol. Int.* **2005**, *25*, 103–107. [CrossRef] [PubMed]
36. Carpenter, L.; Nikiphorou, E.; Sharpe, R.; Norton, S.; Rennie, K.; Bunn, F.; Scott, D.L.; Dixey, J.; Young, A. Have radiographic progression rates in early rheumatoid arthritis changed? A systematic review and meta-analysis of long-term cohorts. *Rheumatology* **2016**, *55*, 1053–1065. [CrossRef]
37. Markusse, I.M.; Akdemir, G.; Dirven, L.; Goekoop-Ruiterman, Y.P.; van Groenendael, J.H.; Han, K.H.; Molenaar, T.H.; Le Cessie, S.; Lems, W.F.; van der Lubbe, P.A.; et al. Long-Term Outcomes of Patients With Recent-Onset Rheumatoid Arthritis After 10 Years of Tight Controlled Treatment: A Randomized Trial. *Ann. Intern. Med.* **2016**, *164*, 523–531. [CrossRef] [PubMed]
38. Allaart, C.F.; Markusse, I.M.; Lems, W.F. What have we learned from BeSt? *Clin. Immunol.* **2018**, *186*, 74–78. [CrossRef]

39. Heimans, L.; Wevers-de Boer, K.V.; Visser, K.; Goekoop, R.J.; van Oosterhout, M.; Harbers, J.B.; Bijkerk, C.; Speyer, I.; de Buck, M.P.; de Sonnaville, P.B.; et al. A two-step treatment strategy trial in patients with early arthritis aimed at achieving remission: The IMPROVED study. *Ann. Rheum. Dis.* **2014**, *73*, 1356–1361. [CrossRef]
40. Heimans, L.; Akdemir, G.; Boer, K.V.; Goekoop-Ruiterman, Y.P.; Molenaar, E.T.; van Groenendael, J.H.; Peeters, A.J.; Steup-Beekman, G.M.; Lard, L.R.; de Sonnaville, P.B.; et al. Two-year results of disease activity score (DAS)-remission-steered treatment strategies aiming at drug-free remission in early arthritis patients (the IMPROVED-study). *Arthritis Res. Ther.* **2016**, *18*, 23. [CrossRef] [PubMed]
41. Akdemir, G.; Heimans, L.; Bergstra, S.A.; Goekoop, R.J.; van Oosterhout, M.; van Groenendael, J.; Peeters, A.J.; Steup-Beekman, G.M.; Lard, L.R.; de Sonnaville, P.B.J.; et al. Clinical and radiological outcomes of 5-year drug-free remission-steered treatment in patients with early arthritis: IMPROVED study. *Ann. Rheum. Dis.* **2018**, *77*, 111–118. [CrossRef]
42. Keystone, E.C.; Breedveld, F.C.; van der Heijde, D.; Landewe, R.; Florentinus, S.; Arulmani, U.; Liu, S.; Kupper, H.; Kavanaugh, A. Longterm effect of delaying combination therapy with tumor necrosis factor inhibitor in patients with aggressive early rheumatoid arthritis: 10-year efficacy and safety of adalimumab from the randomized controlled PREMIER trial with open-label extension. *J. Rheumatol.* **2014**, *41*, 5–14. [CrossRef]
43. Keystone, E.C.; van der Heijde, D.; Kavanaugh, A.; Kupper, H.; Liu, S.; Guerette, B.; Mozaffarian, N. Clinical, functional, and radiographic benefits of longterm adalimumab plus methotrexate: Final 10-year data in longstanding rheumatoid arthritis. *J. Rheumatol.* **2013**, *40*, 1487–1497. [CrossRef] [PubMed]
44. Ruyssen-Witrand, A.; Guernec, G.; Dupont, J.; Lapuyade, D.; Liote, F.; Vittecoq, O.; Degboe, Y.; Constantin, A. Ten-year radiographic and functional outcomes in rheumatoid arthritis patients in remission compared to patients in low disease activity. *Arthritis Res. Ther.* **2023**, *25*, 207. [CrossRef] [PubMed]
45. Bergstra, S.A.; Landewe, R.B.M.; Huizinga, T.W.J.; Allaart, C.F. Rheumatoid arthritis patients with continued low disease activity have similar outcomes over 10 years, regardless of initial therapy. *Rheumatology* **2017**, *56*, 1721–1728. [CrossRef] [PubMed]
46. Markusse, I.M.; Dirven, L.; Gerards, A.H.; van Groenendael, J.H.; Ronday, H.K.; Kerstens, P.J.; Lems, W.F.; Huizinga, T.W.; Allaart, C.F. Disease flares in rheumatoid arthritis are associated with joint damage progression and disability: 10-year results from the BeSt study. *Arthritis Res. Ther.* **2015**, *17*, 232. [CrossRef]
47. Markatseli, T.E.; Voulgari, P.V.; Alamanos, Y.; Drosos, A.A. Prognostic factors of radiological damage in rheumatoid arthritis: A 10-year retrospective study. *J. Rheumatol.* **2011**, *38*, 44–52. [CrossRef]
48. Smolen, J.S.; van der Heijde, D.M.; Aletaha, D.; Xu, S.; Han, J.; Baker, D.; St Clair, E.W. Progression of radiographic joint damage in rheumatoid arthritis: Independence of erosions and joint space narrowing. *Ann. Rheum. Dis.* **2009**, *68*, 1535–1540. [CrossRef]
49. Heckert, S.L.; Maassen, J.M.; Nevins, I.; Baudoin, P.; Steup-Beekman, G.M.; Huizinga, T.W.J.; Bergstra, S.A.; Allaart, C.F. Long-term clinical outcomes in early rheumatoid arthritis that was treated-to-target in the BeSt and IMPROVED studies. *Rheumatology* **2025**, *64*, 1052–1059. [CrossRef]
50. Welsing, P.M.; van Gestel, A.M.; Swinkels, H.L.; Kiemeney, L.A.; van Riel, P.L. The relationship between disease activity, joint destruction, and functional capacity over the course of rheumatoid arthritis. *Arthritis Rheum.* **2001**, *44*, 2009–2017. [CrossRef]
51. Smolen, J.S.; Aletaha, D. Patients with rheumatoid arthritis in clinical care. *Ann. Rheum. Dis.* **2004**, *63*, 221–225. [CrossRef]
52. Aletaha, D.; Smolen, J.; Ward, M.M. Measuring function in rheumatoid arthritis: Identifying reversible and irreversible components. *Arthritis Rheum.* **2006**, *54*, 2784–2792. [CrossRef] [PubMed]
53. Aletaha, D.; Funovits, J.; Smolen, J.S. Physical disability in rheumatoid arthritis is associated with cartilage damage rather than bone destruction. *Ann. Rheum. Dis.* **2011**, *70*, 733–739. [CrossRef] [PubMed]
54. van der Pol, J.A.; Allaart, C.F.; Huizinga, T.W.J.; Bergstra, S.A. Are poor prognostic factors a realistic basis for treatment decisions in patients with rheumatoid arthritis? Lessons from the IMPROVED study. *RMD Open* **2024**, *10*, e004382. [CrossRef] [PubMed]

MDPI AG
Grosspeteranlage 5
4052 Basel
Switzerland
Tel.: +41 61 683 77 34

Journal of Clinical Medicine Editorial Office
E-mail: jcm@mdpi.com
www.mdpi.com/journal/jcm

www.ingramcontent.com/pod-product-compliance
Lightning Source LLC
Chambersburg PA
CBHW041018270926
51850CB00024B/1509
* 9 7 8 3 7 2 5 8 7 1 6 4 3 *